GOVERNORS STATE UNIVERSITY LIBRARY

3 1611 00317 6481

MEDICAL LIBRARY
ASSOCIATION *Guides*

⊲ **W9-BHM-728**

Health
Informatics
for Medical
Librarians

ANA D. CLEVELAND
and
DONALD B. CLEVELAND

GOVERNORS STATE UNIVERSITY
UNIVERSITY PARK
IL 60466

NEAL-SCHUMAN PUBLISHERS, INC.
NEW YORK   LONDON

R
858
.C54
2009

Published by Neal-Schuman Publishers, Inc.
100 William St., Suite 2004
New York, NY 10038

Copyright © 2009 Medical Library Association.

All rights reserved. Reproduction of this book, in whole or in part, without written permission of the publisher, is prohibited.

Printed and bound in the United States of America.

The paper used in this publication meets the minimum requirements of American National Standard for Information Sciences—Permanence of Paper for Printed Library Materials, ANSI Z39.48-1992.

Library of Congress Cataloging-in-Publication Data

Cleveland, Ana D., 1943-
  Health informatics for medical librarians / Ana D. Cleveland and Donald B. Cleveland.
    p. cm. — (Medical Library Association guides)
  Includes bibliographical references and index.
  ISBN 978-1-55570-627-2 (alk. paper)
  1. Medical informatics. I. Cleveland, Donald B., 1935- II. Title.

R858.C54 2009
651.5'04261—dc22

                                                        2009017656

Contents

List of Informatics in Action! xi

Preface xiii

Acknowledgments xvi

Part I: Understanding Health Informatics

1. Introduction and Overview 3
   Ubiquitous Need for Health Information 3
      Relationship Between Healthcare and Information 4
      The Ubiquity of Healthcare Information 4
      Understanding the Information Problem 5
   The Nature of Information 6
   What Is Health Informatics? 8
      Health Informatics as a Discipline 10
      Health Informatics as a Profession 11
   The Vital Role of Health Information Technology 11
      Background of Health and Computers 13
      The Challenges Facing Information Technology in Healthcare .. 13
      Information Technology and People 16
      The Extent of Health Informatics 17
   Applications 18
   Summary 18
   References 18

2. The Environment of Modern Medicine 21
   The Universality of Healthcare 21
   New Healthcare Paradigm 22
   Structure of the Healthcare System 23
      Types of Services 23
      Paying for Healthcare 23
   The People in Healthcare 24
      Physicians 25

Hospitalists 26
Biomedical Engineers 27
Chiropractors 27
Clinical Laboratory Technologists 27
Dentists 28
Dental Assistants 28
Dental Hygienists 28
Health Informationists 28
Licensed Practical/Vocational Nurses 29
Nurse Practitioners 29
Paramedics 29
Pharmacists 30
Physician Assistants 30
Registered Nurses 31
Veterinarians 31
Medical Research 32
Recent Trends 33
Group Medical Practice 34
Managed Care 34
Role of the Patient 34
Outpatient Care 35
Long-term Care 35
Complementary and Alternative Medicine 36
Uninsured People 36
The Internet and Integrated Medical Information Systems . . . 37
Health Informatics Skills and Competencies in the
Twenty-first Century 38
Summary 39
References 40

3. How Informatics Impacts Modern Healthcare **43**
Medical Decision Making 43
The Nature and Importance of Medical Data 44
Desirable Characteristics of Medical Data 44
Data Gathering 44
Documenting Healthcare Operations 45
From Data to Information 46
The Medical Decision-making Process 47
Examples of How Health Informatics Impacts Healthcare 48
Changes in Patient Care 48
The People Factor 53
The Rise of Evidence-based Medicine 53
Telehealth and Access to Healthcare 57

Summary 60
References 61

4. **Major Application Areas** **63**
   Direct Patient Care Informatics 63
      Primary Care Informatics 63
      Nursing Informatics 67
      Dental Informatics 68
      Behavioral Informatics 69
      Public Health Informatics 70
      Veterinary Informatics 72
      Bioinformatics 73
   Support Services Informatics 73
      Pharmaceutical Informatics 74
      Pathology Informatics 75
      Laboratory Informatics 75
      Medical Imaging Informatics 76
      Consumer Health Informatics 77
   Summary 80
   References 81

5. **Health Sciences Librarians and Health Informatics** **85**
   Health Sciences Libraries 86
   The Leadership of the U.S. National Library of Medicine 86
   Impacts of Changes in Health Sciences Libraries 88
      Changing Healthcare Environments 88
      Impact of Computers and Related Information Technologies . . 89
      The Medical Library Assistance Act 90
      Information Needs and Searching Behaviors of
         Healthcare Providers 91
   Intersections of Health Sciences Librarianship and
      Health Informatics 93
      Common Intellectual Base and Operational Theorems 94
      New Roles and Opportunities 95
      Health Information Technology Management 96
      Evidence-based Medicine and the Health Sciences Librarian . . 97
      Patient and Consumer Services 98
      The Informationist 99
      Health Sciences Librarians and Bioinformatics 100
      Education and Training Roles for Health Sciences Librarians . . 100
   Health Sciences Librarians and a Relevant Research Agenda 101
      Health Sciences Librarians and Research 101
      Research Partnerships with Health Informatics 103

Summary 106
References 106

Part II: Mastering Health Informatics

6. The Organization of Medical Knowledge **111**
Organization of Knowledge 111
Knowledge Management and Health Information 112
Medical Terminology 113
Definitions 114
Medical Ontologies 115
Medical Classification and Coding 115
Registries 118
The Medical Literature 120
  Medical Textbooks and Reference Tools 121
  Medical Journals 121
  Trends and Prognosis for Medical Journals 122
Bibliographic Control 126
  Cataloging and Classification 127
  Subject Vocabularies 127
  The Indexing Function 128
Summary 131
References 131

7. Health Information Technology **133**
Managing Healthcare Information with Technology 133
The Expectations of Health Information Technology 134
Networking with Telecommunications 136
Medical Database Management 136
  Database Management Systems 137
  Biomedical Databases 138
The Internet 139
  Health Consumers and the Internet 139
  Web-based Healthcare Information Systems 141
Mobile, Wireless, and Wearable Technologies 142
Artificial Intelligence in the Health Sciences 144
  Expert Systems 145
  Robotics 146
  Natural Language Processing 147
Virtual Reality 147
Connectivity and Interoperability 148
Summary 149
References 150

8. The Electronic Health Record **153**
The Nature of Health Records 153
Problem-oriented Health Records 154
Personal Health Records 155
The EHR 156
Definition 156
Need for the EHR 156
Universality of EHRs 157
Challenges 157
Electronic versus Paper Patient Records 158
Basic EHR Functions 159
The Ideal EHR 159
Selection of an EHR 160
User Interfaces 160
Implementation of the EHR 161
Web-based Systems 161
Issues and Caveats 162
Health Record Information Ownership 163
Trends and Potentials of the EHR 164
A National Health Record 165
Opportunity for the Health Sciences Librarian 166
Summary 166
References 166

9. Healthcare Information Management Systems **169**
Information Management 169
Correct Information at the Right Time 170
Complexity of Healthcare Information Systems 170
Understanding Information Needs and Opportunities 170
Information Resources Management 171
Major Types of Health Information Systems 172
Clinical Information Systems 172
Hospital Information Systems 173
Supportive Health Information Systems 176
Healthcare Information System Analysis 178
Basic Rules for Acquiring an Information Management System .. 179
Successful Information System Implementation 183
Evaluation of an Information System 186
The Role of the Library 187
Summary 188
References 188

10. Medical Imaging **191**
    Introduction 191
    Medical Imaging Basics 192
    Digital Imaging 193
    Imaging and Medical Practice 194
        Imaging Acquisition Modalities 194
        Major Uses of Imaging in Healthcare 197
    Managing Imaging Information 198
        Image Manipulation 198
        Image Transport 199
        Image Organization, Storage, and Retrieval 200
        Image Indexing 200
        Image Access 203
        Image Quality 205
    Picture Archiving and Communication Systems 205
    Emerging Imaging Technologies 206
    Medical Images and the Health Sciences Librarian 207
    Summary 209
    References 209

11. Ethical and Legal Issues in Health Informatics **211**
    Ethics and Medicine 211
        Concept of Professional Ethical Codes 212
        Medical Codes of Ethics 213
        Ethical Concepts Regarding the Patient–
          Healthcare Provider Relationship 214
        Ethics in Medical Research 216
    Ethics and Informatics 217
    Medical Legal Issues 218
        Informed Consent 218
        Information Ownership 219
        Negligence/Malpractice 220
        Product Liability 221
        Fraud and Abuse 222
    Privacy and Confidentiality Issues 222
        Secondary Uses of Patient Data 224
        Health Grid Computing 224
        Health Insurance Portability and Accountability Act of 1996 ... 225
        USA PATRIOT Act and Medical Privacy 226
    Issues for Health Sciences Librarians 226
    Summary 227
    References 228

12. **Bioinformatics and Genomic Medicine** **231**
      Defining Bioinformatics 231
      Areas of Bioinformatics Study 232
      Deoxyribonucleic Acid: The Information Key to Life 233
            Genes and Genetics 234
            The Genome 234
            Genome Mapping 235
            The Human Genome Project 236
            Stem Cell Research 237
            Genetic Testing 237
            Genetic Engineering and Cloning 238
      Genomic Databases 239
      Bioinformatics Applications 241
      Genomic Medicine 242
            Personalized Medicine 242
            Societal Concerns 243
            Impact and Hopes 243
      Role of the Health Information Professional 244
      Summary 246
      References 246

13. **The Age of Health Informatics** **249**
      Education, Research, and Career Paths 249
            Educational Pathways 249
            Continuing Education 252
            Health Informatics Research 252
            Career Opportunities 253
            Professional Associations 254
      Trends and Horizons in Health Informatics 256
            Advances in Health Informatics Technologies 257
            Health Informatics and an Innovative Internet 259
            Emerging Health Informatics Specialties 259
      A Final Word 260
      References 262

Glossary **265**

Index **279**

About the Authors **287**

Informatics in Action!

1.1 Health Information Podcasting 12
2.1 Identifying Informatics Competencies 39
3.1 Telehealth Status 60
4.1 Community Health Literacy Level 79
5.1 Mysterious Drug Interaction 104
6.1 Patient/Consumer Access to Health Records 126
7.1 Applying Web 2.0 Technology 140
8.1 National Network of EHRs 165
9.1 An Integrated Hospital Information Management System 179
10.1 Training PACS Users 207
11.1 Online Copyright Permission System 220
12.1 DNA Property Rights 245
13.1 Emergency Preparedness Information 260

Preface

Healthcare, in all of its ramifications, is information driven. Health informatics—one of the most exciting areas of modern medicine—is an interdisciplinary field and has been defined in many ways. These definitions are discussed in Chapter 1, but a working characterization of health informatics might be stated as *the theoretical framework and practical applications resulting from integrating information technology with the health sciences.* The acquisition, transfer, interpretation, and application of information begin in the physician's office and extend throughout the entire health system, including the clinic, the hospital, the pharmaceutical industry, insurance payers, government agencies, and the patient/consumer.

Healthcare in the twenty-first century faces changes, challenges, and golden opportunities. Costs continue to explode, bringing financial constraints and operations concerns. Demands for quality health services and patient safety have created greater information expectations from professionals and the public. At the same time, the health sciences are standing on the threshold of a new era of discovery and advancement, particularly in the development of genomic medicine and the availability of sophisticated information technologies.

Health informatics is the discipline that will guide healthcare through these new paradigms. The integration of medical librarians into health informatics endeavors is a major step in recognizing their function in information management. Medical librarians are positioned to play a major role in the new directions occurring in the fast-changing healthcare environment.

A basic knowledge of health informatics is essential for anyone seeking to work in the healthcare environment today. The primary intended audiences for *Health Informatics for Medical Librarians* are medical librarians and students in the schools of library and information sciences. Another major audience is librarians in public and special libraries who deal with health information resources and services. Healthcare professionals who need an introductory guide to health informatics will find this book very useful. These professionals use information technology every day and will benefit from learning about the grounded issues of health informatics.

The underlying principle that drives health informatics and medical librarianship together is that information management is at the core of their existence. The premise of the book is that medical librarians have a naturally intrinsic role in health informatics, but to do so they need to have an understanding of health informatics and of the professionals working in this expanding and exciting field.

In 2002, Prudence Dalrymple observed, "What librarians have thus far lacked is the domain knowledge that comes naturally to medical informaticists" (Dalrymple, 2002: 5). We wrote *Health Informatics for Medical Librarians* largely to help alleviate this problem by providing medical librarians with background knowledge of healthcare technology that will help clarify their role as it relates to health informatics.

While the pages that follow cover the major procedures and techniques used in health informatics, the book's primary objective is to introduce health informatics and to describe the medical environment and culture in which health informatics professionals work. We also suggest roles that medical librarians can embrace to become active participants in health informatics.

The conceptual framework of the book is as follows:

- Healthcare and supporting services are information intense.
- Information technology is essential to the success of modern day healthcare.
- Health informatics is the platform for ensuring the success of information technology in healthcare.
- Medical librarians are positioned by both training and professional mission to be an integral part of the health informatics environment.
- In order to fulfill this mission, medical librarians should be well versed in the theoretical foundations and practical applications of health informatics.

The book is structured into two parts. Part I: Understanding Health Informatics defines health informatics and its role in healthcare. We begin by describing the infrastructure and environment of healthcare, including the people who work in the field and their activities. We then discuss how informatics is impacting modern healthcare and include specific examples. We also discuss the major specialty areas of health informatics and present appropriate examples. In the final chapter in Part I, we describe medical librarianship and the potential role of librarians in health informatics.

Part II: Mastering Health Informatics covers specific aspects of health informatics. We begin with the organization of medical knowledge and then discuss health information technology, the electronic health record, and healthcare information management systems. In subsequent chapters we cover medical imaging, ethical and legal issues in health informatics, and bioinformatics and genomic medicine. In the final chapter we summarize various issues in health informatics and describe our vision of the future.

Good health is the most important thing any of us can possess, and it is dependent on quality information. Medicine is an unparalleled setting in which librarians can demonstrate the value of their work. In *Health Informatics for Medical Librarians*, you will find the basic set of tools needed to help improve healthcare and play a key role in the adventure.

REFERENCE

Dalrymple, Prudence W. "The Impact of Medical Informatics on Librarianship." In *Libraries for Life: Democracy, Diversity, Delivery.* 68th IFLA Council and General Conference: Conference Programme and Proceedings (August 18–24, 2002). IR 058 549. Glasgow, Scotland: IFLA. Available: www.ifla.org/IV/ifla68/papers/098-115e.pdf (accessed December 14, 2008).

Acknowledgments

We express our appreciation to the numerous students who took our classes and identified the need for a textbook on heath informatics for medical librarians.

We thank Laurie Thompson, Assistant Vice President for Library Services, University of Texas Southwestern Medical Center Library at Dallas, who approached us on behalf of the Medical Library Association to write a book related to medical informatics. We thank our dean, Herman L. Totten, who supported us with encouragement and resources throughout the project.

We offer a special thanks to Jodi L. Philbrick for her dedication in reading the manuscript and making recommendations that improved the content of the book. We appreciate the discussions we had with her regarding health informatics.

We end with a word of gratitude to the National Library of Medicine for their support throughout our long professional careers. Their vision of health informatics has been an inspiration in all our endeavors.

Part I

Understanding Health Informatics

Chapter 1

Introduction and Overview

This chapter provides an overview and a working definition of the concept of health informatics and its relation to information technology. It briefly describes the evolution of modern health informatics from the initial application of computers in medicine through the next four decades, including the changing perception of the definition of health informatics. The current definition is broad, encompassing all the facets of information creation and management across the spectrum of healthcare. Although health informatics focuses on the vital role of information technology, it also encompasses systems and the people in those systems.

UBIQUITOUS NEED FOR HEALTH INFORMATION

Every moment of the day and night medical events occur all over the world, some routine, others dramatic. On the expressway two cars smash together. In a living room a woman has a heart attack. At a clinic a man is having his annual physical exam, perhaps worried about a high cholesterol level.

In the case of the car accident, the emergency medical service (EMS) personnel arrive and spring into action, and information assessments begin. Are the victims breathing? Do they have a pulse? Are they bleeding? Are the victims conscious? The EMS team administers first aid and attach monitoring devices. They further examine the victims for trauma to the head and neck and to other parts of the body. They gather accident information from police officers and spectators. As soon as it is feasible, the victims are taken to the hospital in an ambulance. On the way the paramedics stay in contact with the emergency room via radio communications, sending information ahead, including electronic data from the monitoring systems.

Meanwhile, in the living room, EMS personnel are assessing the woman having a heart attack and gathering data. At the clinic where the man is getting his annual physical exam, lab technicians are processing tests, and medical personnel are interviewing the patient. In all three of these scenarios, the driving force behind every decision made and every action performed is information. Each step the health team takes is based on knowledge and skills, but no decision is made or action is taken until information regarding the situation is obtained and assessed. Obtaining the needed information may take a few seconds, or a few minutes, or longer, but it is a continuum of information assessment, action, new information, action, and so on until the scenario is played out, whatever the outcome.

Healthcare has always depended on information—accurate, at the right place, at the right time—but the modern age of information technology is changing the way this information is obtained, created, processed, delivered, and applied. The changing infrastructure of health information is promoting a heightened understanding and appreciation of the role of information in every facet of healthcare. In many ways healthcare is being reshaped by information technology, particularly by communication technology and cyberspace.

Relationship Between Healthcare and Information

What is the relationship between healthcare and information? Simply put, information is the fuel that drives healthcare decision making. The healthcare field is information intensive, because quality healthcare depends on quality information. Information is intrinsically inseparable from the operations and decisions made in healthcare.

The healthcare profession has been information driven since the days when a prehistoric doctor asked, "Where does it hurt?" The modern physician may ask the same question but collects further information from examinations, lab tests, and radiology tests and often from stored information resources such as the medical literature and online databases. Throughout the diagnosis, treatment, and follow-up stages, information is the guiding light for actions taken. There are immense information needs in today's primary, secondary, and tertiary healthcare levels and in the complex infrastructure of healthcare-supporting services. In addition to providing direct clinical support, systems also support management, research, and education activities. Obviously, the need for developing sophisticated and robust integrated information systems is the result of the complexity of today's healthcare enterprise.

The Ubiquity of Healthcare Information

Healthcare information has always existed in parallel with medical practice. In prerecorded history, medical information was passed down orally and by demonstration. As soon as writing was invented a medical literature began to evolve, beginning with the cuneiform tablets from ancient Mesopotamia, dating at least as far back as 2500 BC. Many of these early writings were prescriptions and remedies. By 1700 BC, Mesopotamia and Egypt had laws regulating medicine and a substantial number of physician records and case studies recommending actions for treating the sick and wounded. A well-known example is the Edwin Smith Papyrus (2007). Edwin Smith (1822–1906) was an American dealer of antiquities, a money lender, an adventurer, and sometimes a shady character. He recognized that the papyrus was special and bought it in 1862. He tried but was unable to completely translate it. American archaeologist and historian James Breasted successfully translated it in 1930. The papyrus was written around the seventeenth century BC but is believed to be based on material dating back to earlier centuries. The papyrus is a medical account of 48 clinical cases of head and spine trauma, including information on examination techniques, recognizing disease, and prescribing treatments (Edwin Smith Papyrus, 2007). The papyrus demonstrates that doctors were well on the way to creating a medical literature centuries ago, and they continue today.

By the early classical period, records and instructions of medical practice, recordings of human anatomy, and texts of ailments and herbal cures had become sophisticated. In the early centuries AD, physicians were classifying diseases and their descriptions. Around 1000 AD, they began to replace herbal medicines with chemicals, and they recorded these. In the 1600s, the concept of the scientific journal and its accompanying abstracting and indexing tools evolved into a powerful means of disseminating medical information. During the Age of Enlightenment and into the nineteenth century, the basic studies of biology, chemistry, and physics became truly scientific, and the field of medicine incorporated these developments into practice and research. Modern medicine began to emerge.

Today health information systems exist in a complex infrastructure upon which medical science builds and depends. Effective healthcare relies on a clear flow of accurate information, and this is becoming more obvious as the complexity of the healthcare infrastructure continues to increase. Information must be effectively communicated throughout the entire healthcare system, from the individual patient, through the local systems and all personnel in the systems, and finally to globally linked systems. The only way to maintain order and a workable structure is to manage the information systems effectively and efficiently. Information management is a central element for quality healthcare.

Understanding the Information Problem

Providing timely, accurate information to healthcare personnel is more than a technological problem. It is a difficult intellectual problem, which librarians and information scientists have long faced. How is information most effectively and easily packaged, stored, retrieved, formatted, and delivered? How can we use information technology to maximize the success of our endeavors? How do we meld humans and technology into an effective information system?

In this book, the term *information system* is not limited to computer hardware and software. Technology is merely one set of tools. An information system is a structured, purposeful use of many tools. The term *system* encompasses many resources, including people as well as computers (Cowan, 2003). Although technology is a very powerful and indispensable tool, there is more to health informatics than just a computing machine. Information processes begin and end with people.

The challenges faced with managing information are partly the result of the enormous growth of medical science knowledge and the proportional growth of the information generated. Inevitably, every generation complains about an "information explosion." In the September 1841 issue of *The American Eclectic*, the German doctor Wolfgang Menzel (1841: 280) protested against the increasing number of scientific periodicals in Germany:

> Of medical journals, there are forty-three in Germany. It must be granted that different modes of practice require different periodicals. . . . But forty-three journals are an astonishing number. What physician who practices daily can read them all, and to what physician who does not practice can they be useful?

What would Menzel think of MEDLINE? With today's high speed and high capacity computing technology, the sheer volume of the literature is not the basic challenge. A more difficult challenge is to foster mechanisms for integrating communication in the complex healthcare system, which includes healthcare professionals, research scientists, and research institutes, universities, funding agencies, professional associations, publishers, and libraries. How do we best facilitate the transfer of information across such a diverse population? The tasks are to understand how to effectively manage that information and to develop mechanisms to ensure that the information is delivered where and when it is needed. This is not a simple task, but it is one that informatics is vigorously addressing.

THE NATURE OF INFORMATION

A true understanding of informatics begins with a tacit operational definition of the concept of information. The word *information* means different things to different people. To the average person it can refer to such things as facts in books, road signs, what's on TV tonight, ingredients in a candy bar, and medication instructions. This is a normative perception of what information is, but an understanding of health informatics requires a deeper conception of the nature of information and its effects on human activities, including healthcare.

We must look beyond the definition to its *properties*. Just as we can investigate gravity and electricity, we can look into the properties of information. You may not completely understand what gravity is from its definition, but if you jump off the Eiffel Tower, you will surely be able to describe some of its properties.

In this book we define information as *patterns imposed on matter and energy*. Patterns exist in everything in the universe, and organisms bring order to the chaos around them by recognizing the patterns. Patterns are information, and complex patterns create complex information. An example is DNA, which is a complex series of chemical patterns that define life itself in a living organism. Another example is language, which is based on patterns created by humans, and written language is a complex series of patterns of symbols. These patterns are critical. For example, the two sentences "The lion ate the tiger" and "The tiger ate the lion" have the exact same words, but the sentences are entirely different in meaning. The brain recognizes language by recognizing patterns. In fact, if we go to the basic level, the human brain works by neutrons firing off signals in distinct patterns. The brain understands the multidimensional combinations of these patterns and responds by taking the actions required.

Understanding patterns is critical to informatics and to constructing information systems, because computer technology is engineered to recognize and manipulate patterns, all the way from the byte level up to the database. Information classification and structure are based on fundamental, universally recognized patterns.

Moving to the next level, all organisms, from simple cells to human beings, require information in order to make good decisions. Processing information is the way we organize things—our systems and our personal lives. Quality healthcare information allows control over healthcare events, leading to quality outcomes.

One approach to understanding information is to think of it as the critical element in a system, because without information there can be no system. Information gives structure to a system. Health informatics can be thought of as the information engine that structures the healthcare system. However, these structures do not come without planning and implementation via effective information management.

Informatics is more than information retrieval. It also involves the application of information to specific situations. Information management requires interaction between physical records and specific data; identification of the intellectual content of the records and data; the storage, retrieval, and transfer of the records and data; and their projected use. This is true of a library book, an Internet search, or a magnetic resonance imaging scan.

We have been told, rather frequently, that this is the "information age" and that the key to success is knowledge management and connectivity. Two primary factors characterize the information age. The obvious one is the growth in the amount of information created, but closely related to this is the increasing amount of information becoming available in new formats that cannot be handled with traditional techniques. An example of this is the rapid development of digital imaging technology.

Fifty years ago the term *information explosion* first appeared to describe the growth of information. Since then we have had continuous dire warnings that we are going to be overwhelmed with information, but we have managed to keep a certain amount of control, thanks to the incredible development of information technology in ways not even dreamed of in the 1950s. Nowhere is this more evident than in the healthcare field.

WHAT IS HEALTH INFORMATICS?

Health informatics is an interdisciplinary field of researchers, practitioners, and educators from a variety of specialties who are skilled in information technology and focused on enhancing healthcare. It encompasses the management of health information of all forms and at all levels of operation.

With the emergence of a new discipline, especially one highly interdisciplinary in nature, comes problems of what to name the field and how to define it. A consensus must be reached on what comprises its core knowledge and what application directions are necessary to educate new practitioners in the discipline. Health informatics has struggled with this basic problem for many years. The members of a profession are always naturally reluctant to recognize a new interdisciplinary specialty that claims to include their specialty, especially by using some kind of Venn diagram explanation.

The general term *informatics* was first used in Europe in the 1960s and was intended to distinguish itself from library and information science and computer science. About this time, informatics training programs began in France, Germany, Belgium, Poland, and the Netherlands. Such programs were in place in the United States by the 1970s (Felkey, Fox, and Thrower, 2006). The term *informatics* defined the theoretical base and practical applications of the effective collection, organization, management, and use of information. The concept of a theoretical base in the definition is important, because it indicates that the activities are more than *ad hoc* procedures; rather, they involve a logical, hopefully scientific, approach to understanding the basic nature of information in all its natural and manmade forms.

Health informatics, as a subarea of informatics, is generally characterized by an emphasis on technology, particularly information technology, as a fundamental tool for creating, managing, and making available health information. The paper document was the basic information device for many millennia, but in recent decades healthcare information systems began converting to electronic technology and attention is now given to related research and intellectual aspects of health information management.

Health informatics is a recent term, reflecting a broader perception of the field. In the beginning, the concept was narrowly focused on medical computing techniques and expressed in such terms as:

- medical computing,
- medical computing science,
- medical electronic data processing, and
- medical information science.

In the 1960s, the terms *medical computing* and *medical computing science* indicated the interface between the health sciences, particularly clinical medicine, and the computer. The early definitions focused on the application of computers to medicine. Collen (1986) described medical informatics as the application of computer technology to all fields of medicine—medical care, medical teaching, and medical research. By the late 1980s, definitions began to include the need for a scientific base, which was necessary in order for health informatics to be a true discipline. According to the U.S. Department of Health and Human Services (1987: 31), "Medical informatics attempts to provide the theoretical and scientific basis for the application of computer and automated information systems to biomedicine and health affairs. . . . [M]edical informatics studies biomedical information, data, and knowledge— their storage, retrieval, and optimal use for problem-solving and decision- making."

In 1986, the Association of American Medical Colleges (AAMC) published a definition of medical informatics, characterizing it as the study and application of methods and techniques for managing information, particularly in support of medical research, education, and patient care. The definition also identified informatics as interdisciplinary, encompassing different medical science areas and a number of related information disciplines. The ultimate objective of medical informatics, according to the AAMC (1986), is to promote better medical care.

In 1990, Shortliffe and Perreault defined medical informatics in terms of traditional information storage, retrieval, and use of medical information, in particular for supporting medical decision making and problem solving. They also viewed it as interdisciplinary, tied to all basic and applied biomedical sciences, with a common connection to information technologies.

Stead (1994) also defined medical informatics as an interdisciplinary field, and he identified some of the contributing fields. He included the basic health sciences as the starting point, adding techniques and knowledge from biometry, computer science, decision science, library science, and number of other areas. Of particular interest was the inclusion of policy science. Medical information's purpose is to provide support in the solution of problems in healthcare delivery and education.

Värri's (1997) broad definition is that "Healthcare Informatics is the scientific discipline that is concerned with the cognitive, information processing and communication tasks of healthcare practice, education and research, including the information science and technology to support these tasks." In 2004, the National Library of Medicine defined medical informatics as "the field of information science concerned with the analysis and dissemination of medical data through the application of computers to various aspects of health care and medicine" (U.S. Department of Health and Human Services, 2004).

The British Medical Informatics Society (2004) said that medical informatics "can be best understood as meaning the understanding, skills and tools that enable the sharing and use of information to deliver healthcare and promote health." The Society also pointed out that informatics has gone through a number of name changes, which indicates a shift in the conceptualization of the field. In particular, the changes reflect the fact that people now play a more active role in their healthcare. Shortliffe and Blois (2006: 24) then changed the term *medical informatics* to *biomedical informatics* and redefined it "as the scientific field that deals with biomedical information, data, and knowledge—their storage, retrieval, and optimal use for problem solving and decision making."

The broadening of the term *medical informatics* to, for example, health informatics reflects the evolving multidisciplinary nature of information management in healthcare. Health informatics is vastly more than computer science with a medical perspective. It is how we view the role of information and new information technology tools for successful outcomes in healthcare. Health informatics is defined by the problems inherit in all the health sciences, and it derives its methods, techniques, and theories from a number of other disciplines. Health informatics is about systems, the nature of the information, the specifics of a particular application area, the institutional setting, and how humans accept new ways of doing things, especially by recognizing that information is the driving force in the universe and in the specific environments in which they work. Once people understand the true nature of information, technology can exponentially enhance their knowledge and skills.

Goldstein et al. (2007: 8) summarized it well: "Medical informatics tools, technology, and tactics include not only computers and information systems, but also clinical guidelines, formal medical languages, standards, interoperability, and communication systems." Health informatics embraces an extensive range of specific applications, includes the theories and applications of health science information in all its guises, and recognizes that the key element of all activities related to the health enterprise is information. The common thread in the various definitions of health informatics is that information is the bridge between healthcare and information technology. The definitions today are broader in meaning, more inclusive, and more interdisciplinary. For the purpose of this book, we use the broader term *health informatics* to emphasize that it as an interdisciplinary body of knowledge and skills related to every aspect of healthcare.

Health Informatics as a Discipline

Health informatics is both a discipline and a profession. To qualify as a discipline, an area of study must have an extensive theoretical knowledge base and tested application theorems. Health informatics evolved as a separate discipline by adopting and refining techniques from many fields, including the basic sciences, the social sciences, and the humanities. As indicated by the cited definitions, medical informatics began to emerge as a distinct discipline in the 1980s as a support discipline for modern healthcare. Recently, the American Medical Informatics Association (AMIA) announced the establishment of The Academic Forum to promote biomedical and health informatics as a formal academic discipline.

Health Informatics as a Profession

Professions exist because societies need them. Most people have a more or less accurate perception of what a profession is, but there is no absolute consensus or exact definition. In general, a profession is an occupational group that has defined general elements, specific properties, and common operational relations. Information professionals must understand this interrelated structure and, in particular, the relationships among information resources.

In the past few decades health informatics has developed into a medical specialty and thus into a profession. It is evolving into a profession out of diverse, interdisciplinary groups of people who realized the potential of using information technology to manage healthcare information. Today this technology is challenging all of the healthcare professions and enterprises. This phenomenal application of information technology has lead to the rise of experts who call themselves health informatics professionals.

THE VITAL ROLE OF HEALTH INFORMATION TECHNOLOGY

Health information technology consists of the hardware and software used to manage information across the full spectrum of healthcare. Health information technology is impacting healthcare procedures, institutional operations, quality of healthcare, and costs, and it is opening avenues of opportunity hardly dreamed of a few decades ago. Healthcare turned to computers for the same reasons that society in general did—the overwhelming growth of information and the need for faster and more effective storage and access to information. The volume and complexity of medical knowledge long ago exceeded what humans could handle with traditional tools.

In the twenty-first century, healthcare cannot be separated from information technology. Quality healthcare starts with the knowledge and skills of human beings, but technology, especially information technology, enhances and augments that human knowledge and skills. Modern healthcare requires sophisticated and powerful information technology, and this is a major aspect of health informatics. Healthcare concerns every individual and every nation in the world, although global healthcare remains an elusive dream; in too many instances the gap between the haves and have-nots in healthcare remains formidable. Information, or the lack of it, is a central issue in the endeavor to achieve quality healthcare worldwide. Technology allows rapid access and transfer of health information, and it allows global sharing of scarce resources.

Information technology has moved into practically every arena of healthcare, including clinics, laboratories, hospitals, administrative offices, and health insurance companies. It provides healthcare at distances, through telemedicine, to manage healthcare facilities, perform research, education patients and their families, and access supportive resources, including information from global databases. Adopting new health information technologies and finding ways to integrate them into practice "will require a culture shift in the behaviors, beliefs and practices of individual healthcare providers and delivery organizations" (Institute of Medicine, 2008: 18).

The amount and complexity of health information plus the fact that the developing healthcare technology is information based have created an environment of dependency on information technology. The health sciences librarian plays a role in applying new information technologies to healthcare. For an example, see Informatics in Action! 1.1.

INFORMATICS IN ACTION! 1.1

Health Information Podcasting

Location: Nursing School

Problem: A large number of faculty, students, and staff listen to podcasts, mostly on their own computers and iPods. Several faculty members contacted the library to inquire about podcasting services. To date, the library has not explored the use of podcasts to support the curriculum.

People Involved: The information technology librarian, the director of the library, the academic dean of the nursing school, and selected members of the faculty.

Action Taken: Jeannie, the information technology librarian, is well aware of the ubiquity of podcasting. In fact, she bought one the first iPods, but she was surprised when she discovered that there are many podcasts on the Internet related to nursing. These podcasts range from news, lectures, case studies, course-related supplements, to research and more. Also, a multitude of sites feature podcasts. She proposed to the director of the library that they create podcasts, host faculty podcasts on the library's Web site, subscribe to podcasts, develop policies for the library to be a repository of faculty podcasts, and loan iPods as a systematic service for the faculty, staff, and students of the nursing school.

Takeaway: Jeannie was aware of the latest trends in podcasting and realized that the library had an opportunity to develop a new resource for their clientele.

Background of Health and Computers

Information plays a critical role in all activities related to healthcare, including clinical decision making, care management, patient education, public health, and policy making. As emphasized earlier in this chapter, gathering information has always been the first step in medical care, even centuries before electronic computers. For example, the stethoscope was invented to capture information. Information technologies that capture information are likewise invented for the advancement of healthcare, and the healthcare information profession, in many guises, is becoming a central player.

The application of computers to healthcare parallels the application of computers to other industries. By the late 1950s, practitioners realized the possibility of using computers to process medical information. For example, early information specialists developed data processing systems based on punch cards, and in healthcare this allowed statistical compilations of incidences, distributions, and causes of disease (Abdelhak et al., 2007). Early business data processing systems were also adapted to handle medical billing and other administrative functions.

Once hospital information systems were implemented, attention was soon given to handling the complex medical literature. The National Library of Medicine developed a pioneer computerized system of databases and databanks called MEDLARS (Medical Literature Analysis and Retrieval System), which evolved into a number of database collections, search engines, and gateways.

In the early 1970s, information specialists began to create medical decision-making systems for physicians, including medical expert systems. One famous example was MYCIN, developed by Edward Shortliffe and others at Stanford University. This system diagnosed infectious blood diseases and recommended antibiotics for treatment. Yu et al. (1979) reported that MYCIN had an impressive rate of correct diagnoses.

There is no doubt that the remarkable development of information technology in the past two decades is transforming healthcare systems worldwide. With the new millennium came a proliferation of electronic linkages among all healthcare endeavors. As Goodman (1998: 9) states, this linkage is "between and among hospitals, health maintenance organizations, multispecialty groups, insurance companies, clinic, physicians' and nurses' offices, laboratories, research sites, pharmacies, and, indeed, any place that people visit for healthcare or related services and any place that saves information about those visits."

The Internet has fostered change throughout society and most certainly in health informatics. It has empowered many millions of people all over the world in every aspect of life, including healthcare providers and most certainly their patients.

The Challenges Facing Information Technology in Healthcare

The design and implementation of first-class computer-based information systems in any field, including healthcare, is always a challenge. It is especially true in healthcare because of the diversity of people, functions, and expected outcomes involved. The application of new information technologies to healthcare has greatly changed the healthcare delivery environment in the past few decades and promises to do so even more in the decades that lay ahead.

According to Wickramasinghe, Gupta, and Sharma (2005: ix):

> Healthcare in the 21st Century is facing three very large forces of change, namely, an informed and empowered consumer, the need of e-health adaptability and a shift from focusing on primarily curing diseases to the prevention of diseases. In addition to having to contend with these forces, the cost of delivering quality healthcare is increasing exponentially.

All of these forces of changes are about information. Integrating information technology is perceived to be an essential component to meeting the challenges these changes create.

One criticism of this integration is that the healthcare industry has been slow in embracing and applying information technology. According to the critics, healthcare in the United States has always lagged behind other industries in investing in information technology. In 2004, the U.S. Office of the President issued a news release stating that while most American industries were spending approximately $8,000 per worker for information technology, the healthcare industry was spending only about $1,000 per worker. The news release also states that although the U.S. healthcare system is one of the most innovative in the world, its innovation and foresightedness have not been applied to the healthcare information systems, and this has built-in potential for problems. Some technology experts believe that the slow adoption of information technology by the healthcare industry is because of "the high initial cost of the equipment, difficulties in communicating among competing systems, and fear of lawsuits against hospitals and doctors that share data" (Freudenheim and Pear, 2006).

According to Stead and Fickenscher (2008), problems with healthcare information technology applications at the present time are the rapid pace of changes regarding quality and costs, a disconnect between the health industry and what is happening in information technology, and the question of how to use information technology to get aggregated information to people, not just how to automate data processing and medical devices. They maintain that the healthcare industry is still applying procedures and approaches that were developed in the 1970s to an information world that has changed dramatically.

The American Medical Association (2006) identifies seven barriers to the adoption of health information technology:

- Vendor selection and risk of obsolescence
- Cost
- Workflow (e.g., fear of disrupted services and acceptance by those involved)

- Uncertain return on investments
- Standards
- Data exchange model
- Privacy and security

Washington lawmakers continue to urge the healthcare industry to accelerate its use of information technology, insisting that such use will save money and improve care. Others, however, see problems with this, such as how to protect the privacy of medical records. U.S. Congressman John D. Dingell said that expanding electronic healthcare systems "clearly has great potential benefit . . . but it also poses serious threats to patients' privacy by creating greater amounts of personal information susceptible to thieves, rascals, rogues and unauthorized users" (Harris, 2006).

While it is true that healthcare has been lagging in the adoption of information technology, some obvious trends indicate that a massive amount of information technology is being incorporated into the medical field. New healthcare information tools are helping individuals maintain their health, and in the last decades of the twentieth century and into the new millennium, a new generation of healthcare providers is accepting and using the technology.

A continuing major challenge is to enhance quality and efficiency in healthcare delivery. We turn to computers with the expectation of achieving improvements, and we hope they will save money in the long run (Cowan, 2003). However, the first goal in implementing information technology should not be simply to reduce costs. It should be to enhance the quality of healthcare and improve patient safety. The justification of automation is value added to the services provided both in what is being done and in the potential to do things not possible before. Ideally, information technology improves quality of care and reduces costs primarily by making information more accurate and faster to access and by allowing applications that were difficult to realize with traditional manual systems.

Related to quality is the disadvantage that advanced and sophisticated information technology can cause advanced and sophisticated errors and/or abuse. Ironically, information technology can drastically reduce error but also can create its own errors. Anecdotes abound in both cases. For example, Goodman (1999) describes how computers still make mistakes. In one case a computer-controlled radiation therapy machine burned three patients to death with massive overdoses of radiation therapy due to software errors, a faulty micro switch, and confusing error messages. Also, it appears that there was inadequate testing and some negligence by hospital employees. Another case was a PC-based medication dosage system that caused medication errors (Goodman, 1999). Security and error creation and reduction are major challenges in information technology (Institute of Medicine, 2000). These issues are discussed in detail in later chapters.

Healthcare information technology applications must be prepared to meet the changes in healthcare. Stead and Fickenscher (2008) suggest that a number of changes are on the horizon for healthcare in the next 5 to 10 years. First, there will be a shift from expert-based care to system-supported practice. Instead of relying on experts for decision making, personnel will work within the infrastructure of systems for the delivery of healthcare. Second, there will be shift from medicine designed for a general population of patients to medicine tailored to the individual patient. Third, health support will be embedded into a person's environment, coming from many sources, such as education, social networks, and entertainment. Finally, an important impetus for changes in healthcare will come from outside the healthcare world.

Information Technology and People

Major activities of healthcare professionals are gathering data, classifying them into useful information, recording and storing them, and making them accessible. This involves many tasks at many nodes in the system. According to Young (2000: 9), "Healthcare is an information-dependent profession and is profoundly affected by technology. The healthcare professional spends more than 50 percent of his or her time gathering, sharing, analyzing, and seeking information." Today virtually all of these activities can be aided by information technology.

Computer applications are always about people. In the end, it is people who use knowledge plus new information to make decisions. Judgment making by computers is still a primitive science, although computers are powerful aids for human judgment making. The present state of the art and science of decision making is a melding of computer processing power with the knowledge and judgments of human beings.

A sophisticated level of informatics skills is needed by healthcare professionals in order to keep pace with the rapidly developing information technology and the changing medical practice and culture in the twenty-first century. In this age of information technology, healthcare personnel must learn to use information technology.

It is often wondered if computers are destined to replace humans. Computers certainly replace humans in performing certain tedious, routine tasks, but in general computers free humans to operate and make decision on a higher level. Information technology allows activities to be done that are not feasible manually. However, it must be remembered that tools do not define a science or a profession. Tools are only devices that help implement the intellectual and practical activities of societal endeavors. Computers do not define health informatics; rather, they enable healthcare professionals to obtain information in a faster, more efficient way. Technology alone does not make an information system. Technology combined with people make an effective information system.

The information age is a reality in healthcare. It is difficult to imagine a future in healthcare without advance information technology. It is equally difficult to imagine good decision making without direct human involvement.

The Extent of Health Informatics

In the beginning, health informatics was concerned primarily with applying information technology, but this has expanded. It now addresses the basic issues of information processing and the larger phenomena of information itself. It has also broadened the scope of applications. Clinical medicine and nursing had been the primary users of health informatics, but now health informatics is being integrated across the wide spectrum of healthcare (Young, 2000). Information technology has become an inseparable, intrinsic part of healthcare at every point of care and in practically all areas and medical specialties. The importance of information has become obvious to all healthcare professionals.

The Institute of Medicine's Committee on the Quality of Health Care in America identified a number of key areas in which information technology can help improve healthcare delivery. For example, the ubiquitous World Wide Web gives health providers as well as consumers better access to clinical evidence and the latest medical advances. The Internet and other developing technologies allow the collection and sharing of clinical information in many ways and on a scale not possible until now. This sharing of data via databases makes possible workable computer-aided decision-support systems. The Institute of Medicine maintains that clinicians must be trained to use the knowledge tools that support these decision-making systems. These automated systems should lead to the melding of knowledge tools to augment the skills and experience of the clinicians.

Information technology can also have a major impact on reducing errors. This can be achieved "by standardizing and automating certain decisions and by aiding in the identification of possible errors, such as potential adverse drug interactions, before they occur" (Institute of Medicine, 2000).

The Institute of Medicine also maintains that information technology can improve communication between clinicians and patients. It is envisioned that a time will come when patients can routinely obtain test results and exchange information online with their healthcare providers. This will reduce costs to the consumer and will save everybody's time. The IOM points out that changing information technology is bringing a new dimension to the idea of "point of care." Technology has evolved to the point that information can be made available simultaneously in a number of different places. "A patient's record can start at several points (e.g., the clinic, the hospital, the surgeon's report) and can grow and be transferred electronically to other places of need" (Institute of Medicine, 1999). The most important place to be able to quickly access the best information available is at the patient's bedside.

APPLICATIONS

If healthcare informatics is truly a science and/or a profession, then its underlying theoretical principles are the same regardless of any particular application area. The different areas distinguish themselves by their respective procedures and by the nature of their work. Health informatics is discipline specific. Information in each application area incorporates the fundamental characteristics and practice principles of the specific discipline, but the general theoretic base of informatics, as a science, is general whatever the specific application.

Information technology is transforming the healthcare industry. With its expanding nature and its ubiquity, it is no surprise that a new group of people have emerged who define themselves as professionals in a new specialty called health informatics. The next chapter goes into details of the major application areas of health informatics.

Major societal changes always cause concerns, and the rapid development of information technology has generated concerns throughout society, including healthcare. The term *information society* implies an increasing dependency on information for individual and social survival. We have always needed information to survive, but now we seem to be increasingly dependent on the technology for obtaining that information. In 1934, T.S. Eliot asked the questions, "Where is the wisdom we have lost in knowledge? Where is the knowledge we have lost in information?" If he were around today, he might be concerned that in our rush to use technology we will lose some of our the wisdom. In the feeding frenzy of information technology we must not forget the human individual. This concern for the human element is a major issue in health informatics.

In this book, we use the term *health informatics* broadly to encompass the entire enterprise, infrastructure, and supporting disciplines related to health information. Most important are the people who serve and who create and use health information.

SUMMARY

This chapter reviewed the background and basic concepts of health informatics—its origin, definition, and domain of application. The next chapter will discuss the medical environment in which health informatics exists.

REFERENCES

Abdelhak, Mervat, Sasra Grostick, Mary Alice Hanken, and Ellen Jacobs. 2007. *Health Information: Management of a Strategic Resource,* 3rd ed. Philadelphia: Saunders.
American Medical Association. "HIT Overview." Chicago: American Medical Association (September 27, 2006). Available: www.ama-assn.org/ama/pub/category/16682.html (accessed October 12, 2008).

Association of American Medical Colleges. 1986. *Medical Education in the Information Age.* Proceedings of the Symposium on Medical Informatics. Washington, DC: Association of American Medical Colleges.

British Medical Informatics Society. "What Is Medical Informatics?" London: British Medical Informatics Society (2004). Available: www.bmis.org/what_is_mi.html (accessed October 12, 2008).

Collen, Morris. F. 1986. "Origins of Medical Informatics." *Medical Informatics [Special Issue]. Western Journal of Medicine* 145, no. 6 (December): 778–785.

Cowan, Daniel L., ed. 2003. *Informatics for the Clinical Laboratory: A Practical Guide.* New York: Springer-Verlag.

Edwin Smith Papyrus. 2007. In *Encyclopaedia Britannica Online.* Available: http://search. eb.com/eb/article-9032043 (accessed October 12, 2008).

Eliot, T.S. 1934. "Choruses from the Rock." The Columbia World of Quotations. New York: Columbia University Press (1996). Available: www.bartleby.com/66 (accessed October 12, 2008).

Felkey, Bill B., Brent I. Fox, and Margaret R. Thrower. 2006. *Health Care Informatics: A Skills-based Resource.* Washington, DC: American Pharmacists Association.

Freudenheim, Milt and Robert Pear. "Health Hazard: Computers Spilling Your History." *New York Times* (December 3, 2006). Available: www.nytimes.com (accessed October 12, 2008).

Goldstein, Douglas, Peter J. Groen, Suniti Ponkshe, and Marc Wine. 2007. *Medical Informatics 20/20: Quality and Electronic Health Records Through Collaboration, Open Solutions, and Innovation.* Sudbury, MA: Jones and Bartlett.

Goodman, Kenneth W., ed. 1998. *Ethics, Computing, and Medicine: Informatics and the Transformation of Heath Care.* Cambridge: Cambridge University Press.

Harris, Gardiner. "Report Finds a Heavy Toll from Medication Errors." *New York Times,* July 21, 2006.

Institute of Medicine. "Crossing the Quality Chasm: The IOM Health Care Quality Initiative." Washington, DC: National Academies Press (1999). Available: www. iom.edu/CMS/8089.aspx (accessed October 12, 2008).

Institute of Medicine. "To Err Is Human: Building a Safe Healthcare System." Washington, DC: National Academies Press (2000). Available: www.nap.edu/catalog. php?record_id=9728 (accessed October 12, 2008).

Institute of Medicine. 2008. *Evidence Based Medicine and the Changing Nature of Healthcare.* Roundtable on Evidence Based Medicine. Washington, DC: National Academies Press.

Menzel, Wolfgang. 1841. "German Periodicals." *The American Eclectic* 2, no. 5 (September): 269–290.

Shortliffe, Edward and Marsden S. Blois. 2006. "The Computer Meets Medicine and Biology: Emergence of a Discipline." In *Biomedical Informatics: Computer Applications in Health Care and Biomedicine* (pp. 3–45), 3rd ed, edited by Edward H. Shortliffe and James J. Cimino. New York: Springer-Verlag.

Shortliffe, Edward H. and Leslie E. Perreault, eds. 1990. *Medical Informatics: Computer Applications in Health Care.* Reading, MA: Addison-Wesley Publishing.

Stead, William. 1994. "JAMIA—Why?" *Journal of the American Medical Informatics Association* 1, no. 1 (January–February): 75–76.

Stead, William and Kevin Fickenscher. "Healthcare Tech and the World: A Macro Perspective on How Technology Will Impact Healthcare in the Future." Podcast Series: *Healthcare Tech and the World, Perot Health Systems* (June, 2008). Available: www.perotsystems.com/MediaRoom/Podcasts (accessed October 25, 2008).

U.S. Department of Health and Human Services, Public Health Service, National Institutes of Health, National Library of Medicine. "Collection Development Manual." Bethesda, MD: National Library of Medicine (2004). Available: www.nlm.nih.gov/tsd/acquisitions/cdm/subjects58.html (accessed October 12, 2008).

U.S. Department of Health and Human Services, Public Health Service, National Institutes of Health, National Library of Medicine. 1987. *NLM Long Range Plan. Report of the Board of Regents.* Bethesda, MD: National Library of Medicine.

U.S. Office of the President. "President Bush Touts Benefits of Health Care Information Technology." Washington, DC: Office of the Press Secretary (April 27, 2004). Available: www.whitehouse.gov/news/releases/2004/04/20040427-5.html (accessed October 12, 2008).

Värri, Alpo. "The Case for Creating an International Committee for Standardization of Healthcare Informatics." International Healthcare Informatics, Task Group 2 (March 19, 1997). Available: www.cs.tut.fi/~varri/busiplan.html (accessed October 12, 2008).

Wickramasinghe, Nilmini, Jatinder N.D. Gupta, and Sushil K. Sharma. 2005. *Creating Knowledge-based Healthcare Organizations.* Hersey, PA: Idea Group Publishing.

Young, Kathleen M. 2000. *Informatics for Healthcare Professionals.* Philadelphia: F.A. Davis Company.

Yu, Victor L., Bruce G. Buchanan, Edward H. Shortliffe, Sharon M. Wraith, Randall Davis, A. Carlisle Scott, and Stanley N. Cohen. 1979. "Evaluating the Performance of a Computer-based Consultant." *Computer Programs in Biomedicine* 9, no. 1 (January): 95–102.

Chapter 2

The Environment of Modern Medicine

This chapter introduces the environment and organization of modern medicine as a foundation for understanding health informatics. The premise is that health sciences information professionals, including librarians, should clearly understand the infrastructure of the healthcare enterprise if they wish to find and fulfill their role in the rapidly developing field of health informatics.

Health informatics is intrinsically woven into the infrastructure of the health sciences, that is, into the nature and methods of medicine and healthcare services. Understanding the conceptual framework of healthcare is essential to understanding health informatics. This chapter examines modern medicine and the personnel involved.

THE UNIVERSALITY OF HEALTHCARE

Healthcare, of some sort, predates civilization, probably before the medicine men of primitive tribes. Actually, health concerns are not limited to humans, as evidenced by animals expressing attention and sorrow to members of their own species, especially mates and offspring, that suffer from sickness or die. At a more fundamental level, nature has built into all living things, both plants and animals, mechanisms for fighting disease and repairing damaged cells. These mechanisms are a part of the survival instinct.

Since the beginning of the human race healthcare has been an integral part of life itself. In the early records from antiquity it appears that caregivers used a combination of superstition, religion, ritual, and real medicine (Abdelhak et al., 2007). By the time of the ancient Greeks, the invocation of supernatural powers and the use of magic potions had faded (although remnants still exist in the modern world), and medicine began to be based on rational scientific methods. Ancient Greek medicine formed the foundation for modern Western medicine.

Medieval medicine in the Western world did not progress much beyond the medicine of ancient Greece and Rome. The recorded works of classical times remained the basic tenets of medieval medicine. However, in the Middle East, the Middle Ages were a golden age of scientific advances, including health and medicine. Practitioners looked for cures and promoted hygiene.

The Renaissance and the following centuries in the West brought a strong sense of a science-based medicine, and practitioners applied the advances in chemistry and biology to medicine. This opened the door to the scientific age and to modern medicine.

Today, healthcare is being reshaped by a number of elements, such as managed care and other variations in access to healthcare, costs, outcomes and satisfaction, concerns with patient safety, evidence-based medicine, complementary and alternative methods of care, and a demanding health consumer taking an active role in healthcare decisions. Networking and advancing electronic communication technologies are making health information available to all sectors of society, and a systems-based, team approach is becoming the norm. A team approach to healthcare means that health professionals, consumers, and communities work together to improve care and clinical outcomes. At the same time these changes are bringing many concerns regarding, for example, postgenomic medical ethics, privacy, and security. Healthcare has always been an integral part of society, and it has always created societal issues that continually need to be addressed. We discuss some of these societal issues in this book.

NEW HEALTHCARE PARADIGM

During most of the nineteenth century and into the twentieth century, the U.S. paradigm for healthcare generally involved sole practitioners with an office and a small staff. The physician was in charge of the way medicine was practiced in his or her office, and patients and family had limited, if any, input into health care decisions. Traditionally, the medical encounter was physician centered and facility centered; patients made an appointment and went to the doctor's office. This paradigm is, however, changing (Ball, 2003). According to Shine (2002), autonomous practices are shifting to teamwork and systems; solo practices are shifting to group practices and multidisciplinary problem solving.

The twentieth century brought rapid changes in medical theory and practice, and present day forces are reshaping traditional medical practice. The phenomenon of patients interacting with a single physician, usually over a long period of time, has given way to patients interacting with many physicians, specialists, subspecialists, and other healthcare providers. Now healthcare teams consist not only of physicians but also nurses, therapists, social counselors, healthcare insurers, the government, and lawyers. Today's healthcare system, in the United States and elsewhere, is a complex structure "composed of multiple types of facilities, providers, payers, and regulators as well as consumers who are demanding more and better health care" (Abdelhak et al., 2007: 8). The modern paradigm is system structured and managed, driven by information technology, including networking and advanced communication infrastructures.

STRUCTURE OF THE HEALTHCARE SYSTEM

Health informatics is based on an understanding of how the healthcare system is structured, where information is needed, and the nature of the needed information. The healthcare system is a complex maze of subsystems, sometimes overlapping, connected through people and technology. It consists of a broad range of professionals, technical support personnel, and numerous staff at all levels.

Types of Services

Many types of healthcare facilities and services are available to the population, existing in a complex system of therapeutic, remedial, and preventive models. Healthcare services are provided by hospitals, clinics, governments, volunteer agencies, independent healthcare professionals, pharmaceutical and medical equipment manufacturers, and private insurance companies.

The healthcare system offers four broad types of services: diagnosis and treatment, rehabilitation, disease prevention, and health promotion. Traditionally the most used services involved diagnosis and treatment. Usually people waited until they were ill to seek medical attention. However, because recent technologic advances have greatly improved the capacity of the healthcare system to diagnose and treat illnesses, people now seek these services more often. These advances have also increased the complexity and cost of healthcare.

Modern medicine now also focuses on disease prevention, and health promotion, and rehabilitation after illness. Disease prevention is closely related to health promotion. The aim is to promote an understanding of the risks of disease, injury, disability, and death. Modern medicine promotes health literacy and behavior modification in order to eliminate the risks. Health promotion services are designed to help clients reduce the risk of illness, maintain optimal function, and follow a healthy lifestyle. These services are provided in a variety of ways and settings.

Paying for Healthcare

The healthcare system is primarily financed through nongovernmental, private means by either personal funds or health insurance plans. The federal government provides very few direct health services, preferring to develop new, improved services by furnishing funds for programs it wants to see developed and/or expanded. With some exceptions, the federal government has no authority to provide direct services—this is a function of the private sector and the states. The federal government is involved, however, in financing research and individual healthcare for the elderly and indigent via Medicare and Medicaid.

The U.S. Congress plays a key role in the federal activities related to healthcare by passing laws, allocating funds, and conducting investigative work through committees. The most important federal agency concerned with health affairs is the Department of Health and Human Services (DHHS). The principal health-related unit within this department is the Public Health Service (PHS), which has five units within its domain: National Institutes of Health (NIH); Alcohol, Drug Abuse, and Mental Health Administration (ADAMHA); Food and Drug Administration (FDA); Centers for Disease Control and Prevention (CDC); Health Resources and Services Administration (HRSA); and the Agency for Healthcare Research and Quality (AHRQ). State and local governments also provide public health services at the state, county, and city levels.

THE PEOPLE IN HEALTHCARE

The education and practice of the people in healthcare is regulated by agencies, organizations, and legislation. Regulation includes state licensure, certification, and accreditation of educational programs.

In the United States, the healthcare industry employs more people than any other industry, and it continues to grow. The U.S. Bureau of Labor Statistics projects that between 2008 and 2016 three million healthcare jobs will be created (Glod, 2008).

Because the U.S. healthcare industry is so large and complex, it is also very labor intensive. The healthcare system consists of a wide range of professionals, associates, and rank and file personnel engaged in a multitude of different activities; at every level and point in the system, information is the critical element.

Healthcare practitioners work in hundreds of different healthcare environments, ranging from clinics and hospitals to educational institutions, government, and private industry. Practitioners include (in addition to physicians and nurses) audiologists, cardiovascular technicians, dental assistants, home healthcare aids, nuclear medicine technicians, and many others.

Understanding the different levels of healthcare personnel, the nature of their education, and their professional responsibilities is the first step in understanding their information needs. Healthcare informatics professionals must thoroughly understand the healthcare professions and the activities of their personnel.

The following discussion highlights a variety of workers who staff the healthcare infrastructure. While this list is not complete, it does represent the major levels and gives a broad perspective on the complexity of the work force. The discussion is based in part on information in the U.S. Department of Labor Statistics' (2008) "Occupational Outlook Handbook, 2008–09."

Physicians

The American Medical Association (2004) divides the physician's professional activities into *patient care* and *nonpatient care*. Patient care can be given by *office-based practices* or *hospital-based practices*. Office-based practices may have one or two physicians or a group of physicians. Although there is a resurgence of interest in home care, private practice continues to be the most prevalent type. However, managed care is leading many physicians to move toward the integrated group and salaried practice. Hospital-based practice includes individuals who divide their time between a hospital and a private office.

Individuals in a nonpatient care service may have teaching appointments in medical schools or other institutions of higher learning. Some perform administrative tasks, and some are employed by insurance companies, pharmaceutical companies, corporations, voluntary organizations, medical societies, and broadcasting, just to mention a few.

There are two general types of physicians: The MD (Doctor of Medicine) and the DO (Doctor of Osteopathic Medicine). Both types undergo similar training. Both obtain undergraduate degrees and attend four years of medical school. The DO goes to a school of osteopathic medicine, while the MD goes to a school of medicine. Both take licensing exams, have specialties, set up practices, perform surgery, and issue prescriptions. The basic difference between the two groups is that the DO has specific training in osteopathic manipulation on patients. Osteopathic medicine views the body as a whole system, with disease being a total body malfunction. Treatment may involve physical manipulations and recommending a plan to enhance the body's natural healing powers. Osteopathic medicine is a fast growing segment of the healthcare industry.

There are dozens of medical specialties, ranging from those based on major body organs to nuclear medicine, occupational medicine, and public health. The American Medical Association (2008) lists 110 national medical specialist societies. The largest are family practice, emergency medicine, internal medicine, obstetric-gynecology, orthopedics, pediatrics, psychiatry, and surgery.

About one third of MDs and more than half of DOs are primary care physicians. They practice general and family medicine, general internal medicine, or general pediatrics and usually are the first health professionals patients consult. Primary care physicians tend to see the same patients on a regular basis for preventive care and treatment. General and family practitioners emphasize comprehensive healthcare for patients of all ages and for the family as a group.

The basic medical school educational program for physicians lasts four years, usually divided into a preclinical and a clinical part. In the preclinical part the basic sciences dominate the curriculum, with such subjects as anatomy, biochemistry, physiology, microbiology, pharmacology, and pathology. Some schools structure their programs to emphasize the basic sciences, and others present the sciences within the context of their relevance to each organ system in the body. With the latter approach, students from the beginning make medical decisions by studying the interacting of science with the human body.

During the clinical part of the program, students begin to see patients. They take medical histories and are involved in diagnostic and treatment plans. Of course, they are closely monitored by faculty and other personnel involved in the cases.

Teaching methods have changed in recent years, with a movement toward problem-based learning (often using evidence-based medicine procedures, which are discussed in Chapter 3). The formal lecture format is being replaced by the case study approach and small-group learning experiences. Another major shift is the increased use of computer technology, two examples being computer-assisted learning and virtual reality simulations. After students finish the four-year program and an internship, they often follow up with residency training, which can vary from three to seven years, according to the specialty.

After completing his or her education, a physician has to obtain a license to practice. The requirements for licensing are (1) graduating from an accredited medical program and (2) passing a licensing examination. Each state has its own laws and rules for licensing. The following Web sites present more detailed information about medical education:

- American Medical Association (AMA). Available: www.ama-assn.org (accessed October 14, 2008)
- Association of Medical Student Association (AMSA). Available: www.amsa.org (accessed October 14, 2008)
- Association of American Medical Colleges (AAMC). Available: www.aamc.org (accessed October 14, 2008)
- Career MD (residency resource for medical students). Available: www.careermd.com (accessed October 14, 2008)
- National Resident Matching Program (NRMP). Available: www.nrmp.org (accessed October 14, 2008)
- Fellowship and Residency Electronic Interactive Database. Available: www.ama-assn.org/ama/pub/category/2997.html (accessed October 14, 2008.

Hospitalists

In recent years, a new type of physician has emerged: the "hospitalist" or inpatient specialist. These physicians are employed full time by a hospital, where they maintain an office, equipment, and support staff and receive a salary. They generally come from the ranks of internal medicine.

It should be made clear that a hospitalist is a physician. The distinguishing characteristic of hospitalists is that their primary focus is the general medical care of patients in a hospital. Their basic activities are patient care, but they also teach and do research, all of which is related to hospital medicine (Society of Hospital Medicine, 2008).

There have always been physicians who focused on inpatients, but in the past decade the number of doctors practicing as hospitalists has increased dramatically. More jobs are currently available in this area than in any other area of internal medicine (Society of Hospital Medicine, 2008).

The advantage of this type of service is that patient care is immediately and consistently coordinated throughout the patient's hospital stay. Proponents of the hospitalist model believe that it also improves quality of care and saves costs. The downside is that some patients don't like being assigned a new physician during a critical time in their healthcare. In addition, there is the potential for lack of communication between the inpatient physician and the patient's primary care provider.

Biomedical Engineers

By combining biology and medicine with engineering, biomedical engineers develop devices and procedures that solve medical and health-related problems. Many conduct research, together with life scientists, chemists, and medical scientists, on the engineering aspects of the biological systems of humans and animals. Biomedical engineering is different from health informatics in that the biomedical engineer is basically concerned with machines and devices.

Chiropractors

Chiropractors diagnose and treat patients whose health problems involve the body's muscular, nervous, and skeletal systems, especially the spine. The chiropractic approach to healthcare is holistic, stressing the patient's overall health and wellness.

Most states require at least two years of undergraduate education to enter a chiropractic program, although more states are now requiring a full four years. All states require a Doctor of Chiropractic degree from an accredited four-year program. In addition, most states require a four-part examination in order to be licensed. Some chiropractic colleges offer specializations (e.g., sports injuries, rehabilitation, orthopedics) through postdoctoral training.

Clinical Laboratory Technologists

Clinical laboratory technologists play a crucial role in the detection, diagnosis, and treatment of disease. They analyze body fluids, tissues, and cells. The basic education requirement for a medical or clinical laboratory technologist is a bachelor's degree in medical technology or in one of the life sciences. An alternative is a program that combines course work, specialized training, and on-the-job experience. The education program is heavy in science and laboratory technical skills.

Dentists

Dentists diagnose and treat tooth and oral tissue problems. They also perform corrective surgery on gums and supporting bones to treat gum diseases. To be licensed as a dentist, candidates must complete a program at a dental school accredited by the American Dental Association and pass an examination. Dental school programs are usually four years long and consist of courses in the basic sciences and a clinical part in which students treat patients while under the supervision of licensed dentists. Graduates receive a Doctor of Dental Surgery (DDS) or a Doctor of Dental Medicine (DMD). Candidates must pass a written and practical examination. The written portion may be taken from the Nation Board Dental Examinations or from the a state dental board, and the practical part is taken at the state level. Postgraduate programs are available for those who want to specialize (e.g., cosmetic dentistry).

Dental Assistants

Dental assistants perform auxiliary services related to dental work. Duties may include simple patient care, laboratory work, and office duties. Dental assistant training has primarily been provided on the job, but more two-year colleges and trade schools are now offering training programs. The American Dental Association's Commission on Dental Accreditation accredits dental assistant programs. The community college programs are two years long and grant an associate degree, but most other programs are one-year long and grant a certificate or diploma. The programs require classroom and laboratory work and practical experience in dental schools, clinics, or dental offices.

Dental Hygienists

Dental hygienists examine teeth and gums and perform other technical duties. They also educate patients on good oral hygiene. Licensure is granted in accordance with the individual state requirements.

Most accredited dental hygiene programs lead to an associate degree, a certificate, or a bachelor's or master's degree. Higher degrees are required if the dental hygienist wishes to teach or work in public or school health programs. To be licensed, candidates must graduate from an accredited dental hygiene program, successfully complete the written National Board Dental Hygiene Examination, and pass the regional or state clinical board exam.

Health Informationists

The National Library of Medicine defines informationists as information specialists who have received graduate training and practical experience that provides them with a disciplinary background both in medical or biological sciences and in information sciences/informatics. The cross training provides informationists with a unique perspective on the acquisition, synthesis, and application of information to problem solving and program development in their chosen area.

Careers in health informatics require formal education and training, and there are a number of pathways for achieving this. Those with clinical experience and no information technology expertise, or those with degrees in such fields as computer science or health sciences librarianship, should pursue postgraduate training that focuses on health informatics.

Licensed Practical/Vocational Nurses

Licensed practical/vocational nurses (LPN/LVN) provide basic bedside care for the sick, injured, convalescent, and disabled under the direction of physicians and registered nurses. They take vital signs, treat bedsores, prepare and give injections, apply dressings, and so on.

Usually a high school diploma is required to enter an approved practical nursing program. These programs exist mainly in technical or vocational schools and in community colleges. Other avenues are programs in high schools, hospitals, and colleges. The programs last about a year and include both classroom study of basic nursing care and practical experience. For licensing, all states require the passing of a national exam called the NCLEX-PN exam after successful completion of a state-approved training program.

Nurse Practitioners

A nurse practitioner (NP) is a special type of registered nurse who maintains a close relationship with physicians in patient care, providing a wide range of services, including some generally given by the physicians, and sometimes serving as a patient's regular healthcare provider. NPs focus on individualized care. Some NPs conduct research and are involved in patient advocacy. They work in widely diverse environments, including physician offices, community health centers, home care agencies, hospice centers, hospitals, and nursing homes.

After becoming a registered nurse, the NP candidate must obtain a master's degree and receive training in the diagnosis and management of common medical conditions. The State Boards of Nursing regulate NPs, and each state has its own licensing criteria. NPs can also apply for national certification from the American Nursing Association or other professional nursing boards such as the American Academy of Nurse Practitioners.

Paramedics

People's lives often depend on the quick reactions and competent care of emergency medical technicians and paramedics. These specialists respond to medical emergencies and care for patients before the patients reach a health facility. They work in numerous settings that require quick medical responses, such as ambulance services, fire departments, private businesses, and industrial settings.

Paramedics need both formal training and certification. Training is offered in tiers, including basic, intermediate, and higher levels. Classroom work is interspersed with work time in ambulances and/or emergency rooms. These programs take up to two years and end with an associate degree in applied sciences. The training prepares the graduates to take the National Registry of Emergency Medical Technicians Exam and to become registered. Some states require this national registration, and other states have their own registration systems.

Pharmacists

Pharmacists dispense drugs prescribed by physicians and other health practitioners and provide information to patients about medications and their use. They advise physicians and other healthcare providers on the selection, dosages, interactions, and side effects of medications. Pharmacists must understand the use, clinical effects, and composition of drugs, including their chemical, biological, and physical properties. Most pharmacists work in a community setting, such as a retail drug store, or in a hospital or clinic. They also give advice about durable medical equipment and home healthcare supplies. In general, pharmacists are taking a more active role in counseling consumers about their medications. Most pharmacists keep confidential computerized records of patients' drug therapies to ensure that harmful drug interactions do not occur. These professionals play an essential role in consumer health education, and they are becoming more actively involved as agents of change in community health.

To be licensed, pharmacists must graduate from an accredited college of pharmacy, serve an internship, and pass a state examination. Pharmacy programs typically require a minimum of six years of postsecondary study, and graduates receive a Doctor of Pharmacy (PharmD) degree. After obtaining the degree, graduates may take the licensure examination of a state board of pharmacy. Pharmacists may do postgraduate work toward master's and PhD degrees.

Physician Assistants

Physician assistants (PAs) provide healthcare services under the supervision of physicians. They should not be confused with medical assistants, who perform routine clinical and clerical tasks. PAs are formally trained to provide diagnostic, therapeutic, and preventive healthcare services, as delegated by a physician. Working as members of the healthcare team, they take medical histories, examine and treat patients, order and interpret laboratory tests and X-rays, make diagnoses, and prescribe medications.

PAs must complete an accredited program and pass a national exam. Generally, these programs are in schools of allied health, four-year colleges, or medical schools. Also, many of these programs have clinical teaching affiliations with medical schools. The course of study includes basic science, health sciences, and supervised clinical training. In most cases a master's degree is awarded, although a few programs offer bachelor's or associate degrees. In addition to obtaining a degree, graduates must pass the Physician Assistant National Certifying Examination, which is administered by the National Commission on Certification of Physician Assistants. The exam is opened only to graduates of an accredited program. Those who wish to become a specialist can enter a postgraduate program.

Registered Nurses

Registered nurses (RNs) work to promote health, prevent disease, and help patients with health-related concerns. They are advocates and health educators for patients, families, and communities. When providing direct patient care, they observe, assess, and record symptoms, reactions, and progress, assist physicians during treatments and examination, administer medications, and assist in convalescence and rehabilitation. There is a wide diversity of types of nurses depending of the work setting, and specialties focus on disease, ailment, or condition; organ or body system type; or population. RNs can combine specialties from more than one area, such as geriatric oncology.

Hospital nurses form the largest group of nurses. Most are staff nurses, who provide bedside nursing care and carry out medical regimens. *Office nurses* care for outpatients in physicians' offices, clinics, surgical centers, and emergency medical centers. *Triage nurses* assess the severity of the patient's concerns (e.g., symptoms) and then guide the patient to the appropriate level of care. This service is usually offered at a healthcare facility. *Nursing home nurses* manage the care of residents with conditions ranging from a fracture to Alzheimer's disease. *Home health nurses* provide periodic services to patients at home. *Public health nurses* specialize in community health. They work in government and private agencies and clinics, schools, retirement communities, and other community settings. *Occupational health nurses* provide nursing care at worksites to employees, customers, and others with minor injuries and illnesses.

RNs must graduate from an accredited nursing program and pass a national licensing examination known as the NCLEX-RN in order to obtain a nursing license. There are a number of educational pathways, including a bachelor's of science in nursing (BSN), an associate degree in nursing (ADN), and a diploma. The bachelor's degree is from a regular four-year college program. The associate degree offered by community colleges takes two to three years, and the diploma program obtained in hospitals takes three years. There are master's degrees and postmaster's degree for nurses wanting to become administrators, teachers, or researchers. Nursing programs include formal course work and supervised clinical experience in healthcare sittings.

Veterinarians

Veterinarians specialize in animal medicine and play a major role in the healthcare of pets, livestock, and zoo, sporting, and laboratory animals. Some veterinarians use their skills to protect humans against disease carried by animals and conduct clinical research on human and animal health problems. Most veterinarians perform clinical work in private practice. More than half of private practice veterinarians predominately, or exclusively, treat small animals.

Veterinarians in clinical practice diagnose health problems, vaccinate against diseases such as distemper and rabies, medicate animals suffering from infections or illnesses, treat and dress wounds, set fractures, perform surgery, and advise owners about feeding, behavior, and breeding.

Veterinarians must complete a four-year program from an accredited college of veterinary medicine and obtain a Doctor of Veterinary Medicine (DVM) degree. Not all veterinary schools require a bachelor's degree, but they do require a large number of undergraduate credit hours, with an emphasis on the sciences. Graduates must pass a national board examination to obtain a license before they can practice. Veterinarians can obtain board certification in a specialty by completing a three- to four-year residency program.

This list of specialties is by no means exhaustive but rather representative of the nature of the personnel involved in healthcare. Others include community health educators, nutritionists, physical therapists, psychologists, nuclear medicine technologists, healthcare social workers, health services managers, cardiovascular technologists and technicians, and diagnostic medical monographers.

MEDICAL RESEARCH

Since humans became conscious of themselves as entities, they have tried to understand their existence and answer puzzling questions. For this purpose, humans created religion, philosophy, and eventually science. All professions have a theoretical base, that is, an extensive set of general principles and understandings that come from experience and from research. Scientists developed a variety of procedures for observations and analysis known collectively as the *scientific method*. Using the scientific method to learn new knowledge is called *research*. Research is the driving force that advances medical science and its supporting disciplines. Olson (2000: 236) identifies three broad categories of research in healthcare:

> Three broad categories of research are carried out in healthcare organizations: clinical, administrative, and educational research. Within each category, both basic and applied investigations are conducted. **Basic research** has no immediate or practical goal, but it establishes a reservoir of data, theoretical explanations, and concepts that can be utilized in applied research. **Applied research** is aimed at solving specific problems. **Clinical research** is carried out in any setting in which patient care is provided and involves examining outcomes relating to those services.

Clinical research is costly and subject to rigid ethical controls. Funding comes primarily from the government and industry. Government funding has been extensive for many years, but also substantial monies come from the pharmaceutical industry and other businesses that have economic interests in healthcare. Also, organizations and philanthropic foundations provide funds.

In addition, administrative research addresses the operations of systems that deliver healthcare services, including work flow efficiency, utilization of resources, outcome evaluations, and cost. Educational research addresses the effectiveness of educating healthcare professionals, including curriculum and education delivery formats and methods. In recent years educational research has included patient education and how to make the patient more a part of the healthcare process.

Information professionals are key players in all phases of research. Research builds on the existing knowledge base of a discipline, and that knowledge base is preserved in the literature. This is where the information professional steps to the forefront of the research process. Because information technology plays a major role in research, health informatics experts are involved at the basic level.

RECENT TRENDS

Recent changes in healthcare include medical advances, the relationship between these advances and information technology, and the recognition of the critical role that information plays throughout the healthcare endeavor. New trends in medicine include more group medical practices, managed care, increased role of the patient, outpatient care, long-term care, complementary and alternative medicine, the growing uninsured population, and the burgeoning use of the Internet and integrated medical information systems.

Another trend is the linkages among public health protocols, preventive medicine, and the development of personalized medicine, which is being encouraged by the rise of genomic research and applications. In other words, the new goal is "wellness" in individuals and in the population (Joiner, 2006).

Furthermore, health management, from small clinics to the most complex health organizations, is increasingly being structured around the "systems approach." This approach usually involves some form of information technology, but the concept embraces more than technology. It involves the entire infrastructure of the organization, including people and all the resources engaged in the healthcare services.

In *Crossing the Quality Chasm: A New Health System for the 21st Century*, the Institute of Medicine (2001) listed five significant changes occurring in healthcare: (1) the shift from acute to chronic care, (2) the move to expand evidence-based medicine and the use of information technology, (3) the increased use of teams in clinical practices, (4) the increasing complexity of delivery arrangements, and (5) changing patient–clinician relationships. We discuss some of these paradigm shifts in more detail.

Group Medical Practice

Group practice is when a number of physicians band together, usually on the basis of specialization, to provide patient care. Often the groups share facilities and have centralized management. Many people believe that healthcare has become so complex that it takes carefully assembled and organized teams to give quality care at a profitable level. The ideal group practice is composed of physicians who have the same philosophy of healthcare and its delivery, and group practice has been criticized for not achieving this. Critics say that group practice is more of a business model, not a healthcare service model (Enthoven and Tolen, 2004).

Managed Care

The *MedlinePlus Dictionary* (U.S. Department of Health and Human Services, 2005) defines managed care as "a system of providing health care (as by an HMO or a PPO) that is designed to control costs through managed programs in which the physician accepts constraints on the amount charged for medical care and the patient is limited in the choice of a physician." *Managed care* is a broad term that encompasses care provided by various health maintenance organizations (HMOs), preferred-provider organizations (PPOs), and other health plans. Managed care is a system based on the idea of prepaid membership rather than fee for service. The system usually includes a group of providers who offer a specific health plan. Patients join the plan and pay in advance. Managed care emphasizes prevention, accessibility, and overall primary care with minimized specialist care. The advent of managed care has lowered costs and excessive use of services in the past few decades but has compromised the role of the physician and, to some extent, eroded patient trust in the system (Ball, 2003).

PPOs have the advantage over HMOs in that patients can received treatment outside a list of preferred of doctors, and they receive at least partial reimbursement, usually around 90 percent, of the expenses. Both HMO and PPO providers believe that their customers should have more health information. This is a signal to health informatics professionals that customers are capable of making informed decisions related to their healthcare and the economics involved in those decisions.

Role of the Patient

A strong interest in the role of the patient in healthcare has emerged in recent year in part due to the general societal consumer movement in the United States and to the more universal coverage of health matters in the media. Consumer awareness has moved into healthcare, especially the idea that patients should not be passive observers of their own health, simply taking medications on time and remembering doctor appointments, but should make needed lifestyle changes and take some responsibility for good health. They should become partners with the healthcare providers.

The changing role of the patient also includes the concept of patient empowerment. Patients should be empowered to make their own choices. The idea is that everyone has the basic right to make choices and assume responsibility for outcomes regarding their health.

Outpatient Care

In the past two decades, patient care has shift from inpatient to ambulatory. According to the Centers for Disease Control and Prevention, ambulatory care is increasing in large part because of information technology. Clearly, information technology can enhance the quality and management of ambulatory services, which in turn will result in their expanded use.

The emphasis, especially in managed care, is on more outpatient care and shorter hospital stays. According to Abdelhak et al. (2007), four factors are driving this shift:

1. Technology allows services to be provided in outpatient settings.
2. Government and other payers now offer reimbursement incentives for outpatient services.
3. Managed care is based on outpatient services.
4. The consumer movement encourages patients to seek ambulatory care.

In the past few decades both the types of outpatient services offered and number of patients utilizing them have increased. This is a response to economic pressures, but in addition medical advances and techniques have made it possible for many patients to have shorter hospital stays. Hospitals have been redesigning their service infrastructures to focus on outpatient care.

A key element in successful outpatient care services is communication between health care providers and the patients and their families. Clearly, increased health literacy is a significant factor in the trend toward more outpatient care.

Long-term Care

As the average life expectancy continues to increase, the number of people over age 65 and the healthcare challenges associated with this population are growing. The term *long-term care* covers many situations, including home care, assisted living, and nursing homes, and services range from simple custodial care to intensive medical care. In 2008, 9 million people over 65 needed long-term medical care (U.S. Department of Health and Human Services, 2008). Because of the rapidly increasing number of elderly people and rising healthcare costs, some estimates project that by the year 2012 approximately 12 million people in the United States will need long-term care.

Complementary and Alternative Medicine

Interest in complementary and alternative medicine (CAM) continues to increase in the general population and in clinical medicine. In 1998, the National Institutes of Health established the National Center for Complementary and Alternative Medicine (NCCAM).

CAM is defined by the NCCAM (2008) as "a group of diverse medical and health care systems, practices, and products that are not presently considered to be part of conventional medicine." Complementary medicine is combined with conventional medicine, whereas alternative medicine is used instead of conventional medicine.

According to a survey on alternative medicine use in the United States published in the *Journal of the American Medical Association* in 1998, 42 percent of the population used at least one alternative therapy in 1997. Users were more frequently women than men (49 vs. 38 percent), and 50 percent were in the 36–49-year age bracket. Fifty-one percent had a college education, and 48 percent had incomes over $50,000. This study gives quantitative support to the impression that more patients are turning to nontraditional forms of health care. Clearly, the attention being paid to alternative medicine is appropriate, at least in terms of the magnitude of its use (Eisenberg et al., 1998).

There is an exponential increase in the use of alternative and complementary therapies. "In 2001, Americans invested US $50 billion in this form of health care, according to John Weeks, editor of *The Integrator*, a newsletter tracking 'the business of alternative medicine,' with 40% of American adults turning at some point to alternative medicine" (Willinsky and Quint-Rapoport, 2007: e19). There is no formal consensus of what constitutes alternative and complementary therapies, but in general they include biologically based practices (e.g., dietary supplements), mind–body medicine (e.g., meditation), and physical manipulation–based practices (e.g., massage).

In January 2005, the Institute of Medicine released *Complementary and Alternative Medicine in the United States*, a report that discusses the scientific and policy implications of the widespread use of CAM. There is a movement toward integrative medicine whereby professionals in conventional and complementary medicine work together to provide patients with the safest and most appropriate treatments. As evidence of the effectiveness of CAM builds up in the literature, healthcare providers will be more likely to incorporate CAM into their practices.

Uninsured People

Over 47 million Americans are without health insurance, and the number is growing. People are paying for healthcare services with credit cards and getting into debt at an alarming rate. About half of all personal bankruptcies are caused by high medical bills. Surprisingly, most of the people who go bankrupt do have health insurance, but it doesn't cover the expenses (Associated Press, 2005). Families are more and more turning to credit cards, and this has a snowballing effect because credit card interest rates are exorbitant. Low and middle income people have 46 percent more credit card debt if they are incurring medical expenses (Consumer Action, 2007).

More and more kids are being "left behind" when it comes to having adequate healthcare. Government initiatives to insure children have increased in recent years. In most states uninsured children in families of up to four can get some insurance if the family earns less than $34,100 (U.S. Department of Health and Human Services, no date). The issue continues to be debated every time new appropriation bills come up before the U.S. Congress.

Economic troubles and the growing costs of healthcare have caused some businesses to drop employee health coverage plans; and some workers can't afford the plans that are offered. While most uninsured individuals are from low income groups, the uninsured stretch across all income levels. Related to this is the sky-high cost of prescription drugs, which greatly affects the uninsured. Many consider the problem of the medically uninsured a major crisis in the United States.

The Internet and Integrated Medical Information Systems

The use of the Internet in the healthcare industry has exploded and continues to accelerate day by day. Every facet of healthcare is affected, including healthcare services, access to the professional/nonprofessional literature, telemedicine, and health commercial enterprises, consumer information. Healthcare professionals, supporting staff, patients, insurers, educators, researchers, government agencies, commercial enterprises, and others are turning to the Internet. Clearly, the Internet is becoming interwoven into the fabric of healthcare, not only in the United States, but globally.

The concept of integrated medical information systems has been around for a number of years, but the rapid development of communication systems and other information technology has greatly increased the movement toward integrated medical information systems. The common goal of most healthcare information systems today is to integrate all electronic systems throughout an organization and with other healthcare facilities as needed. These systems are designed around advanced telecommunication technology that allows linkage of patient information at all levels and interaction of all administrative and support systems in the organization(s). Integrated systems reduce duplication of work, bring faster information access, and vastly enhance reporting and legal compliances. Major vendor systems on the market are integrated systems, and there is a movement to build these systems on an Internet platform. This movement raises issues of interoperability and standards for communication and data transmission.

Integrated health information systems have positively impacted patient safety, global health, home healthcare, implantable eCare, and emergency preparedness and response systems. A major topic in the past decade or more has been the emergence of electronic medical records. Recent healthcare literature reflects a growing interest in the implementation of these systems. Chapter 8 is devoted to the electronic medical record.

HEALTH INFORMATICS SKILLS AND COMPETENCIES IN THE TWENTY-FIRST CENTURY

Technology is of little use without skilled humans who know where, when, and how to use it. Health informatics is the study of how health information is created, structured, and effectively distributed to those who need it. It deals with the total spectrum of health information from its creation to its final applications. Hence the general competencies and skills required in health informatics include not only the ability to analyze medical information but also the ability to communicate that information as medical knowledge.

Some essential skills are prerequisite for clinician informatics professionals, in addition to medical knowledge. The informatics professional must know how to keep up with the growing body of medical knowledge, including understanding the scientific process and interpreting the statistical-based research that is universal in medical research. The informatics professional must be able to interpret uncertain clinical data and to detect inconsistencies and defects in methodology and procedures in research. Finding evidence and mining the information are basic competencies required of these professionals.

The informatics professional needs to be able to analyze and structure clinical decisions in terms of risks and benefits and to adapt and apply clinical knowledge to specific situations. Finally, the informatics professional needs to be able to communicate with all those he or she deals with and be capable of selecting and utilizing the most appropriate method (e.g., face-to-face interview, telephone, e-mail, or text messaging) for doing this (Coiera, 1998). The preceding skills discussed by Coiera, and others, in the late 1990s, focused on practicing clinicians who are pursuing a career in health informatics. However, health informatics has grown beyond a clinical situation to encompass much more, and it continues to broaden its scope into areas that were not previously considered part of health informatics. For instance, the National Health Service in the United Kingdom has included all its information technology services, including information technology support, under the jurisdiction of health informatics.

Today, the field of health informatics is diverse and the skills and knowledge required vary according to the job, but there are a number of broad requirements: (1) knowledge of information technology, especially in healthcare applications; (2) understanding of the principles of information organization,

INFORMATICS IN ACTION! 2.1

Identifying Informatics Competencies

Location: Newly established medical school

Problem: Administrators are creating an informatics department at a newly established medical school. The faculty and administrators want to ensure that the students have the informatics competencies needed to be successful in clinical practice and medical research.

People Involved: Curriculum committee and the informationist from the library.

Action Taken: Max, the informationist, holds a PhD degree in health informatics and a master's degree in library and information sciences, with a concentration in health sciences librarianship. He decided to use a quantitative approach to address the uncertainty regarding what competencies and skills should be taught to medical students. He used the bibliometric technique known as *Bradford's Law* to analyze the catalogs of informatics programs as well as the recommendation reports from informatics associations in order to identify the most current competencies being taught. He charted the distribution into a Bradford-like curve, which grouped consensus competencies and skills at the high end of the distribution curve.

Takeaway: Max drew on his educational experiences in an informatics program and on his familiarity with bibliometric techniques from information science to identify the current focus and concentration of informatics competencies and skills perceived to be needed by clinicians and medical researchers.

retrieval, and use; (3) understanding of the principles of system analysis and design, (4) in-depth understanding of the healthcare enterprise in all its guises; and (5) excellent communication skills, both oral and written.

The skills and competencies needed in health informatics change with trends and developments in the healthcare field and in informatics practices. For example, presently there is a trend to "consumer informatics, measuring and improving quality in health, team and interpersonal skills, and data mining could be among tomorrow's core competencies and knowledge requirements" (Huang, 2007). Also, as the fields of genetics and genomic medicine advance, health informatics professionals will need to become proficient and knowledgeable about bioinformatics data and their applications to healthcare.

SUMMARY

It is not possible to fully understand health informatics without understanding the healthcare infrastructure, including the people involved and what they do. To provide useful information in any form or for any purpose, it is essential to have a clear perspective of the environment where that information is created, transferred, and used. With this background, the next chapter discusses how health informatics impacts modern medicine.

REFERENCES

Abdelhak, Mervat, Sara Grostick, Mary Alice Hanken, and Ellen Jacobs. 2007. *Health Information: Management of a Strategic Resource,* 3rd ed. Philadelphia: Saunders.

American Medical Association. "Choosing a Specialty." Chicago: American Medical Association (April 24, 2008). Available: www.ama-assn.org/ama/pub/category/2375.htm (accessed October 15, 2008).

Associated Press. "Medical Bills Make up Half of Bankruptcies." New York: MSNBC (February 2, 2005). Available: www.msnbc.msn.com/id/6895896 (accessed October 15, 2008).

Ball, Marion J. 2003. *Consumer Informatics: Applications and Strategies in Cyber Healthcare.* New York: Springer-Verlag.

Coiera, Enrico. 1998. "Medical Informatics Meets Medical Education: There's More to Understanding Information Than Technology." *Medical Journal of Australia* 168: 319–320.

Consumer Action. "Medical Bills on Credit Cards." San Francisco: Consumer Action (March, 2007). Available: www.consumer-action.org/radar/articles/medical_bills_on_credit_cards1 (accessed October 15, 2008).

Eisenberg, David M., Roger B. Davis, Susan L. Ettner, Scott Appel, Sonja Wilkey, Maria Van Rompay, and Ronald C. Kessler. 1998. "Trends in Alternative Medicine Use in the United States, 1990–1997." *Journal of the American Medical Association* 280, no. 18 (November 11): 1569–1575.

Enthoven, Alain C. and Laura A. Tolen. 2004. *Toward a 21st Century Health System: The Contributions and Promise of Prepaid Group Practice.* San Francisco: John Wiley and Sons.

Glod, Maria. 2008. "A Head Start for the Medical-Minded: High Schools Offer More Classes in Growing Field." *The Washington Post,* October 4. Available: www.washingtonpost.com/wp-dyn/content/article/2008/10/03/AR2008100303365_pf.html (accessed March 13, 2009).

Huang, Qi Rong. 2007. "Competencies for Graduate Curricula in Health, Medical and Biomedical Informatics: A Framework." *Health Informatics Journal* 13, i2 (June): 89(15). Available: http://jhi.sagepub.com/cgi/content/abstract/13/2/89 (accessed October 19, 2008).

Institute of Medicine. 2001. *Crossing the Quality Chasm: A New Health System for the 21st Century.* Washington, DC: National Academies Press.

Institute of Medicine. 2005. *Complementary and Alternative Medicine in the United States.* Washington, DC: National Academies Press.

Joiner, Keith. "Message from the Vice Provost of Medical Affairs and Dean." Tucson: College of Medicine, University of Arizona (2006). Available: www.medicine.arizona.edu/dean.cfm (accessed October 19, 2008).

National Center for Complementary and Alternative Medicine. "What Is CAM?" Bethesda, MD: U.S. Department of Human and Health Services, National Institutes of Health (August 27, 2008). Available: http://nccam.nih.gov/health/whatiscam (accessed October 19, 2008).

Olson, Suzan. 2000. "Information Becomes Knowledge Through Research." In *Informatics for Healthcare Professions,* edited by Kathleen Young. Philadelphia: F.A. Davis.

Shine, K.I. 2002. "Health Care Quality and How to Achieve It." *Academic Medicine* 77, no. 1: 91–99.

Society of Hospital Medicine. "Definition of a Hospitalist." Philadelphia: Society of Hospital Medicine (2008). Available: www.hospitalmedicine.org/AM/Template. cfm?Section=General_Information&Template=/CM/HTMLDisplay.cfm& ContentID=14048 (accessed October 15, 2008).

U.S. Department of Health and Human Services. "Insure Kids Now!" Washington, DC: U.S. Department of Health and Human Services (no date). Available: www. insurekidsnow.gov (accessed October 15, 2008).

U.S. Department of Health and Human Services. National Clearinghouse for Long-term Care Information. "Understanding Long Term Care." Washington, DC: U.S. Department of Health and Human Services (October, 22, 2008). Available: www.longtermcare.gov/LTC/main_site/understanding_Long_Term_care/Basics/Basics.aspx (accessed March 15, 2009).

U.S. Department of Health and Human Services. Public Health Service. National Institutes of Health. National Library of Medicine. "Managed Health Care." In *MedlinePlus Medical Dictionary.* Bethesda, MD: National Library of Medicine (February 4, 2005). Available: www.nlm.nih.gov/medlineplus/mplusdictionary. html (accessed October 15, 2008).

U.S. Department of Labor Statistics. "Occupational Outlook Handbook, 2008–09." Washington, DC: U.S. Department of Labor Statistics, Office of Occupational Statistics and Employment Projections (2008). Available: www.bls.gov/oco (accessed October 14, 2008).

Willinsky, John and Mia Quint-Rapoport. 2007. "How Complementary and Alternative Medicine Practitioners Use PubMed." *Journal of Medical Internet Research* 9, no. 2 (April–June): e19.

Chapter 3

How Informatics Impacts Modern Healthcare

This chapter discusses how informatics is impacting and changing modern healthcare. While it is not possible to detail the total range and depth of this impact, the examples presented illustrate in general how informatics is fusing into the infrastructure of healthcare.

The adoption of information technology by an organization usually effects major changes in its supporting systems and in the routines and outlooks of the people involved. The changes may bring mixed emotions of fear and uncertainty but also expectations of increased quality and efficiency. There is no doubt that technology, especially information technology, has caused profound changes in the healthcare enterprise.

MEDICAL DECISION MAKING

To understand how health informatics impacts modern medicine, it is necessary to understand the processes of medicine, particularly the decision-making culture and protocols. Medical decision making is the process of reducing ambiguities and overcoming the problems of conflicting or inadequate information in order to properly diagnose and prescribe treatment. The general process is similar to the decision-making process that is used in the daily routines of life. In medicine the process is based on knowledge and skills, and in modern times it usually involves some sort of technology—laboratories, machines, and information systems.

Medical decision making is an iterative procedure of data collection, hypothesis generation, and interpretation, which may go through more than one cycle. The first hypothesis may be a general judgment that is then refined. At the heart of the entire process are data gathering and information synthesis.

Medical decision making is rarely an exact science but consists of science, experience, and subjective inputs, often unique to individuals. It is essential that decision makers have the requisite knowledge and decision-making skills, but it is equally important to recognize when additional information is needed and to know how to acquire that information. It could be said that this is the essence of health informatics.

The Nature and Importance of Medical Data

Information for decision making begins with data. Medical data are a collection of individual pieces of datum, such as blood pressure, temperature, and heart rate, usually recorded over a period of time. Data can be numbers, textual information, or narrative. They can be recorded as electronic markings or images. The uninterrupted facts, numbers, symbols, or images are then sorted, classified, and related to some knowledge structure in order to become information, which is used for decision making.

Healthcare is information based, and information is derived from interpreting data within a known medical context. It follows that medical data are the fundamental elements in medical decision making, including diagnosis, treatment plan, and protocols for the general welfare of the patient. In addition to using data for immediate care giving, data are used by organizations, providers, consumers, and accrediting and regulatory bodies. At the administrative level in a healthcare organization, data-based information is essential to health management and operations.

Some medical decision making appears to be simple and routine and some complex, but all decision making is threatened by missing or imperfect data. Decisions that appear to be straightforward may be biased by faulty data.

Desirable Characteristics of Medical Data

Medical data have the same characteristics as all data, but they also have their own. They are particularly related to the healthcare of humans or other animals and therefore are highly dynamic; that is, they can change moment by moment. Those changes usually have high significance to the healthcare professional monitoring the situation.

To be optimally used, there are a number of desirable factors that characterize medical data, usually related to its form and quality. Tan (2001) listed some major desirable medical data characteristics (see Table 3.1).

Data Gathering

Data are gathered from patients, laboratories, nurses, family members, admissions offices, and other sources. Although specific situations vary, some pieces of information are typically gathered for the medical record. First is the patient's medical history. If this is a continuing patient, then previous history is reviewed and new information is added. Sometimes, errors in the history may be corrected. Questions are asked, such as how and when did the current ill-

Table 3.1. Major Desirable Data Characteristics

Data Characteristics	Description
Accessibility	Available and can be extracted
Accuracy	Error-free
Appropriateness	Contain sufficient detail to support decision making
Comprehensibility	Easy to read and understand; well-formatted
Comprehensiveness	Inclusive and support information needs
Consistency	Not self-contradictory
Relevance	Related to decisions to be made
Reliability	Credible and valid
Timeliness	Available at the right time
Usefulness	Presented in an easy-to-use format

From: Tan, Joseph K. *Health Management Information Systems: Methods and Practical Applications*, 2nd ed. 2001: Jones and Bartlett Publishers, Sudbury, MA. www.jbpub.com. Reprinted with permission.

ness develop and are there any collateral diseases that are present or existed in the past? Also, related family and demographic information is obtained.

Next are the symptoms. When did they begin, and how have they been dealt with? Has anything been tried that provided relief, and are there any circumstances that aggravate the symptoms?

The healthcare provider has to record all physical signs observed during the examination. At this point, pertinent radiological tests, lab tests, and other related information are recorded. Medications being taken are entered, and comments on any side effects are recorded. Finally, the recorder needs to mention the reasoning behind any patient management decisions that have been made (Shortliffe and Barnett, 2006).

Documenting Healthcare Operations

Medical documentation refers to the entire range of documentation in a healthcare organization. These data are used for many other purposes in addition to direct care of patients. For example, all healthcare organizations file legal and financial reports. These reports must be completely and accurately documented both in patient records and in the operational reports of the organization.

Ideally, documentation begins as a byproduct of patient care. As the patient progresses through the healthcare process—entrance into the system, diagnosis and treatment, and finally exit from the process—an ongoing record is kept of what occurred. This compilation of events is the basis of documentation for the patient and, in a larger sense, for the operation of the healthcare organization.

Leiner et al. (2003: 9) provide a checklist of the objectives of medical documentation:

- Support patient care (to remind staff of and communicate information, to help organize the care process).
- Fulfill external obligations (legal requirements, accreditation, and reimbursement regulations).
- Support administration (planning, controlling, and funding the healthcare institution's services).
- Support quality management (enabling critical reflection and systematic monitoring of processes).
- Support scientific research (enabling patient selection and statistical analysis).
- Support clinical education (providing information for critical review and case examples).

Typical sources of documentation data include the following:

- Physician input
- Nursing input
- Laboratory reports
- Control and budgeting
- Admission/discharge information
- Financial accounting information
- Education and research information
- Patient medical records unit
- Library and other information units

The amount of documentation produced by healthcare services is enormous. For example, a typical large hospital may generate 6 or 7 million or more documents a year. This documentation is the lifeblood for all the internal and external operations of a healthcare organization. Information technology tools and information professionals are indispensable to the management of this documentation.

From Data to Information

Health informatics has impacted the processes of gathering, aggregating, sharing, and reporting of data. Before they can be used, data must evolve into information. It is possible to have stacks of data, but no information. Healthcare information can be viewed as a metamorphosis from data. The transformation begins with the input of patient data, either historical or currently gathered. These data are enhanced by knowledge-based information, for example, from the medical literature, and then analyzed by healthcare experts. Through these processes, data become the information that drives decision making and planning for patient care. Finally, the data join conglomerate data that are used for community healthcare and policy making. The same data and metamorphosed information may be used for different purposes by a number of different groups within the health environment (Abdelhak et al., 2007). The need for many members of a healthcare organization to draw on the same data is one reason for the trend toward integrated information systems.

Information fuels healthcare endeavors. Timely and accurate information is essential at every part of the healthcare continuum from the patient to the highest level of healthcare management. The quality of the information depends on the quality of the data that generate it.

The Medical Decision-making Process

The medical decision-making process is usually not an "all at once," single point in time event. It is a step-by-step procedure involving information gathering, analysis, and refinement. The decision making may also involve a patient and the family (Hersh, 2003). The basic model consists of the following:

- Observation
- Diagnosis
- Treatment

As noted earlier, the process begins with recording the patient's history or reviewing it in existing records, and new data are collected from examinations and lab tests. These data are used to make decisions regarding the nature of the problem and the therapy needed. Often the health problem is not clear cut, and the data may suggest different causes and thus different courses of action. In this case, a search for more information may be in order. Consulting colleagues and various information systems, examining the patient further, and ordering more laboratory tests may supply additional information. Physicians may turn to the literature for synthesis and interpretation of data in order to deal with care problems. In some cases, the situation may not allow time for further searching, or it may be impossible to collect more data.

The most common process of medical decision making is known as the *hypothetico-deductive method* of problem solving. Initial observation and data lead to one or more hypotheses of the medical situation. The hypotheses may be accepted, rejected, or refined for another cycle of data collection.

In practice, the process is flexible, with built-in subjective decision making along the way. It is more than following a formal set of logical operations, such as "If this. . . then this." Clearly, guidelines and rules are useful, but decision making is more than a quantitative set of steps. According to Merck Research Laboratories (2004):

> [M]ost patients have some feature that distinguishes them from the groups presented in such formal guidelines. Guidelines cannot adequately represent variations among patients with different demographics, co-morbidities, and histories. Guidelines can aid in the management of many clinical problems, but the clinician must always use appropriate clinical judgment and interpret conflicting data that fall between the rules.

It may be more realistic to think of decision options in terms of probabilities. This approach has lead to the development of mathematical tools that can be used as computer algorithms to assist with decision making. Today's decision-making process may include more formalization and algorithms, such as decision-making theory and artificial intelligence, including expert systems. Theoretical decision-making models exist and have been tested, but the average physician does not usually sit down with a patient and calculate a Markov model of the prognosis. However, computer software now offers the possibility of making such a scenario practical.

Finally, it should be remembered that accurate, timely, and appropriate information enhances the potential of good decision making but does not guarantee it. The final decision is the responsibility of humans.

EXAMPLES OF HOW HEALTH INFORMATICS IMPACTS HEALTHCARE

The examples of how informatics has impacted modern healthcare are too numerous to mention or discuss in their entirety. This section presents some of the most highly visible areas and illustrates their impact.

Changes in Patient Care

Healthcare informatics and the accompanying information technology have instigated profound changes in patient care. The utilization of information technology, directed by a growing cadre of healthcare informatics professionals, is bringing healthcare into a new era of quality patient care. Some representative examples are highlighted.

INFORMATION AND QUALITY CARE

One of the major observations made in the landmark report of the Institute of Medicine (IOM) in 2001 was that the "chasm" in healthcare quality was the result of four situations: (1) a lag between progress in research and change in medical practice, (2) a system geared for acute care when most health needs are related to chronic care, (3) inadequate use of information technology, and (4) payment structuring that provides little incentive to improve quality.

All four items are related in someway to information, but items 1 (research into applications) and 3 (lack of optimal use of information technology) are situations specific to health informatics. In the years since the IOM (2001) report was released, the rate at which the recommendations have been implemented is disappointingly slow. However, progress has been made in medical record keeping, patient involvement in medical decision making, dissemination of information to the lay public, diagnostic tools, patient safety, and information retrieval of medical information for the healthcare professional and the public.

Clearly, quality patient care begins with quality information. As we entered the twentieth-first century, the quality of healthcare became a major topic of discussion, all the way from the individual patient up to the highest levels of government and the corporate world. Society has become uneasy about the current quality of care, especially the performance of healthcare personnel. Some issues include the following:

- Productivity and profitability versus excellence in care
- Liability and the practice of defensive medicine
- Definition and assessment of professional competence

In addition to the IOM, many other agencies and organizations are expressing concern about quality care. For example, in December 2003, the Agency for Health Research and Quality (AHRQ) began publishing *The National Healthcare Quality Report*, which, according to the agency, is the first national comprehensive effort to measure the quality of healthcare in the United States. This report contains information about the quality of health services for seven types of clinical conditions: cancer, diabetes, end-stage renal disease, heart disease, HIV (human immunodeficiency virus), AIDS (acquired immunodeficiency syndrome), mental health, and respiratory diseases. The report also includes data about maternal and child health and nursing home and home healthcare and patient safety. This is an example of an effort to identify and measure disparities in access to and use of healthcare information by different populations.

There are many barriers to achieving quality healthcare. From the viewpoint of information professionals, these problems are very often related to information—either lack of it or errors in it. Quality in healthcare is not determined solely by physicians—it requires the involvement of all the personnel in a healthcare system and their access to quality information.

PATIENT SAFETY AND MEDICAL ERRORS

Patient safety and its connection to medical error is a persistent issue in the healthcare field and continues to be a topic of discussion, debate, and concrete efforts to address it. *Patient safety* is a broad term defined as "freedom from accidental injuries stemming from the processes of health care" (Sutker, 2008: 9). Collecting safety data is related to the operational structure of an organization. First, data are collected on the medical processes as they are being carried out. Safety breaches can occur as healthcare providers go about their duties. Later, an examination of results and outcomes can reflect safety breaches that were not necessarily detected at the procedural stage, for example, a patient developing an infection contracted during surgery. These data should be linked, analyzed, and reported among the healthcare personnel involved.

Medical error and patient safety are closely tied to the concept of standards of care. For example, in November 2003, the IOM's Committee on Data Standards for Patient Safety issued the report *Patient Safety: Achieving a New Standard for Care* as part of the healthcare quality initiative that began with the report *To Err Is Human: Building a Safer Health System* (IOM, 2000). Since 2003, The Joint Commission has published the "National Patient Safety Goals," which has contributed greatly to the adoption of safety practices in healthcare organizations. *Patient Safety* calls for a more uniform data standard in healthcare, which will lead to more integration of the information technology infrastructure into the healthcare environments. Without a doubt, such standards will impact the quality of patient care. Uniform data standards enable healthcare providers and patients to have real-time access to clinical results and medical records in efficient and safe ways, for example, the electronic transmission of a patient's records from one hospital to another when he is treated in both. The adoption of such standards requires the cooperation of the government, the healthcare industry, and the patients.

The literature carries diverse opinions of exactly what is a medical error. The most often quoted source is James Reason, who has published a number of papers on the topic. Reason (2000) says that there are two approaches to the problem, the person approach and the system approach. The person approach focuses on the errors of individuals, blaming them for forgetfulness, inattention, or moral weakness. The system approach concentrates on the conditions under which individuals work and tries to build defenses to avert errors or mitigate their effects.

Medical errors can be thought of as being either errors of commission or errors of omission. An error of commission "involves doing something incorrectly, like misreading a label. . . . Errors of omission involve not doing something that should have been done" (Sutker, 2008: 10). Faulty communication is an underlying cause 65 percent of the time (The Joint Commission, 2007).

A medical error is injury or harm caused by medical management rather than by the natural health problem or physical situation of the patient. In 2000, the IOM released the report *To Err Is Human: Building a Safer Health System*, which states that medical errors probably cause an unacceptable number of deaths per year. More deaths are caused by medical errors than by highway accidents and breast cancer combined (Harris, 2006).

One obvious factor in medical error is poor communication caused by vague terminology. If a patient says that she is in pain, what kind of pain is she referring to, and what is the degree of pain? This type of communication problem can occur at any step in the healthcare provision process.

Another major type of error can occur during the medication process—procuring the drug, prescribing it, dispensing it, administering it, and monitoring its impact. The potential for error is inherent in each one of these steps, and most of the errors are information related, caused by lack of information, inaccurate information, inaccessible information, or misunderstood information. The occurrence and prevention of errors in medication, as in most areas of medical error, can be traced to the information factor. Almost 80 percent of medication errors result from lack of access to medication information or to information about the patient (Felkey, Fox, and Thrower, 2006).

Medication errors harm 1.5 million people and kill several thousands each year in the United States, costing the nation at least $3.5 billion annually according to the IOM. Recognizing the enormity of this problem, the IOM studied the prevalence of medication errors and formulated a national agenda for reducing them. The report, *Preventing Medication Errors,* states that such errors are common and costly to patients, the healthcare industry, and the nation, and it outlines a comprehensive approach to decreasing them (Institute of Medicine, 2006).

Reviewing medical errors is not new. For example, The Joint Commission has reviewed key error occurrences for years. When it comes to reviewing errors, some of the issues are who should do the review, what information is needed, and what the best way is for reporting errors.

The IOM (2006) strongly recommends electronic information technology as a major tool for reducing errors in information transfer and use. In response to the IOM's reports health officials and hospital groups pledged to do better in error prevention, but many of the most important efforts have been slow to take hold (Harris, 2006).

The authors once heard a lecture by a renowned surgeon who told the audience, seriously, that the audience could not imagine how hard it is for a surgeon to be sure that he is amputating the correct leg because the patient is all covered up! To be fair, several of his colleagues in the audience strongly protested this statement, but this episode illustrates a worrisome attitude toward medical error that sometimes exists in the healthcare profession.

Without doubt, information is at the heart of a large part of medical error. Human error will never be exorcised from civilization, because humans can fail even when they have the best information before them. On the other hand, almost always they will fail if they have no information or when they act on invalid and faulty information.

ASSESSING BLAME FOR THE MEDICAL ERROR

When things go wrong, the first impulse is to find someone to blame. The blame must be assigned to people—computers cannot be sued—but the truth is that assigning blame is not a simple task.

Medical error becomes murky when technology is involved. If the technology fails, is the manufacturer of that technology to blame, or the vendor who installed it, or the healthcare personnel who used it? In the early years of automation, the standard response to system failure was to blame the computer. For decades, individuals, businesses, and organizations liked to blame the computer, but time and technological developments have made this excuse obsolete, at least in the sense of the reliability of the technology. It is generally agreed that the major cause of medical error is bad healthcare policy and/or faulty procedures, not individuals (Institute of Medicine, 2000).

SOLUTIONS

A major first step in trying to control medical error is to design a *superior information system*. There are many major and minor systems in healthcare that need careful analysis, such as scheduling, operations, billing, handling of lab tests, dispensing medication, and checking for drug interactions.

Communication failure is a common factor in medical error, and one of the major promises of information technology is to improve communications. Bates and Gawande (2003) identified three ways that information technology helps mitigate adverse events caused by error: (1) it helps to prevent errors and thus adverse events in the first place, (2) it promotes a more rapid response when adverse events occur, and (3) it provides documentation and feedback about the adverse events. Research shows that information technology can reduce the frequency of errors of different types and probably the frequency associated with adverse events (Bates and Gawande, 2003).

Bates and Gawande (2003) also believe that improved access to reference information and increased provision of instant information at the point of care will reduce medical error. Information technology provides what they call "forcing functions." Forcing functions are restricting the way tasks may be performed. For example, if doctors have to type in orders it will eliminate the problem of illegibility.

EVALUATION OF HEALTHCARE

Evaluation is the process of identifying and collecting data by careful appraisal and establishing criteria by which to assess and determine both the quality of the service and the degree to which the service accomplishes stated goals and objectives. Attitudes toward the evaluation of healthcare provision have changed profoundly. Most healthcare professionals and their patients would like to have a fail-proof way to measure the effectiveness of the healthcare given, but there is no such thing as a perfect and proficient way to evaluate healthcare services and outcomes. However, because of economic and legal pressures and a growing assertiveness on the part of patients and their families, methods of evaluation are increasingly important.

During recent years, health services and organizations have begun to make their reports available to the public. Healthcare professionals and organizations have realized that they can no longer conceal information about the quality of services. The public is demanding to know where and how they can check on a healthcare service before committing themselves. The federal government has an initiative called Hospital Consumer Assessment of Healthcare Providers and Systems (HCAPS), which provides a standard survey for measuring patients' perceptions of the care they are getting. In terms of evaluation and published information on quality of service, healthcare is entering a new age.

The growth of the Internet has given patients access to large amounts of medical information, including information that evaluates healthcare organizations, services, and personnel, as well as information related to financial stability, strong points, and problems of healthcare facilities. Also, much evaluative information exists in print form, and the news media constantly report anecdotes. Modern society is seriously interested in evaluating the entire spectrum of healthcare. Some evaluation methods are fraught with subjective facets but a great deal of thought is being given to the problems, and some workable methods, such as outcome measurement, have been developed.

Humankind is moving toward a new frontier of patient care. The road signs are marked with the word *information.*

The People Factor

Implementing new information systems impacts the organization and the people in the organization. New technology and new ways of doing things always mean changes, both major and minor.

Health organizations are often large and complex, involving hundreds of subsystems, operations, and people. Success or failure in implementing information technology depends highly on issues of managing people and melding technology into a compatible organizational structure. Technological change usually means organizational change. It is essential to success that the people accept the change and obtain the necessary training to use it. People are afraid of change primarily because they do not know how it will impact their jobs. Information technology does eliminate certain tasks (thus jobs), but it also creates new ones. Those who are unwilling or incapable of learning new skills must be shifted to other tasks or they may have to leave the organization. Computer applications usually mean the elimination of low-skill jobs. For example, electronic medical record systems imply no more file clerks.

Without a doubt, the introduction of information technology into the healthcare environment is moving the work situation into a mode of ubiquitous instant access to information. The latest technology is small, powerful, mobile, and often wireless, making information available anywhere and at anytime. This impacts the way organizations are structured and the way people do things.

The Rise of Evidence-based Medicine

A major impact of health informatics is the development of evidence-based medicine (EBM). EBM introduces a new dimension to accessing, assessing, and integrating medical knowledge into clinical practice.

The kernel idea of EBM has been around for many years, but the term itself and the formulation of its procedures are only about 25 years old. In the late 1970s and early 1980s, a group of physicians at McMaster University in Hamilton, Ontario, were bothered by existing assumptions made by clinical practitioners and felt that the medical literature was haphazardly utilized. The need for structured and logical methods to identify the "best" research available became obvious. From this came the idea of *critical appraisal* of the literature, which then evolved into *clinical epidemiology* and finally into *evidenced-based medicine* (EBM). The procedures were refined, guidelines were developed, and techniques were tested.

The core concept is that medical decisions should be based on the best available evidence related to the situation at hand. It is a method for linking a healthcare situation with the current medical literature related to it. The consensus in the literature then becomes a major factor in the immediate decision making.

Traditionally, clinical decisions were made on the basis of the expertise of the decision maker. Prior to the EBM movement, the decision maker was expected to be up to date and informed about his or her field and thus well qualified to make decisions. EBM is about the specific, most current knowledge needed to treat an individual patient, and the goal is operational as the focus is on melding this knowledge with professional expertise. The objective is to view each patient as a special case in light of the latest research and the experiences of others.

In the beginning, EBM asserted that nonevidence-based inputs such as intuition, personal experience, and expert opinion should be deemphasized, but more recently the position has shifted. Now the focus in on integrating evidence-based approaches with other valid inputs.

EBM is more than a typical search of the literature to compile a list of citations to be read in the order that they are found, although literature searching is at the heart of EBM. It is a more systematic and scientific approach, sorting clinical research according to the strength of the research, thereby weeding out the various types of biases that can occur.

In order to know the "best" research available, healthcare practitioners have traditionally read the literature, taken continuing education courses, and attended professional meetings. Only recently have health professionals addressed the idea of how to systematically identify the best research out of the enormous volume of new information created daily.

EVIDENCE-BASED MEDICINE PROCEDURES

The premise of EBM is that more and better evidence is needed for medical decision-making and that the best evidence in the research literature can be identified and extracted. Of course, the question naturally arises: What is evidence? We define evidence as something that furnishes proof. There is no such thing as absolute evidence, and human judgment will always be necessary to evaluate the so-called evidence. Therefore, we further maintain that the concept of evidence-based procedures means that practitioners use the latest professional interpretation of research in the immediate domain of concern.

EBM procedures consist of five general steps:

1. Formulate the question or questions that need to be answered to satisfy the healthcare need of a specific patient.
2. Retrieve the necessary information to answer the questions with a systematic search of the relevant literature
3. Read and critically assess the retrieved information to answer the questions.
4. Implement the findings.
5. Evaluate the process to ascertain if optimal outcomes have been obtained for the patient and the healthcare system.

Straus and Sackett (1998: 342) formulated it slightly differently:

1. Convert the need for information into clinically relevant, answerable questions.
2. Find, in the most efficient way, the best evidence with which to answer these questions (whether this evidence comes from clinical examination, laboratory tests, published research, or other sources).
3. Critically appraise the evidence for its validity (closeness to the truth) and usefulness (clinical applicability).
4. Integrate the appraisal with clinical expertise and apply the results.
5. Evaluate your performance.

Over the years a number of professional associations and individuals have published their "guidelines." The following example of a typical "checklist" for EBM clinical reviews is adapted from Siwek et al. (2002):

- There exists new and relevant information about the topic of concern.
- More than one source for evidence-based reviews on the topic is checked.
- The sources are comprehensive assessments, such as those included in MEDLINE and the Cochrane Collaborations Database.
- Studies are both statistically and clinically significant.
- The reviews cover recent developments, other viewpoints, and any controversies.
- Major points concerning diagnosis and treatment are highlighted.

A number of excellent Web sites regarding EBM, with links to further resources such as guidelines for using EBM procedures, include the following:

- Evidence-Based Medicine Resource Center. Available: www.ebmny.org/cpg.html (accessed October 19, 2008)

- Karolinska Institutet. Available: www.mic.ki.se/EBM.html (accessed October 19, 2008)
- HealthLinks, University of Washington. Available: http://healthlinks. washington.edu/ebp (accessed October 19, 2008)

EVIDENCE-BASED MEDICINE CRITICS

EBM has critics, some very outspoken (Holmes et al. 2006), but most healthcare professionals view it as one major resource in a large tool kit. It must be understood that there is more to medical decision making than just evidence, no matter how "best" it is. According to Hersh (2003: 7):

> Evidence alone, however, is not sufficient for decisions. Both patients and clinicians may have personal, cultural, or other preferences that influence how evidence will be applied. The healthcare professional may also have limited training or experience to be able to apply evidence, such as a physician not trained as a surgeon or not trained to perform a specific treatment or procedure. There are other constraints on decision making as well. There may be legal or other restrictions on what medical care can be provided. There may also be constraints of time (patient far away from the site at which a specific type of care can be provided) or financial resources (patient or entity responsible for paying for the care cannot afford it).

Sometimes the opposition to EBM stems from a lack of understanding of the EBM concept. It is not a radically new method, totally quantified, mechanized, or impersonal. All of the human factors are still a vital part of EBM. The concept simply emphasizes the availability of systematic tools for procedurally finding the latest and best knowledge of the variables involved in a specific medical event. The use of EBM procedures in their strictest, most formalized form is clearly not the major paradigm in the practice of medicine, but the techniques are being applied successfully.

LINKING EVIDENCE-BASED MEDICINE TO THE CONCEPT OF BEST PRACTICE

There is a trend toward linking evidence-based medicine to the concept of best practice. *Best practice* is a specific action or actions based on quantitative and qualitative evidence of success. In evidence-based methods, healthcare professionals find, appraise, and use research findings as the basis for clinical decision. The development of EBM has adopted the term *best practice* as a rationale for EBM, and now the term is being connected with the delivery of quality of healthcare.

The idea of best practice is widespread today. Best practice ideas did not originate with the health sciences, but are ubiquitous across many sectors. As early as 1919, Frederick Taylor, the famous management consultant, declared that in any enterprise there is always a best way to do things, and the idea is still prevalent in modern business practices (Kanigel, 1997).

The vision of best practice is idealistic but at the same time can be operationally practical. It is idealistic in the sense that everybody involved in a system wants to have the best outcomes possible, regardless of the approach. The operational actions related to obtaining this, however, must involve formal and informal procedures to implement quantitative and qualitative methods to establish concrete expectations and then evaluate if those outcomes were successful. Clearly, EBM is a tool for doing this.

EBM continues to be a highly visible topic in medical schools' curricula and in the healthcare literature. It is critical that information professionals have a clear understanding of the principles of EBM. It is not an ivory tower intellectual abstraction; rather, it is a tool that gives a practical operational approach to medical decision making. It is a systematic and evaluative way to look at the most current research, but it is *not* a substitute for individual clinical experience, knowledge, and skills. We discuss the role of the medical librarian in the EBM process in detail in Chapter 5.

Telehealth and Access to Healthcare

Telehealth is another highly visible example of the impact of informatics on healthcare. *Telehealth* is an inclusive term that implies the use of telecommunication and other information technologies to provide healthcare in its many forms to distant points. It acknowledges and incorporates the cultural factors, education, ethnicity, and other facets of the healthcare situation. Telehealth is a concept for healthcare delivery, consisting of people, systems, and specific procedures.

Telemedicine is an early term meaning the application of information technology, particularly interactive audio and video communication, to interact with patients in remote areas. *Telecare* was a spinoff from telemedicine, meaning the delivery of care to people external to an institution, usually in their homes. Later the term *e-health* was coined to depict Internet-based care.

Telehealth uses multimedia communication technologies to deliver healthcare across geographical distances, time, and cultural barriers, providing data gathering, diagnosis, treatment, patient monitoring, and consultation. Among the services it provides are imaging, home care, and emergency support (Kim et al., 2008).

In one sense telehealth has been around for a long time, as in the use of the telegraph and later the telephone to request and receive medical advice. By the turn of the twentieth century people were experimenting with transmitting images electronically (Sharpe, 2001). The modern concept of telehealth, however, began in the 1960s when computer and communication technologies began to change the ways in which society communicates and health professionals responded by trying new ways to deliver remote distance healthcare.

Telehealth has rapidly developed from a curiosity into a full-grown healthcare delivery enterprise. There are many reasons for the growth of telehealth in the last two decades, including the exponential development of information and telecommunication technologies. Unforeseen technological advances, mass production, and lowering costs gave a lift to telehealth and it potentials. The impetus was twofold (Sharpe, 2001: 1):

1. The social imperative to increase access to health care for those underprivileged and underserved
2. The economic imperative to decrease the cost of such care for all healthcare

Telehealth continues to expand both in technological techniques and in widespread applications. It is encompassing the full spectrum of available technology, including databases, imaging, telemetry, robotics, telephones, fax, and interactive audio and video communications, and it has great potential for global health applications.

TELEHEALTH APPLICATION AREAS

Telehealth started with radiology. With the development video, health professionals created video images and sent them electronically to points of need. In 1948 radiological films were sent over telephone lines. In the 1950s teleradiological systems were being tried, and by the 1960s the federal government was promoting a number of related projects. Now it is routine to send X-rays, CT scans, and MRIs to networked healthcare facilities. When videoconferencing was instigated, real-time exchanges were possible between healthcare providers and remote patients or between health professionals separated by distance. "Distance" is relative; it can refer to somewhere thousands of miles away, or across town, or across the hall.

One of the early and major uses of telemedicine was patient monitoring, which became the vehicle for *telehomecare*. Basically, telehomecare allows homebound patients to communicate with healthcare providers through telecommunications and videoconferencing. Monitoring systems send data to the healthcare provider, and the patient and the doctor may have a "virtual visit." These devices monitor such things as heart functions, blood pressure, asthma alerts, insulin-dependent diabetes, and many others (Damigou et al., 2006).

Sharpe (1999) identified some of the services and resources related to telehealth: (1) access to remote health care practitioners in real time; (2) retrieval and transmission of medical records and data; (3) consultation, assessment, and management of previously diagnosed physical or mental illnesses or conditions; (4) identification and diagnosis of new illnesses; (5) implementation and management of medical regimens and treatment for those illnesses; (6) ongoing remote monitoring of the effectiveness of the regimens and the patients' responses and statuses; and (7) patient and caregiver education and support. In recent years other services have been added, such as care for prison-based populations, patient education, and continuing education for healthcare providers.

Telehealth is also effective in mobile emergency and trauma situations, often providing stabilization and continued monitoring of patients before and during transportation to a health facility.

Another interesting application of telehealth is telepsychiatry, where mental healthcare is delivered via telecommunication technology. Telepharmacy is also a viable application. Pharmacists use videoconferencing, the Internet, and e-mail to communicate with patients, and routine activities like refilling prescriptions are done via the Internet all over the United States.

A special avenue for telehealth is electronic communication. In this age it is natural for patients to want to communicate with their healthcare providers via e-mail and text messaging. These methods can be used to make and verify appointments, fill prescriptions, obtain laboratory results, clarify treatments, and provide patient education. Maintaining data security and confidentiality of electronic communications requires caution. Toward this end, the American Medical Association (2004) published its *Guidelines for Physician–Patient Electronic Communication* (1995–2008), and others organizations have issued their own as well.

CONCERNS WITH TELEHEALTH

Rapid advances in information technology are making real what a few years ago were just ideas. The primary advances are the Internet and other sophisticated telecommunication systems, particularly regarding speed, capacity, and high quality image transfer. Governments are beginning to fund telehealth endeavors, as are entrepreneurs seeing money-making opportunities.

Concerns with telehealth applications, however, still need to be resolved. For example, there are no clear, universal standards of care for services delivered via telemedicine. As a result, a number of organizations have created their own standards and guidelines.

The American Nurses Association defined its standards for all telehealth efforts in *Core Principles on Telehealth* (1999) and *Developing Telehealth Protocols: A Blue Print for Success* (2001). In general, the *Core Principles* maintain that care delivered with telehealth technology should be no different in quality from any other type of healthcare service. The principles begin by stating that basic standards of professional conduct are not altered because care is delivered with distant technology, and healthcare providers cannot deliver services by telehealth technology that would otherwise be illegal or unauthorized. The principles also point out that the integrity and therapeutic value of the patient/healthcare practitioners should not be diminished by the use of telehealth technology. The list of principles ends by stating that a systematic and comprehensive research agenda must be developed and supported by government agencies and by health care professions for ongoing assessment of telehealth service (American Nurses Association, 1999).

INFORMATICS IN ACTION! 3.1

Telehealth Status

Location: Medical professional association

Problem: The medical association realizes that the future of telehealth endeavors has not been adequately analyzed on a broad scale in the United States.

People Involved: Officials of the medical association and Dr. Joan Smithers, a health sciences librarianship professor at a well-known iSchool.

Action Taken: Dr. Smithers is known for her expertise in survey research, especially in using the Delphi method. She was hired to investigate telehealth for the medical association. She conducted a Delphi study involving experts in the field of telehealth. The experts were senior level managers of telehealth programs with at least five years of experience and included vice-presidents, chief executive officers, chief information officers, and executive directors. The results of the study provided a clearer picture of the current status of telehealth and future trends in the field.

Takeaway: The association appropriately turned to an expert, Dr. Smithers, in health informatics, survey research, and health sciences librarianship for the study they needed.

The use of telehealth to deliver healthcare services also involves legal and ethical concerns. The major issues are licensing, medical malpractice, and standards of care. Licensing is a problem because each state does its own licensing of health professionals, and this can get complicated when telehealth crosses state and national boundaries, as it often does. Malpractice resolution can be hindered when a patient is in one state and the healthcare provider is in another state. Which state laws have jurisdiction? Another concern is the resistance of healthcare professionals who are wary of long distance care. Finally, there are the ever-present concerns of costs, avenues for the reimbursement for services, rapidly changing information technology, and the need for computer and health literacy.

Despite all the concerns, telehealth has developed into a major area of healthcare. It has the potential to improve quality of care and to expand the variety of healthcare services available to a diverse population, particularly the underserved worldwide. Telehealth is an innovative way to use information technology, and the informatics professional is playing a pivotal role.

SUMMARY

This chapter presented major examples of how health informatics is changing modern healthcare. The examples are by no means exhaustive, but they highlight the powerful impact that is being felt throughout the healthcare enterprise. The next chapter goes into detail about the major application areas of health informatics.

REFERENCES

Abdelhak, Mervat, Sara Gnostic, Mary Alice Hansen, and Ellen B. Jacobs. 2007. *Health Information: Management of a Strategic Resource,* 3rd ed. St. Louis: Saunders/ Elsevier.

American Medical Association, Young Physicians Section. "Guidelines for Physician–Patient Electronic Communication." Chicago: The American Medical Association (December, 2004). Available: www.ama-assn.org/ama/pub/category/2386.html (accessed November 4, 2008).

American Nurses Association. 1999. *Core Principles on Telehealth.* Washington, DC: American Nurses Publishing.

American Nurses Association. 2001. *Developing Telehealth Protocols: A Blue Print for Success.* Washington, DC: American Nurses Publishing.

Bates, David W. and Atul A. Gawande. 2003. "Improving Safety with Information Technology." *New England Journal of Medicine* 348, no. 5 (June 19): 2526–2534.

Damigou, Dionisia, Fotini Kalogirou, and Georgios Zarras. 2006. "Use of Telemedicine Systems and Devices for Patient Monitoring." In *Handbook of Research on Informatics in Healthcare and Bioinformatics* (pp. 221–228), edited by Athina A. Lazakidou. Hershey, PA: Idea Group Reference.

Felkey, Bill B., Brent I. Fox, and Margaret R. Thrower. 2006. *Health Care Informatics: A Skills-based Resource.* Washington, DC: American Pharmacists Association.

Harris, Gardiner. "Report Finds a Heavy Toll from Medication Errors." *New York Times,* July 21, 2006.

Hersh, William R. 2003. *Information Retrieval: A Health and Biomedical Perspective,* 2nd ed. New York: Springer-Verlag.

Holmes, David, Stuart J. Murray, Amelie Perron, and Genevieve Rail. 2006. "Deconstructing the Evidence-based Discourse in Health Science: Truth, Power, and Fascism." *International Journal of Evidence-based Health Care* 4, no. 3 (September): 180–186.

Institute of Medicine. Agency for Healthcare Research and Quality. "The National Healthcare Quality Report, 2005." Available: www.ahrq.gov/qual/nhqr05/nhqr05.htm (accessed October 19, 2008).

Institute of Medicine. 2003. *Patient Safety: Achieving a New Standard for Care.* Washington, DC: National Academies Press.

Institute of Medicine. "Preventing Medication Errors." Washington, DC: National Academies Press (2006). Available: www.nap.edu (accessed October 19, 2008).

Institute of Medicine. Committee on Quality of Health Care in America. 2000. *To Err Is Human: Building a Safer Health System.* Washington, DC: National Academies Press.

Institute of Medicine. Committee on Quality of Health Care in America. 2001. *Crossing the Quality Chasm.* Washington, DC: National Academies Press.

The Joint Commission. "National Patient Safety Goals." Oakbrook, IL: The Joint Commission (2009). Available: www.jointcommission.org/patientsafety/national patientsafetygoals/ (accessed March 15, 2009).

The Joint Commission. "Sentinel Event Statistics." Oakbrook Terrace, IL: The Joint Commission (September 2007) Available: www.jointcommission.org/sentinelEvents/ statistics (accessed October 25, 2008).

Kanigel, Robert. 1997. "Taylor-made (19th-century Efficiency Expert Frederick Taylor)." *The Sciences* 37, no. i3 (May): 1–5. Available: www.ams.sunysb.edu/ ~weinig/Taylor-made.pdf (accessed March 18, 2009).

Kim, Jinman, Zhiqong Wang, Tom Widon Cai, and David Dagan Feng. 2008. "Multimedia for Future Health-smart Medical Home." In *Biomedical Information Technology* (pp. 497–512), edited by David Dagan Feng. Amsterdam: Elsevier.

Leiner, Florian, Wilhelm Gaus, Reinhold Haux, and Petra Knaup-Gregori. 2003. *Medical Data Management: A Practical Guide.* New York: Springer-Verlag.

Merck Research Laboratories. "Clinical Decision-making." In *The Merck Manual.* Whitehouse, NJ: Merck Research Laboratories (2004). Available: www.merck. com/mmpe/index.html (accessed October 19, 2008).

Reason, James. 2000. "Human Error: Models and Management." *BMJ* 320: 768–770. Available: www.bmj.com/cgi/content/full/320/7237/768 (accessed October 19, 2008).

Sharpe, Charles C. 1999. *Medical Records Review and Analysis.* Westport, CT: Auburn House.

Sharpe, Charles C. 2001. *Telenursing: Nursing Practice in Cyberspace.* Westport, CT: Auburn House.

Shortliffe, Edward and G. Otto Barnett. 2006. "Biomedical Data: Their Acquisition, Storage, and Use." In *Biomedical Informatics: Computer Applications in Health Care and Biomedicine* (pp. 46–79), 3rd ed., edited by Edward H. Shortliffe and James J. Cimino. New York: Springer.

Siwek, Jay, Margaret L. Gourlay, David C. Slawson, and Allen F. Shaughnessy. 2002. "How to Write an Evidence-based Clinical Review Article." *American Family Physician* 65, no. 2 (January): 251–258.

Straus, Sharon E. and David L. Sackett. 1998. "Getting Research Findings Into Practice: Using Research Findings in Clinical Practice." *BMJ* 317, no. 7154 (August 1): 339–342.

Sutker, Williams L. 2008. "The Physician's Role in Patient Safety: What's in It for Me?" *Baylor University Medical Center Proceedings* 21, no. 1: 9–14.

Tan, Joseph K.H. 2001. *Health Management Information Systems: Methods and Practical Applications*, 2nd ed. Sudbury, MA: Jones and Bartlett Publishers.

Chapter 4

Major Application Areas

The previous chapters outlined the general structure of modern healthcare, described the major healthcare professionals, and provided examples of how informatics has changed healthcare services. This chapter discusses major application areas of health informatics that emerged as the field developed. Although specific application areas can be delineated and discussed, due to the interdisciplinary nature of health informatics, there is considerable overlap and interaction among the different areas and often the distinctions are blurred. The examples in this chapter include medical specialty areas that have a recognized professional component called *informatics.* This may be a subspecialty or a standard component of a specialty area recognized by a professional organization. Usually the informatics area has a substantial presence in the literature.

Health informatics has transcended its initial applications by the clinical physician and radiology center and now includes activities ranging from top administration of healthcare organizations to everyday operations. In the past decade informatics has spread into practically every medical specialty area and subarea.

The evolving theories and foundation of informatics are the same across all the health sciences. Even though there is a diversity of applications, there is a theoretical common denominator, with the same basic principles, despite a wide range of specific and localized applications. This chapter discusses some of the major application areas, although the list is not exhaustive.

DIRECT PATIENT CARE INFORMATICS

Because healthcare begins with people, it was natural for healthcare informatics to begin with direct patient care and the services related to this care. This section describes some of the direct patient care informatics areas.

Primary Care Informatics

Patient care encompasses the facilities, resources, and personnel needed to provide healthcare services to individual patients. These resources include physicians, nurses, therapists, nutritionists, social workers, laboratories, machines, and pharmacies, and other entities.

Patient care is generally divided into three levels; (1) primary care, (2) secondary care, and (3) tertiary care. Primary care is the broad-based care of the patient's general health. Secondary care is generally defined as care by a specialist, and tertiary care is related to care at special facilities with advanced technology (e.g., at institutions involved in research and other related activities).

Usually, primary care is the first point of contact for those needing health services. It is an ambulatory situation and most likely involves comprehensive and continuing basic care. de Lusignan (2003: 304), in the introduction to an extensive paper, stated that "primary care informatics is an emerging academic discipline that remains undefined" and then proceeded to develop a definition of primary care informatics as "the scientific study of data, information and knowledge, and how they can be modeled, processed or harnessed to promote health and develop patient-centered primary medical care. Its methods reflect the biopsychosocial model of primary healthcare and the longitudinal relationships between patients and professionals."

Information gathering and processing are paramount in primary care. They begin with an assessment of the patient, followed by reassessment from time to time, continuing until the patient no longer needs care—a longitudinal input of changing information that is essential to effective clinical decision making. There are two general types of information that define a patient's situation, which sets the stage for care. First, exactly who is involved in the care, what kind of information will these various professionals need, and how will this information be obtained? Second, what kind of information will each attending professional generate and from where will the information be obtained?

Primary care is characterized by information exchange among a host of medical personnel, patients, and family members. The healthcare provider expends a great amount of time and resources in obtaining patient information, but also, this is the point of care where patients want information, often anxiously. Many times the patient does not get the answers sought. According to Little (2007), a physician seeing 25 patients per day will generate approximately 15 clinical questions; approximately two-thirds of these questions will go unanswered; and one-half of the answers will directly impact patient care. Clearly, there is a vast information need at the point of care for all concerned. There are many overlaps between general health informatics and primary care informatics, but the difference is the focus on the unique specifics of basic primary care. In particular, primary care informatics focuses on, among other things, the development of information technology systems for patient evaluation, electronic patient records, standards, clinical management, patient education, and physician information technology education.

CLINICAL INFORMATION SYSTEMS

One of the earliest efforts in clinical informatics was the development of electronic information systems. Clinical information systems are information technology–based support systems for clinical point of care and usually include patient records, decision-support software, clinical guidelines, drug information, and communication links, both internally and externally. Clinical information system tools include networking, wireless communication, and handheld devices.

All three levels of patient care (primary, secondary, and tertiary) informatics are concerned with clinical information systems. These systems link to systems outside of the point of care, such as in laboratories and imaging centers, and to local and distant hospital management systems, although this is not universal. These clinical information systems structure patient and operational information and provide immediate and easy access, thereby enhancing the quality of care.

There are several types of clinical information systems, representing many levels of sophistication and applications. Making appropriate choices when obtaining and implementing a clinical information system depends on understanding what needs to be done and on the variety and complexity of healthcare information systems on the market. All of these systems can be grouped into two general categories: administrative systems and clinical decision-making support systems.

Administrative systems assist managers and administrators in making and implementing operational decisions. Their major function is to monitor and report on operations. Information is gathered from subsystems and is used for cost analysis, evaluation, planning, and day-by-day operations. Clinical decision-support systems assist those concerned with patient care decisions.

The clinical information system gathers data from patient records, lab reports, the pharmacy, nurse reports, and other sources. Whenever a person seeks help with a health problem, the interaction involves many information systems. When the patient comes to a healthcare facility is recorded. Then blood tests and other tests are ordered and reported (laboratory and radiology information systems). Decision-support systems may be used to help the physician make a diagnosis and prescribe a care plan. Medication may be ordered (pharmaceutical information systems). Follow-up visits may be scheduled (physician's office information system and the patient's medical record). An information system is involved at every step of the process.

When developing a clinical information system it is essential to remember a fundamental principle of implementing any computer-based system—there are always trade-offs. On the one hand is the desire to have the best technology possible, and on the other hand is the necessity that the system reflect information needs of the users and that the users know how the system works. Also, there is no such thing as a generic system that covers all situations. Systems need to be tailored to the specific clinical purposes and services offered by the organization and to the needs of physicians, staff, and patients.

A lot of time and resources are being spent on implementing clinical information systems, but there are a few downsides. For example, implementation costs can be a barrier to many healthcare organizations. Despite all the attention currently being given to privacy and security issues, problems remain and challenges continue. Also, many clinicians say they do not have the time during patient encounters to interact with a computer-based system. However, in general, these systems are proving effective and are enhancing healthcare on many levels.

The following are two examples of modern clinical information systems:

- Centricity Perinatal Clinical Information System. Available: www. gehealthcare.com/usen/perinatal/products/clininfo_system.html (accessed October 19, 2008). This system aids in perinatal documentation from prenatal management to postpartum, nursery and discharge. It also includes patient education. According to the Web site, it "automates documentation of the full spectrum of perinatal care." The system produces a single, continuous file of the entire patient record from start to finish.
- InteGreat. Available: www.igreat.com/productdescriptions.cfm (accessed October 19, 2008). Several modules of this system are available, including electronic health record, automated prescription generation and management, imaging management, clinical documentation, educational management, and disaster recovery backup.

CLINICAL PRACTICE GUIDELINES

The Institute of Medicine defines clinical practice guidelines as "systematically developed statements to assist practitioners and patient decisions about appropriate health care for specific clinical circumstances" (Field and Lohr, 1990: 38). The purpose of guidelines is to enhance decision making and improve patient outcomes in healthcare. Such guidelines are "a solution to inappropriate variations in care, medical errors, high costs, and poor-quality heath care" (Ebell and Siwek, 2006: 1840). A vast number of clinical guidelines were developed in the past decade, ranging across the entire spectrum of healthcare and including EBM, specific diseases, prevention measures, consumer use, and education. A few examples of guidelines include the following:

- "Screening for Osteoporosis in Men: A Clinical Practice Guideline from the American College of Physicians." Available: www.medicalnewstoday. com/articles/106479.php (accessed October 19, 2008)
- "Evidence-based Interventions to Improve the Palliative Care of Pain, Dyspnea, and Depression at the End of Life: A Clinical Practice Guideline from the American College of Physicians." Available: www.ngc.gov/

summary/summary.aspx?ss=15&doc_id=12149&nbr=6246 (accessed October 19, 2008)

- "Diagnosis and Treatment of Low Back Pain: A Joint Clinical Practice Guideline from the American College of Physicians and the American Pain Society." Available: www.annals.org/cgi/content/full/147/7/478 (accessed October 19, 2008)
- "American Association of Clinical Endocrinologists Medical Guidelines for Clinical Practice for the Management of Diabetes Mellitus." Available: www.aace.com/pub/pdf/guidelines/DMGuidelines2007.pdf (accessed October 19, 2008)

Guidelines are created by medical associations, specialty groups, government bodies, local health organizations, and many others. The National Guideline Clearinghouse (NGC) provides comprehensive information on evidence-based clinical practice guidelines.

Although the number of published guidelines continues to increase, there is no consensus on the effectiveness of the guidelines on medical practice. They have, however, proved useful in patient–physician relationships, especially in involving the patient in decision making, and they are increasingly being used in ligation situations.

A number of initiatives were launched to promote guidelines, such as the American Hearth Association's *Get with the Guidelines Program* (GWTG). The American Heart Association created GWTG in 2001 to improve the quality of care of patients hospitalized with cardiovascular diseases. The participating hospitals reported "statistically significant and clinically relevant improvements in the use of key evidence-based therapies . . ." (Fonarow, 2008). Unfortunately, there is little research on how effective the standards of practice and guidelines are and what impact they are having, good or bad, on medical practice. In the meantime, the standards and guidelines keep being produced and published.

Nursing Informatics

Nursing informatics is the application of informatics principles to the education, research, and services of the nursing profession. Clearly, nurses are directly concerned with human actions, reactions, and relationships. For this reason, an emphasis is put on the use of technology to support and enhance these interactions.

Since the 1980s, nursing has been active in informatics and its informatics has developed in parallel with other areas of health informatics. As early as 1980, nurses defined nursing informatics as "the application of computer technology to all fields of nursing—nursing services, nurse education, and nursing research" (Scholes and Barber, 1980: 73). In 1992 the American Nursing Informatics

Association was established and in 1994 defined itself: Nursing informatics is the specialty that integrates nursing science, computer science, and information science in identifying, collecting, processing, and managing data and information to support nursing practice, administration, education, research and the expansion of nursing knowledge (American Nurses Association, 1994: 3).

In 2001, the American Nurses Association's *Scope and Standards of Nursing Informatics* defined nursing informatics as a specialty that "facilitates the integration of data, information, and knowledge to support patients, nurses, and other providers in their decision-making in all roles, and settings. This support is accomplished through the use of information structures, information processes, and information technology" (McCormick et al., 2007: 19).

In the beginning, like informatics in other areas, nursing informatics focused on technology, including hardware, software, and systems analysis and design. Over the years the emphasis has broadened from strictly computer applications and now includes a holistic view of managing data, information, and knowledge relevant to nursing. Now efforts are directed toward elucidating the underlying concepts and theoretical basis for informatics, especially in the area of information storage and access, and incorporating information tools and techniques from other application areas.

The general research goal of nursing informatics focuses on using nursing information systems to strengthen the quality of clinical care. Specific areas include clinical data management, processes and outcomes of care, clinical decision making, terminology structures, and the reliability and validity of clinical language to nursing assessments, diagnosis, interventions, and outcomes. Nursing informatics is also concerned with measuring the effectiveness of the existing information structures that undergird the processes of decision making by nurses in clinical situations. Other topics include security (e.g., signatures and encryption), privacy and confidentiality, promotion of standards, community health, and use of geographic information systems (McCormick et al., 2007). In addition, there is also research interest in patient relationships with the healthcare providers and the choices of treatment. This may include the participation of patients and family in decision making.

Nursing informatics is about technology but it is much more than that. It is about human relations.

Dental Informatics

Dental informatics is the branch of health informatics that uses information technology and information science principles to improve dental practice (including patient care and education), conduct research, and promote professional education. Over 85 percent of dentists have computers in their offices, and a good portion of these professionals use the Internet and other information technologies in their practice (Schleyer et al., 2006). Computers are rapidly becoming another tool for the practicing dentist, and computer skills are becoming a requisite for today's dentist and staff.

Dental informatics is composed of four general areas: (1) practice applications, which include patient records, chair side computing, teledentistry, and decision-support systems; (2) research, including standardization of dental vocabulary, data mining, genetic studies, and imaging; (3) physician and staff education, including educational software and distance learning, and patient education; and (4) management, which includes office administrative systems and quality assessment systems.

The dental informatics specialty has evolved, rather slowly, over the past 40 years, and has developed a core literature, skilled informatics professionals, and educational programs. Between 1975 and 2003, over 600 papers were published about dental informatics; the literature is growing at a rate of about 50 papers annually, which shows a steady evolution of the specialty (Schleyer, 2003). Particularly notable is the contribution being made to genetic, proteomic, epidemiologic, and other databases. Also, the recent rapid advances in computer technology, capture technologies, visualization techniques, and display devices have revolutionized radiology and imaging in dentistry.

Dental professionals believe that one of dentistry's greatest informatics challenges is the acute shortage of researchers, educators, practitioners, and research resources. Dental informatics professionals are urging the augmentation of the research capacity in dental informatics, pointing out the need to recruit and train a strong cadre of dental informaticians (Schleyer, 2003).

Schleyer (2003) offers five recommendations for the improvement of dental informatics: (1) create a more focused, worldwide community of dental informaticians; (2) get more biomedical informaticians interested in dental problems; (3) provide career opportunities and career paths for dental informatics researchers; (4) address grand challenges together as a community, and (5) recruit subsequent generations of dental informaticians. The Dental Informatics Online Community, an e-community, was recently created to connect the small community of dental informatics professionals and to foster a greater awareness of dental informatics (Spallek et al., 2007). Without a doubt, dental informatics is moving into the mainstream of dentistry.

Behavioral Informatics

Behavioral medicine is a broad, interdisciplinary field that addresses a wide range of issues related to illness, wellness, and good health. In a sense, behavioral healthcare is concerned with both the body and the mind. It draws on psychosocial, behavioral, and biomedical knowledge bases that are relevant to healthcare. Its primary professional association is the Society of Behavioral Medicine, whose special interest groups include aging, behavioral informatics, cancer, child and family health, complementary and alternative health, evidence-based behavioral medicine, integrated primary care, and obesity and eating disorders. Behavioral health services are a large industry. According to the World Health Organization, behavioral health problems account for 15 percent of the cost of health care in the world, including the United States; this is more than the costs of all cancers (National Institute of Mental Health, 2009). More than 5,000 U.S. organizations, including group practices, hospital-based systems, and community health centers, provide services (Dewan et al., 2002).

The Society of Behavioral Medicine (2007a) defines health informatics along the same lines as do other areas of health informatics, but it broadens the definition to be more inclusive of the people served, emphasizing the importance of individuals, families, communities, and populations.

The Behavioral Informatics special interest group of SBM focuses on the impact of information and communication technology on health behavior outcomes and processes. According to their working definition of behavioral informatics, it "incorporates the study of the use of these technologies by patients and health care providers as well as the design, implementation, and evaluation of behavior change interventions delivered through advanced technologies" (Society of Behavioral Medicine, 2007b).

Behavioral healthcare has been slow in adopting information technologies, but times are changing. In the beginning, like a number of other healthcare areas, computers were used in behavioral healthcare for billing and other office management tasks. In the 1990s, behavioral health personnel began to design automated outcome analysis systems, and this motivated them to pursue other applications. In the past decade there has been interest in decision-making systems and other mainstream informatics tools. A substantial amount of software exists for behavioral healthcare professionals, including general disease management systems and applications in the various subareas of behavioral care.

One notable area of behavioral informatics is its concern with adequate provision of behavioral health services to rural areas. Approximately one-fourth of the U.S. population lives in rural areas, where typically there is a shortage of healthcare professionals. Over 55 percent of the counties across the country have no psychiatrists, psychologists, or social workers. This has led to the development of behavioral telehealth, including e-mail and Internet searches, as well as real-time exchanges with healthcare providers via video and teleconferencing for health assessment, diagnosis, intervention, consultation, supervision, and education. Members of the behavioral care community recognize the ongoing need for information technology and application systems.

Public Health Informatics

Public health is concerned with the health of human populations and encompasses the total spectrum of healthcare through direct clinical and community services. It is related to issues that go beyond clinical events and looks at the "patient" as being the entire population. Public health focuses on the major threats and challenges facing the health of communities, especially medical care, environmental impacts, and disaster management care. It attempts to organize people and resources to promote disease prevention, safety from injury, and the quality of health in the population at large.

The diversity of public health workers—including physicians, nurses, environmental health specialists, social workers, nutritionists, health information professionals, health educators, epidemiologists, statisticians, public health informaticians, and public health information managers—results in a wide range of information needs. Health informatics is fundamental to the activities of public health services, and this has resulted in the creation of the subarea of public health informatics. Public health informatics integrates public health with information technology. It is about the management of a complex information infrastructure related to global health issues. Public health informatics focuses on the information needed to provide a profile of the general health and welfare of the population and on the systems for collecting data and converting it into information. Data gathered from disparate sources is compiled, organized, and synthesized.

As in health informatics, two primary concerns regarding data gathering are to filter for quality and to keep the data current. The privacy, confidentiality, and security of the data are a persistent challenge (Koo, O'Carroll, and La Venture, 2001), and public health informatics has assisted in developing safe methods for the exchange of data among the users.

O'Carroll (2003: 8–9) lists four "principles" that distinguish public health informatics from other informatics subareas:

- The primary focus of public health informatics is on applications of information science and technology that promote the health of populations as opposed to the health of specific individuals.
- The primary focus of public health informatics is on applications of information science and technology that prevent diseases and injury by altering the conditions or the environment that put populations of individuals at risk.
- Public health informatics applications explore the potential for prevention at all vulnerable points in the causal chains leading to diseases, injury or disability; applications are not restricted to particular social, behavioral, or environmental contexts.
- As a discipline, public health informatics reflects the governmental context in which public health is practiced.

Concern about the problems and needs of public health services related to global health has grown in recent years. The National Center for Public Health Informatics (NCPHI) at the Centers for Disease Control and Prevention

(CDC) provides leadership in the application of informatics to public health practice and research. Another information service in the public health sector is the CDC's Immunization Information Systems (IIS), also known as the "Immunization Registries." These registries consolidate immunization information from disparate sources around the country into one source and keep track of what immunizations children have had, thus making sure children get only the immunizations they need.

Another type of information system in public health is the disease surveillance system; one example is the World Health Organization (WHO)'s Global Outbreak Alert & Response Network (GOARN). GOARN is a technical collaboration among institutions and networks of human and technical resources for rapid identification, confirmation, and response to outbreaks of international importance. It provides an operational framework to keep the international community constantly alert to the threat of diseases (World Health Organization, 2008). HealthMap is another example of a real-time surveillance system that aggregates reports on infectious disease outbreaks (Freifeld and Brownstein, 2008).

Public health is information centered, and information technology is a powerful and essential tool with which to improve the management of information. Public health informatics in the coming years will become a major area of informatics.

Veterinary Informatics

Veterinary informatics is the subarea of health informatics that focuses on how veterinary medical information is generated, managed, communicated, and applied as knowledge to support effective and efficient decision making (Bellamy, 1999). Without doubt, veterinary medicine and human health are entwined. Veterinary informatics draws heavily on informatics from human medicine, for the obvious reason that veterinary medicine has the same scientific roots and similar applications.

The original objectives of the Association for Veterinary Informatics focused on direct computer applications:

- To extend the use of computers in veterinary medicine
- To provide a forum for the exchange of ideas about the use of computers in veterinary medicine
- To provide educational material about the use of computers in veterinary medicine

Information technology is now commonplace in veterinary practice, including practice management systems, medical imaging, quality and cost management, and decision-support systems. However, some veterinary informatics professionals lament that information technology is not being incorporated fast enough and remains rather narrowly focused. According to Smith-Akin et al. (2007), "Veterinary informatics remains an embryonic field with relatively few publications. With the exception of radiology/imaging, published articles are primarily focused on non-clinical areas such as hardware/programming and information retrieval."

Veterinary medicine is actively integrating digital imaging. Veterinarians are beginning to adopt information technology systems that bring evidence-based, clinical information to the point of care when it is needed.

Veterinary informatics is being incorporated into bioinformatics, stem cell research, and genetic engineering as cloning research becomes more important in veterinary medicine. A famous example is Dolly the Sheep, which was cloned from a mammary cell in 1996 at the Roslin Institute in Scotland. Since that time, numerous animals have been cloned, large as well as small—horses, cows, dogs, cats, and, of course, mice.

Veterinarians are interested in stem cell research for the same reasons it is important in human medicine: finding cures for diseases and physical abnormalities and understanding the very basics of life itself. Veterinarians are also interested in educational research and application. For example, virtual reality projects are underway to support teaching veterinary medicine, and some projects are used to develop and test methods with which to evaluate educational outcomes. As in others areas of health informatics, veterinary informatics are increasingly being adapted into all these research areas, and veterinary informatics professionals sense a need for a larger cadre of basic researchers.

Bioinformatics

Bioinformatics is the application of information technology to create, manage, interpret, and use data obtained from complex biological phenomena. Its tools include sophisticated modeling with advanced numerical methodologies. The recent burgeoning of bioinformatics as a field of study is due in part to the growth of research in genomic sequencing and related areas. The data generated by such research are complex, requiring high-performance information technology and competent, skilled professionals.

Some of the major areas of study in bioinformatics are sequence analysis and genome annotations, biodiversity measurements, high-throughput image analysis, comparative genomics, prediction of protein structures, and analysis of gene expression. Bioinformatics is of particular importance to the health sciences in many ways and by extension to health information professionals. Chapter 12 is devoted entirely to bioinformatics and genomic medicine.

SUPPORT SERVICES INFORMATICS

Healthcare has a complex structure of support services for patient care that are essential to the healthcare processes. Most of these areas are primarily concerned with supplying vital information to the patient care providers, and health informatics has enormously enhanced this facet.

Pharmaceutical Informatics

Pharmaceutical informatics (also called *pharmacy informatics* and sometimes *pharmacoinformatics*) is a subset of health informatics that deals with the study, research, and implementation of information technology and its applications to pharmaceutical theory and practice. It is concerned with the research and applications of information technology and systems to the practice of pharmacy and studies ways to maximize the effectiveness and efficiency of this practice.

In 2006, the Healthcare Information and Management Systems Society (HIMSS) established the Pharmacy Informatics Community (PIC) for HIMSS members with a role in pharmacy informatics. The PIC group formulated the following definition (Healthcare Information and Management Systems Society, 2006):

> Pharmacy informatics is the scientific field that focuses on medication related data and knowledge within the continuum of healthcare systems including its acquisition, storage, analysis, use, and dissemination in the delivery of optimal medication-related patient care and health outcomes.

Pharmacy professionals view themselves as having a broader role than the one usually perceived by the general public. Pharmacy is a major, indispensable part of the healthcare system. In particular, pharmacy professionals discover, develop, produce, and distribute drugs, and, of equal importance, they create and disseminate drug-related and other health information to patients and healthcare providers.

Pharmacy informatics has rapidly become involved in designing, implementing, and monitoring information systems and technologies to reduce medication errors and manage the medication delivery process. Medication errors are a major problem in modern healthcare, and, pharmacists obviously can play a major role in reducing these errors. The pharmaceutical industry is currently focused on redesigning systems and methods for better medication delivery. Clearly, this is a task for the informatics professional.

Pharmaceutical informatics research and applications including medication management, computerized prescription orderings, clinical medication documentation, pharmacy automation (including robotics), decision support for medication processes, workflow, adverse drug events, management of drug information, government compliance information, and marketing. Some pharmacy professionals believe that although the healthcare industry is seeking ways to improve safety and quality of care, only a small fraction of U.S. pharmacy students are receiving in-depth exposure to the principles and practice of pharmacy informatics. The problem seems to be the slowness with which the practitioners are turning to informatics techniques and technology. When the practitioners embrace the technology, the educational programs will begin to reflect this (Flynn, 2005). Pharmacists are aware of the need to embrace informatics applications. In 2007, the American Society of Health-System Pharmacists issued a statement defining the pharmacist's role in informatics. Pharmacists can "provide medication-management use cases to help with system builds, testing and troubleshooting and can assist in developing interfaces to disparate applications and systems" (Siska and Meyer, 2008).

Pathology Informatics

Pathology is an information-dominated specialty, and all areas of pathology use computers, in some way, to help manage this information. There are a number of subareas of pathology informatics. For example, the Association for Pathology Informatics (API) focuses on data gathering processes and procedures for examining, reporting, and storing large complex sets of data that are generated in different types of labs, such as clinical, anatomic pathology, and research. Modern information technology is a priority of the API (Association for Pathology Informatics, 2006).

Pathology informatics is a crucial element in healthcare services and research. Every medical department and clinic needs accurate, secure, and rapid delivery of pathology data. The data must be integrated with radiology data, other lab reports, clinical trial databases, epidemiologic databases, and so forth, and they must be organized and formatted to meet the needs of the users of the information (Berman, 2006). Healthcare professionals are increasingly recognizing the need for medical professionals to understand the concepts of pathology informatics.

An example of research and applications in pathology informatics is the Johns Hopkins Pathology Data Warehouse. This system integrates data from laboratory information systems at two hospitals (Johns Hopkins Hospital and Bayview Hospital) and aggregates data from point-of-care testing devices. The data warehouse was designed to store test results for long periods of time to support both daily inquiries and long-term research (Taylor and Nichols, 2000).

Another example is the Shared Pathology Informatics Network (SPIN), which uses the Internet to construct a virtual database that allows investigators to locate appropriate human tissue specimens for their research. This large cooperative project is coordinated by two consortia, Harvard/UCLA and Indianapolis/Pittsburgh. Its current focus is on developing information systems for delivery (Braun, 2005). Pathology was a pioneer in the creation of health informatics and it continues to be closely involved in the evolution of informatics.

Laboratory Informatics

Laboratory informatics is about resource management across all types of laboratories, including pathology, but also many other medical-related and non-medical labs. These laboratories are located in a wide variety of settings, including hospitals, clinics, government, academic institutions, research organizations, industry, agriculture centers, and pharmaceutical companies.

The purpose of laboratory informatics is to maximize laboratory operations. It focuses on information technology and systems to enhance laboratory activities and processes, particularly in the areas of analysis, products, research and development, and personnel and workflow management. It includes "data acquisition, lab automation, data processing, specialized data management systems (such as chromatography data systems), laboratory information systems, scientific data management (including data mining and data warehousing), and knowledge management including the use of electronic laboratory notebooks" (Perry, 2004: 421).

Around 70 percent of the information used in patient care comes from clinical and anatomical pathology laboratories, and the movement toward the electronic health record, with its accompanying needs for high-quality, integrated, and efficiently delivered information, is driving the integration of informatics principles and technology into laboratories. Laboratory managers know they must understand what information is and how it is created and managed (Cowan, 2003). Like other areas of health informatics, laboratory informatics is advancing rapidly and is building a research and applications foundation.

Medical Imaging Informatics

Medical imaging informatics (sometimes called *radiological informatics*) is a highly interdisciplinary field, drawing on general informatics, physics, engineering, biological science, healthcare operations, and imaging technology. It is concerned with the full-range of imaging processes—creation, acquisition, organization, storage, retrieval, interpretation, and transfer to points of use. Medical imaging informatics develops, implements, and evaluates information technology for clinical medical imaging (Geis, 2007).

Andriole (2006) stated that radiological informatics "encompasses concepts touching every aspect of the medical imaging chain from image creation . . . [to] display and interpretation. . . . [T]he value of imaging in medicine care can be enhanced through the seamless integration of information technology tools, enabling knowledge delivery at the point of care." Imaging informatics originated as an intersection of imaging technology with clinical informatics. In the beginning, medical imaging was concerned primarily with the application of biophysics and engineering to enhance the technical aspects of imaging and had little to do with the evolving field of health informatics, but this has changed (Kulikowski, 1997). Presently it is concerned with the basic principles of imaging information management and their integration with specific healthcare principles and procedures.

Imaging informatics can be looked at from several viewpoints. For example, its primary objective is to provide enhanced, sophisticated technology and procedures for direct patient care. Along with laboratory informatics, it supplies basic information for diagnosis, care, and prognosis. On the other hand, the growing imaging knowledge base (and related technology) is opening new frontiers for research in the biological and medical sciences.

The wide range of research avenues in medical imaging informatics include computer graphics and visualization, image database management, software engineering, artificial intelligence, cognitive processes, and modeling. One example is the study of the brain using imaging technology. Some of the popular imaging technologies, such as computed tomography, magnetic resonance imaging, functional magnetic resonance imaging, and positron emission tomography, are both answering questions about the brain and revealing new mysteries. Because medical imaging plays such a major role in today's healthcare, Chapter 10 discusses it in more detail.

Consumer Health Informatics

The consumer movement in the last four decades of the twentieth century has affected attitudes toward and changes in healthcare. We are increasingly looking at health from the consumer's perspective, which is leading to both a new dimension in healthcare and a more demanding public. Patients and their families began to understand that they are consumers of services and products offered for sale, often at an expensive price. As a result, they started to demand more direct and personal involvement in decision making and particularly better access to information. Patients shifted from being passive recipients of care given by a knowledgeable clinician to being active collaborators with the healthcare providers (Brennan and Starren, 2006). This gave rise to the concept of consumer health.

Consumer health is about providing the general public with information about health and the healthcare services available to them. Consumer health *informatics* attempts to maximize this process, and it focuses on the design and implementation of systems that collect related information and funnel it to consumers and to those healthcare professionals who are advocates of consumer health issues.

A NEW PARADIGM FOR HEALTH CONSUMERS

There is a paradigm shift in the relationship between care providers and patients due in part to the rise of consumerism, news media coverage of health topics, and the Internet. Over the years patients have fought for the right to obtain information about their conditions, the right to know their choices, and the right to be involved in the decision-making process. These have been achieved to a large extent, but the sobering fact is that there is now an enormous amount of information, many viable options, and the decision-making is not as straightforward as consumers perceived. It is often a difficult responsibility, and patients and their families are realizing the complexity of the process. In a *New York Times* article, Jan Hoffman (2005), pointed out the complexity of information and resources and entities that modern patients face: "The job of being a modern patient includes not only decision making of course, but often coordinating doctors, medical records and procedures, as well as negotiating with insurance companies, who are often the ultimate arbiters over which treatment options will be covered."

THE UBIQUITY OF CONSUMER HEALTH INFORMATION

Numerous sources of information are available to health consumers, in both electronic and print formats. Healthcare facilities, such as hospitals and doctor offices, often produce pamphlets and other patient-oriented publications. Government agencies publish materials written specifically for the general public. Libraries, especially public libraries, carry health books, journals, and other print and electronic items appropriate for the public of all ages.

With the rapid expansion of available consumer health information came concerns about the accuracy, timeliness, and integrity of this information. Traditionally, patient health information was filtered through the healthcare providers. Patients and their families were told only what the providers thought they ought to know. The medical information often was presented strictly from the perspective of the medical providers, because they were the only ones with access to this specialized information. However, times have changed. One of the reasons that consumers turn to information resources on their own is because they feel frustrated with the lack of health information they are receiving from their healthcare providers. At times, consumers seek additional health expertise from qualified healthcare professionals, and at other times they seek information outside the traditional settings, often for financial reasons, including lack of adequate insurance coverage. The ultimate reason people seek health information is not necessarily so they can act as their own physicians; rather, most people just want to be better informed.

CONSUMER HEALTH TERMINOLOGY

Consumer health terminology is a subarea of consumer health informatics that has received attention. There is a great difference between the languages used by clinicians and by lay public, and some research efforts seek ways to bridge this gap. The Consumer Health Vocabulary Initiative project is an example of a multidisciplinary effort to study the lexical forms used by the lay person and how to most effectively mesh these forms with professional health terminology. If lay consumers are going to receive and understand consumer health information, they must be able to communicate (Consumer Health Vocabulary Initiative, 2006; Zeng et al., 2007).

HEALTH LITERACY

Healthcare professionals, including those working in consumer health informatics, have become concerned with the general population's level of health literacy, which they believe is a vital part of the healthcare process. A high level of health literacy would indicate that individuals have the means and the ability to both obtain and understand basic health information and the services that are available to them. According to the U.S. Department of Health and Human Services' (2000) report, called *Healthy People 2010*, a person's level of health literacy often is a strong demographic indicator of his or her health. Without such literacy, people have less capacity to obtain the basic health information and services that they need. Health literacy is a major problem that needs to be addressed. Clearly, health literacy is significant to the trend toward more outpatient care, because patients and their families need to understand health instructions when they leave the healthcare facility.

Most patients try hard to understand the information given by healthcare providers, but research shows clearly that there are often gaps in communication between what health providers are saying and what the patients actually understand. According to the American Medical Association (2008), "The inability for patients to understand medical information is preventing physician/patient communication, decreasing the quality of medical treatment for an estimated 89 million Americans."

INFORMATICS IN ACTION! 4.1

Community Health Literacy Level

Location: Medium-sized rural community

Problem: Community leaders, including healthcare professionals, are concerned about the health literacy level of the community.

People Involved: The mayor appointed a community committee, composed of the director of the public library, a hospital librarian, educators, healthcare professionals, and selected citizens.

Action Taken: A subcommittee, chaired by the director of the public library, was formed and consisted of the head of the hospital library, educators, citizens representing diverse groups in the community, and selected healthcare professionals. Mai, the hospital librarian, took the lead in gathering examples of community health literacy efforts around the country. The subcommittee recommended several options to improve the health literacy of the community. The public library director and the hospital librarian identified possible funding sources for health literacy programs and wrote a report. The proposal was presented to the community committee for action.

Takeaway: The hospital librarian played a central role in the effort to address a communitywide problem related to health literacy. She was knowledgeable about potential funding agencies.

The Joint Commission (2007: 5) stated that "addressing health literacy issues is not the sole burden of those providing health care services. There are implications as well for health care policymakers, purchasers and payers, regulatory bodies, and consumers themselves." The lack of health literacy is not confined to a single population group but cuts across all ages, races, and income and education levels. People with limited health literacy will do the wrong things or not do anything at all, and in the end, this is dangerous to their health. People with limited health literacy have substantially high medical costs, up to four times greater than with patients with literacy skills, resulting in expenditures of many billions of dollars to the healthcare system.

A major problem is that most patients with limited health literacy skills hide this lack of knowledge and understanding from their healthcare providers because they are ashamed or too shy to ask for help. Sometimes they are not aware of the need for information. On the other hand, more and more patients want to be informed and involved in their health care, and they want to play a major role in the decisions about their own health. According to McKenna (2003: 16), research shows that patients who actively participate in their own care with various means are more likely to be:

- Compliant with medication and treatment regimens
- Satisfied with the medical care they receive
- Likely to experience improved clinical outcomes

Health literacy is not the sole responsibility of the health consumer; it is also a responsibility of the healthcare profession. "[H]ealth literacy goes beyond the individual. It also depends upon the skills, preferences, and expectations of health information and care providers: our doctors; nurses; administrators; home health workers; the media; and many others" (Institute of Medicine, 2004). Health literacy is an information problem and a challenge and responsibility of health informaticians.

Consumer health informatics offers an exciting window of opportunity for information professionals. As more people come to use communication technology to finding information, a new consumer culture in health is developing. Healthcare informatics and health sciences librarians will play a major role in this important area.

SUMMARY

This chapter described selected major application areas of health informatics. It is not unusual for a new discipline to define itself by its developing applications and activities, and this is true of health informatics. Health informatics started as an application of computers to medical processes, but early practioneers soon realized that there was a larger concept involved: information. Information is a complex idea, and the creation and management of information is one of the world's largest industries. Health informatics is about the management of health information and about the people who create, distribute, and use this information.

It is perhaps a bit disconcerting that health informatics has splintered into a long list of subapplications like the ones discussed in this chapter, but this is a perfectly natural turn of events. Although there is an embryonic theoretical base, it remains true that health informatics is about applications. These applications will lead to the improvement and advancement of heathcare to all people.

REFERENCES

American Medical Association. "Health Literacy." Chicago: AMA Foundation (October 14, 2008). Available: www.ama-assn.org/ama/pub/category/8115.html (accessed November 5, 2008).

American Nurses Association. 1994. *The Scope of Practice for Nursing Informatics.* Washington, DC: American Nurses Publishing.

Andriole, Katherine P. "An Introduction to Radiological Informatics, Business Briefing: Future Directions in Imaging." Boston: Harvard Medical School Center for Evidence-based Imaging (2006). Available from Touch Briefings: www.touch briefings.com/download.cfm?fileID=7554 (accessed March 18, 2009).

Association for Pathology Informatics. "What We Do." Bethesda, MD: Association for Pathology Informatics (2006). Available: www.pathologyinformatics.org/mission. htm (accessed November 5, 2008).

Bellamy, James E.C. 1999. "Veterinary Informatics—Why Are We Dragging Our Feet?" *Canadian Journal of Veterinary Medicine* 40 (December): 861–863.

Berman, Jules J. "Welcome." Bethesda, MD: Association for Pathology Informatics (2006). Available: www.pathologyinformatics.org/welcome.htm (accessed November 5, 2008).

Braun, Jonathan. 2005. "Shared Pathology Informatics Network (SPIN)." Bethesda, MD: American Society for Investigative Pathology (2005). Available: www.asip. org/mtgs/EB05/braunabs.htm (accessed November 5, 2008).

Brennan, Patricia F. and Justin B. Starren. 2006. "Consumer Health Informatics and Telehealth." In *Biomedical Informatics: Computer Applications in Health Care and Biomedicine* (pp. 511–536), 3rd ed., edited by Edward H. Shortliffe and James J. Cimino. New York: Springer.

"Consumer Health Vocabulary Initiative." Boston: Decision Systems Group, Brigham and Women's Hospital, Harvard Medical School (2006). Available: http:// consumerhealthvocab.org (accessed November 5, 2008).

Cowan, Daniel F. 2003. *Informatics for the Clinical Laboratory: A Practical Guide.* New York: Springer-Verlag.

de Lusignan, Simon. 2003. "What Is Primary Care Informatics?" *Journal of the American Medical Informatics Association* 10, no. 4 (July–August): 304–309.

Dewan, Naakesh A., Nancy M. Lorenzi, Robert T. Riley, and Sarbori R. Bhattacharya. 2002. "Behavioral Health and Informatics: An Overview." In *Behavioral Health-*

care Informatics (pp. 3–8), edited by Naakesh A. Dewan, Nancy M. Lorenzi, Robert T. Riley, and Sarbori R. Bhattacharya. New York: Springer-Verlag.

Ebell, Mark H. and Jay Siwek. 2006. "Improving Practice Guidelines in AFP." *American Family Physician* 74, no. 11 (December 1): 1840–1841.

Field, Marilyn J. and Kathleen N. Lohr, eds. 1990. *Clinical Practice Guidelines: Directions for a New Program Institute of Medicine (IOM)*. Washington, DC: National Academies Press.

Flynn, Allen J. 2005. "The Current State of Pharmacy Informatics Education in Professional Programs at US Colleges of Pharmacy." *American Journal of Pharmaceutical Education* 69, no. 4 (Article 66): 490–494.

Fonarow, Gregg C. "The American Heart Association's Get with the Guidelines Program: Key Findings and Lessons Learned." Washington, DC: National Guideline Clearinghouse (November 3, 2008). Available: www.guideline.gov/resources/commentary.aspx?file=Get_with_the_Guidelines.inc (accessed November 7, 2008).

Freifeld, Clark and John Brownstein. "HealthMap: Global Disease Alert Map" (February, 2008). Available: www.healthmap.org (accessed November 7, 2008).

Geis, J. Raymond. 2007. "Medical Imaging Informatics: How It Improves Radiology Practice Today." *Journal of Digital Imaging* 20, no. 2 (June): 99–104.

Healthcare Information and Management Systems Society. "Pharmacy Informatics." Chicago: Healthcare Information and Management Systems Society (2006). Available: www.himss.org/asp/topics_pharmacyInformatics.asp (accessed November 5, 2008).

Hoffman, Jan. "Awash in Information, Patients Face a Lonely Uncertain Road." *New York Times*, August 14, 2005. Available: http://query.nytimes.com/search/sitesearch?query=jan+hoffman+2005&submit.x=16&submit.y=13 (accessed November 5, 2008).

Institute of Medicine. "Health Literacy: A Prescription to End Confusion." Washington, DC: The National Academies Press (February 10, 2004). Available: www.iom.edu/?id=31489 (accessed November 5, 2008).

The Joint Commission. *"What Did the Doctor Say?: Improving Health Literacy to Protect Patient Safety."* Oakbrook Terrace, IL: The Joint Commission (February 2007). Available: www.jointcommission.org/PublicPolicy/health_literacy.htm (accessed November 5, 2008).

Koo, Denise, Patrick O'Carroll, and Martin LaVenture. 2001. "Public Health 101 for Informaticians." *Journal of the American Medical Association* 8, no. 6 (November–December): 585–597.

Kulikowski, Casimar. 1997. "Medical Imaging Informatics: Challenges of Definition and Integration." *Journal of the American Medical Association* 4, no. 3 (May–June): 252–253.

Little, David R. "Health of the Population: Medical Informatics Applications." In *Today's Primary-care Informatics News*. Washington, DC: American Medical Informatics Association (April 24, 2007). Available: http://pciwg.amia.org (accessed November 5, 2008).

McCormick, Kathleen A., Connie J. Delaney, Patricia Flatley Brennan, Judith A. Effken, Kathie Kendrick, Judy Murphy, Diane J. Skiba, Judith J. Warren, Charlotte A. Weaver, Betsy Weiner, and Bonnie L. Westra. 2007. "Guideposts to the Future—An Agenda for Nursing Informatics." *Journal of the American Medical Informatics Association* 14, no. 1 (January–February): 19–24.

McKenna, Mindi K. 2003. *High Tech Medicine: Building Your Medical Practice with Computers and the Internet.* Kansas City, MO: Fordham University Press.

National Institute of Mental Health (NIMH). "Statistics." Bethesda, MD: National Institute of Mental Health (2009). Available: www.nimh.nih.gov/health/topics/statistics/index.shtml (accessed March 18, 2009).

O'Carroll, Patrick W. 2003. "Introduction to Public Health Informatics." In *Public Health Informatics and Information Systems* (pp. 3–15), edited by Patrick W. O'Carroll, William A. Yasnoff, M. Elizabeth Ward, Laura H. Ripp, and Ernest L. Martin. New York: Springer.

Perry, Douglas. 2004. Laboratory Informatics: Origin, Scope, and Its Place in Higher Education." *JALA* 9, no. 6 (December): 421–428.

Schleyer, Titus K.L. 2003. "Dental Informatics: A Work in Progress." *Advanced Dental Research* 17 (December): 9–15.

Schleyer, Titus K.L., Thankam P. Thyvalikakath, Heiko Spallek, Miguel H. Torres-Urquidy, Pedro Hernandez, and Jeannie Yuhaniak. 2006. "Clinical Computing in General Dentistry." *Journal of the American Medical Informatics Association* 13, no. 3 (May–June): 344–352.

Scholes, Maureen and B. Barber. 1980. "Towards Nursing Informatics." In *MEDINFO: 1980* (pp. 7–73), edited by Donald A.B. Lindberg and Shigekoto Kaihara. Amsterdam, the Netherlands: North-Holland.

Siska, Mark H. and Gerald E. Meyer. 2008. "Pharmacy Informatics: Aligning for Success." *American Journal of Health-system Pharmacy* 65 (August): 1410–1411.

Smith-Akin, Kimberly A., Charles F. Bearden, Stephen T. Pittenger, and Elmer V. Bernstam. 2007. "Toward a Veterinary Informatics Research Agenda: An Analysis of the PubMed-indexed Literature." *International Journal of Medical Informatics* 76, no. 4: 306–312.

Society of Behavioral Medicine. Milwaukee, WI: Society of Behavioral Medicine (2007a). Available: www.sbm.org (accessed November 5, 2008).

Society of Behavioral Medicine. Behavioral Informatics SIG. Milwaukee, WI: Society of Behavioral Medicine (2007b). Available: www.sbm.org/sig/behavioral_informatics (accessed November 5, 2008).

Spallek, Heiko, Jeannie Yuhaniak Irwin, Titus Schelyer, Brian S. Butler, and Patricia M. Weiss. 2007. "Supporting the Emergence of Dental Informatics with an Online Community." *International Journal of Computerized Dentistry* 10, no. 3 (July): 247–264.

Taylor, Merwyn G., and James H. Nichols. 2000. "JHMI Data Warehouse." Baltimore: Johns Hopkins University (July 2000). Available: http://pathology2.jhu.edu/Informatics/JHMI_Data_Warehouse.htm (accessed November 5, 2008).

U.S. Department of Health and Human Services. "Healthy People 2010: Understanding and Improving Health," 2nd ed. Washington, DC: U.S. Government Printing Office (2000). Available: www.healthypeople.gov/Publications (accessed November 5, 2008).

World Health Organization. "Global Outbreak Alert & Response Network." Geneva, Switzerland: World Health Organization (2008). Available: www.who.int/csr/ outbreaknetwork/en (accessed November 5, 2008).

Zeng, Qing T., Tony Tse, Guy Divita, Alla Keselman, Jon Crowell, Allen C. Browne, Sergey Goryachev, and Long Ngo. 2007. "Term Identification Methods for Consumer Health Vocabulary Development." *Journal of Medical Internet Research* 9, no. 1 (January–March): e4. Available: www.pubmedcentral.nih.gov/articlerender. fcgi?tool=pmcentrez&artid=1874512 (accessed November 5, 2008).

Chapter 5

Health Sciences Librarians and Health Informatics

This chapter addresses the question, where does the health sciences librarian fit into the scheme of health informatics? The question is not how health sciences librarians can become more like health informatics professionals, which is not a meaningful goal. Health informatics and health sciences librarianship are two distinct disciplines with their own missions, skills, and place in the healthcare enterprise, but they intersect in a dynamic, symbiotic way.

The early chapters of this book described the basic tenets and characteristics of health informatics, which should be fundamental in any health sciences librarians' professional education. This chapter examines some of the ways in which the two disciplines meet, interact, and work with each other. To understand the interaction of health informatics and health sciences librarianship, it is necessary to understand the environments of both. Of course, the two disciplines work under the same general environment—healthcare. Over the past few decades both have evolved from being rather narrowly focused to having broader visions of mission and purpose. For example, health informatics was aimed at clinical providers and a few related support functions, while libraries aimed at being bridges between health information and healthcare providers. In the new millennium, both health informatics and health sciences libraries have become support services for physicians and all related health professionals, educators, students, business entities, consumers, government, and others. Public health and global health problems are areas of concern for both health informatics and health sciences librarianship. The scope of mission, technological emphasis, and research objectives have changed for both disciplines. The quest is to examine where these two information professions can become partners.

HEALTH SCIENCES LIBRARIES

There are numerous types of health sciences libraries, such as hospital libraries, academic health sciences libraries, consumer health libraries, veterinary libraries, mental health libraries, public health libraries, and pharmaceutical libraries. These libraries evolved in conjunction with the developing medical profession in the United States. Their mission has always been to provide quality medical information to health professionals, and this has involved the development of sophisticated medical literature bibliographic systems, including the use of information technology, and the insight and foresight of many strong and motivated pioneers in the field.

Librarians in any type of library perform two essential activities. They obtain and maintain up-to-date information resources (both local and virtual), and they manage access to these resources for their clientele. Librarians design and operate systems that acquire, organize, store, and retrieve "on demand" information. The purpose is to serve as a bridge between the creators of knowledge and the users of knowledge. In health sciences libraries the challenge is: How can systems be built that quickly provide accurate information to busy people working in chaotic places? (Taylor, 2006). The complexity of this operation and its need for skills and intellectual savvy are not usually apparent to the general public.

Perry, Roderer, and Assar (2005) define health sciences librarianship as applying organization and management technologies to biomedical scholarly communications. While this is still a major tenet, health sciences libraries have expanded beyond this to increase their service domain to patients, consumers, and, in many cases, the general public. Perry, Roderer, and Assar pointed out that librarianship is more than just the management of an institution called a library. Librarianship concerns itself with users of information and how the information is used. It is concerned with the *purposes* for which users intend to apply information. Understanding the intended use of the information is a key factor in the information provider's approach to finding the appropriate information.

THE LEADERSHIP OF THE U.S. NATIONAL LIBRARY OF MEDICINE

The U.S. National Library of Medicine (NLM) is one of the most prestigious and well-known biomedical libraries in the world. NLM is at the forefront of promoting the symbiosis of health sciences librarianship and health informatics.

The library has over 9 million books, journals, and other formats of information. However, the size and quality of NLM's collection is only one of its assets. NLM is known for its pioneering and adventurous leadership in research support and in innovative programs and outreach to the healthcare enterprise and to individual citizens.

NLM evolved from a library established in the Office of the Surgeon General of the Army in 1836. It actually began to be a viable tool in 1865 when John Shaw Billings, MD (1838–1913), was appointed supervisor. Billings was a successful physician, involved in many areas of endeavor. During the Civil War he served in a number of major battles and also found time to organize hospitals in Washington, DC. After the war he reorganized the library and museum of the Office of the Surgeon General and was active with the National Board of Health. He continued his work in planning hospitals, including the one at Johns Hopkins University. However, he is best remembered for his librarianship and for turning the collection at the Surgeon General's Office into the prestigious National Library of Medicine.

Over the years, NLM has been a leader in developing information access systems. In the 1880s, under Billings' direction, *Index Medicus,* a subject/author guide to the medical literature, was created. This was a formidable undertaking— humans, not computers had to do the task. *Index Medicus* spawned diverse information retrieval tools over the years, such as MEDLARS (Medical Literature Analysis and Retrieval System), MEDLINE, and the current PubMed Central, which allows public access to a large repository of medical journals.

Of particular interest is NLM's involvement in informatics. NLM is a major bridge in the connection and interoperability of health sciences librarians and health informatics. An important milestone for NLM was the opening of The Lister Hill National Center of Biomedical Communications in 1980 as NLM's research and development component. The Lister Hill National Center for Biomedical Communications explores the uses of computer, communication, and audiovisual technologies to improve the organization, dissemination, and utilization of biomedical information. Currently the center is applying modern communications technologies to healthcare-related projects involving, for example, telemedicine, test bed networks, virtual reality, and the Unified Medical Language System. The Visible Human Project® has created, in complete anatomical detail, three-dimensional representations of the male and female human body, resulting in a large digital image library. *Profiles in Science* is the center's Web site that provides access to the laboratory notes, photographs, and correspondence of notable American scientists (National Library of Medicine, 2007).

In 1988 the National Center for Biotechnology Information (NCBI) was established and has taken on the task of developing information services for biotechnology, including how to best store and make accessible data related to human genome research. "NCBI is a recognized leader in basic research in computational molecular biology, and is also responsible for developing innovative computer solutions for the management and dissemination of the rapidly growing volume of genome information" (National Library of Medicine, 2007).

NLM has been a strong supporter of health informatics in numerous ways, through grants, training, and outreach programs with focuses available for health sciences librarians. An example of training is a course held annually at Woods Hole, Massachusetts, at the Marine Biological Laboratory, for 30 specially selected applicants in the health professions, research, and librarianship. It is a one-week intensive course in medical informatics, providing hands-on experience in a wide range of informatics areas (National Library of Medicine, 2008). Truly, the NLM plays a major, active role in health informatics.

IMPACTS OF CHANGES IN HEALTH SCIENCES LIBRARIES

As discussed in Chapter 2, the healthcare environment has been changing dramatically in the past few decades, and this has effected changes in health sciences librarianship and in the role of the health sciences librarian. When a domain of users changes their environment and *modus operandi*, their information needs change. Some of the major changes are discussed in the following sections.

Changing Healthcare Environments

One of the most ubiquitous changes in healthcare has been the move to information technology at all levels. Technology has permeated all clinical and administrative aspects of healthcare. As a result, it is imperative that the health sciences librarian embrace this technology, especially in terms of how it impacts the delivery of library information services. Health sciences librarians have a commendable history of using technology.

A major impact has been the move toward end-user searching. This reflects changes in medical education and in the practice of medicine as well as the presence of the Internet and a new generation of young people who consider using computers to be second nature. Today's healthcare providers and those in training are developing information skills; they know how to search for information in this "digital and networked world" (Groen, 2007: 148). Health sciences librarians are the obvious professionals for teaching online searching skills both in the library and in the student's own environment.

Another example of change that impacts health sciences librarians is the explicit recognition in recent decades that information management is a key factor in quality healthcare and patient safety. Among others, The Joint Commission on Accreditation of Healthcare Organizations (JCAHO), also known as The Joint Commission, is very much concerned about these issues, and information management is a key concept in their accreditation endeavor. In fact, one of the chapters in the Joint Commission's annually updated *Comprehensive Accreditation Manual for Hospitals (CAMH): The Official Handbook* is devoted to information management.

A hospital is a complex organization, and it is dependent on a multidimensional array of information about care, treatment, and services. Managing this information requires careful planning and execution of the plans. Information management should support decision making, ensure patient safety, and improve performance throughout the organization (Medical Library Association, 2007). Quality assessment and improvement are information driven, and information management is what librarians do.

Another impact on libraries of the changes in healthcare is the growing emphasis on consumer health. As discussed in Chapter 4, consumer health is information driven and thus its growth is affecting the health sciences librarian. Empowered consumers see the library as another resource for finding the health information they need and expect the librarians to find types of information that in the past were not perused by consumers.

A final example is the explosive growth of medical information and knowledge. The exponentially increasing volume of medical knowledge is profoundly affecting library information delivery services and is one of the driving forces in the move to digitalization of health sciences libraries. It would be impossible to cope with this knowledge growth without information technology. Health sciences librarians must expand their mission, goals, and personal skills in order to remain partners in the changing healthcare environment, especially with the push toward integrating advanced information management technologies into healthcare in all its facets.

Impact of Computers and Related Information Technologies

Computers have profoundly impacted libraries, as they have all other segments of society. Today's society is in the midst of an information revolution equivalent to that of Gutenberg's time (Groen, 2007). Health sciences libraries were among the first in the new revolution to utilize information technologies of all kinds. Decades ago these libraries were engaged in cooperative agreements with each other, using the technology of the time to do such things as share cataloging information and form interlibrary loan agreements. Health sciences libraries were among the first to implement computer-based bibliographic automation, such as MEDLARS. In 1943, NLM was distributing microfilm copies of documents and in the 1950s was using punch card systems for creating indexes. By the 1960s, these index publishing processes had migrated to computers (McKnight, 2005).

With the advent of large-scale, tape-driven batch processing systems, libraries started creating computer-generated catalogs and indexing databases. Soon random access became ubiquitous, the microchip for storage and processing was invented, and microcomputers evolved. Parallel and related to these developments was the move to timesharing computing and the creation of the Internet. A major intellectual milestone in the evolution of computers came around 1970 when it was recognized that computers are much more than calculating machines—they are powerful devices for communication. The incredible birth and growth of computers as a major force in society all occurred in a very brief time span of about 50 years.

Health sciences librarianship is a profession concerned with both the basic premises of services and the vehicles and systems to deliver those services. Health sciences libraries have moved beyond being the traditional depositories of retrospective literature; they now have a presence in cyberspace and use nontraditional formats and virtual library concepts. The concept of services has become more diversified and broader, and the systems are becoming digital, virtual, and health information technology driven. Today, health sciences librarians realize that health sciences information resources are evolving into digitalized form, and the day when this transfer will be complete is not too far away. Along with digitalization is the move to make information increasingly available through networks and sophisticated communication devices.

Technology allows direct access by users from their offices, at the patient's bedside, in their homes and cars, in cyber cafes, and in remote areas across the globe. Web 2.0 and Web 3.0 are enabling new paradigms of how information and people should be interoperable and interconnected in ways not perceived a decade ago.

Health sciences librarians must continue to evaluate and monitor what their roles will be in this climate of change. They have a history of adopting and adapting new technology, and this tradition is as active now as it ever was. From time to time librarians have felt that their value has been undervalued by healthcare providers and that there is a perception problem on the part of the providers of the role the librarians play. Health sciences librarians are often frustrated because the services and resources they are providing are not fully recognized. Groen (2007: 260) believes that librarians must examine themselves and get the right people into the profession: "It is incumbent on the medical library profession to identify the necessary knowledge and skills that are required to fill this need and to recruit into the profession of medical librarianship those individuals who posses the potential to fill this role." The ideal recruit will have more than a minimal background in the biomedical sciences and subsequently will resonate more with health sciences professionals.

In the 1990s articles appeared in the literature predicting that information technology would make libraries nonrelevant and would soon lead to the demise of librarianship. The exact opposite has happened. Libraries embraced the technology, changed their sense of mission, and are thriving in the cyberspace age. As Mark Twain purportedly said, "The reports of [our] death have been greatly exaggerated."

The Medical Library Assistance Act

The Medical Library Assistance Act (MLAA) greatly affected health sciences libraries. The MLAA was passed by the U.S. Congress in October 1965 as a response to the growing concern that there was a gap between the information needs of the healthcare providers and the resources of the health sciences library (Cummings and Corning, 1971). This legislation gave a needed boost to medical libraries around the country.

The MLAA mandated the following programs (Cummings and Corning, 1971: 378):

1. Construction of facilities
2. Training in medical library sciences
3. Special scientific projects
4. Research and development in medical library science and related fields
5. Improvement and expansion of the basic resources of medical libraries and related instrumentalities
6. Establishment of regional medical libraries
7. Biomedical publications, and
8. Regional branches of the National Library of Medicine

The MLAA is closely tied to the services and activities of the NLM. Between 1965 and 1970, $43 million in grants and contracts were awarded to support core library activities and facilities improvement. A major purpose of the MLAA was to upgrade the nation's medical libraries by establishing local interrelations in a formal way. The Act gave NLM the responsibility for a grant program that created the Regional Medical Library Network, which is now known as the National Network of Libraries of Medicine (NN/LM). The network is the basic infrastructure that provides equal access to biomedical information by all health professionals across the country. NN/LM includes eight regional medical libraries and about 4,762 "primary access" libraries. For the most part, the regional libraries are located at medical schools or academic health sciences centers, and the primary access libraries are at hospitals. "The Regional Medical Libraries . . . exhibit and demonstrate NLM's products and services at national, regional and state health professional and consumer oriented meetings; provide training and consultations; coordinate the basic network services . . . [and] work to improve the supporting infrastructure for health sciences libraries . . . " (National Library of Medicine, 2007).

Information Needs and Searching Behaviors of Healthcare Providers

Health informatics and health sciences librarianship are about the delivery of health-related information to those who need it—healthcare providers, consumers, and the general public. The needs of consumers are discussed in Chapter 4; this section focuses on the needs of healthcare providers.

The delivery of information to health providers is a two-sided coin. One side is the *need* of the user and the other side is *how* the user finds the information, which is called *information-seeking behavior*. Information delivery begins with a clear understanding of who the users are, what they do, and what specifically they need.

Because of the wide range of healthcare professions, the users are numerous and varied and have a multitude of different needs. For example, healthcare providers have large numbers of clinical questions and little time to find and understand the answers. Some of the more general categories of information needs include the following:

- Information on a specific patient
- Information on a specific disease or condition
- Information related to alternative causes of a symptom
- Laboratory or radiology reports interpretations
- Treatment information (including complementary and alternative treatments)
- Drug information
- Information on new procedures
- New technology
- Standard references, such as the definition of a term
- Patient education resources
- Social and professional issues related to practice

The information needs of physicians are important for many reasons but probably most important is that information is a key to quality healthcare and to reducing medical errors. When healthcare providers encounter an event of uncertainty, they often require additional information in order to make a decision. If the information is not available, the possibility of an error being made is increased. Sometimes physicians are not even aware of gaps in their knowledge and their corresponding information needs.

Understanding the information needs of physicians—and all other healthcare providers—is the first step in providing information services. The goals and operations of the systems in which these professionals work must be clearly understood, particularly their specific and concrete information needs. Without this understanding, medical decision making cannot be optimized.

Medical decision making remains at the heart of what healthcare providers do, and in the past few years notable changes have occurred because of the advancements in the management of health information, including, for example, new ways for accessing the medical literature and the steady improvements in expert systems. The main drawbacks are convincing healthcare providers of the usefulness and possibilities of the new tools and, more important, ensuring that the implementers truly understand the needs of the users. "Unfortunately, medical information science has not acquired a formal understanding of the information needs of physician" (Woolf and Benson, 1989: 372).

Woolf and Benson's observation can be extrapolated to the healthcare enterprise in general. Although it has been two decades since Woolf and Benson's study, the literature still focuses on developing information technology, not on understanding the user's information needs.

The second side of the coin is information-seeking behavior. Case (2002: 76) stated that "information seeking is a taken-for-granted concept, a catchall phrase that encompasses a variety of behaviors seemingly motivated by the recognition of 'missing' information." Information professionals and systems designers need to do much better.

Many studies describe how users obtain information. Taylor (2006) lists a number of basic groups of resources that doctors typically turn to: (1) colleagues in person, (2) colleagues through electronic means, (3) books, (4) books through electronic means, (5) journals, and (6) journals through electronic means. Clinicians who use electronic information resources use a variety of searching techniques (McKibbon, Friedman, and Crowley, 2007).

Studies show that approximately one half of clinical questions can be answered from the clinical record. One quarter are answered from textbooks or journals, and about one quarter are patient specific and require in-depth synthesis from various knowledge resources (Bennet et al., 2005).

Turning to colleagues is an easy, usually fast, way to find answers. Studies show that this happens approximately 35 percent of the time. Standing in the doorway of a colleague or calling one on the phone can be a fruitful way to exchange ideas and elaborate to make things more clear. Of course, there are downsides. The colleague may not know any more about the question than the inquisitor.

INTERSECTIONS OF HEALTH SCIENCES LIBRARIANSHIP AND HEALTH INFORMATICS

Health informatics has changed dramatically during its short life span, evolving from basic applications of computers to clinical processes to a broader understanding of human needs for information. The much older profession of health sciences librarianship has also changed, and the changes in both professions are drawing them closer together in many aspects.

Librarianship has always been literature focused. In the beginning it was primarily concerned with the custodianship of books. Around the turn of the twentieth century, the paradigm shifted; reference work evolved, and librarianship became service oriented. The resources and professional expertise of the health sciences librarian are still basically centered on the published literature, and while this remains a major function, they must embrace the full infrastructure of health science information and understand that health information is much more than the literature.

As health informatics moved beyond its narrow focus on computers, the intellectual and theoretical bases moved closer to the knowledge domain of medical information science and librarianship. At the same time, health sciences librarianship broadened its sense of mission and became one of the leaders of applying information technology in all its forms. A common ground between the two fields is emerging, because clearly both are concerned with the effective and efficient creation, transfer, and use of quality information at the right place and at the right time.

Common Intellectual Base and Operational Theorems

The intellectual base and operational theorems of health informatics and health sciences librarianship converge at a number of points, offering opportunities for collaboration in the common cause of managing knowledge for the healthcare professions. Without a doubt, in the changing health information environment the health sciences librarian must: (1) master the skills expected of the twenty-first century librarian and (2) understand the basics of health informatics. Those librarians who understand health informatics will have a powerful tool to use in their interactions with today's health informatics professionals and other healthcare professionals.

Both fields have the mission to provide information services to the vastly diverse range of personnel who make up the healthcare enterprise, and there are similarities and differences in how this is done. Health informatics is about communication, systems, networking, devices and instruments, human psychology, economics, and, of course, information technology in all its forms. It is about understanding healthcare and the people who provide it and about the organizations that provide the platforms for healthcare delivery. The modern health informatics world works within this broad context, and librarians who want to be a part of this must retool themselves and move beyond "managing containers of information" (Giuse et al., 1997: 58).

All professions, including the health professions, depend on their knowledge bases, created through centuries by research and experience, and the knowledge bases must be effectively managed. Healthcare information systems, traditional and electronic, contain knowledge-based resources and people managing the system who have the skills to organize, retrieve, and transfer the information. Organizing, preserving, and providing access to professional knowledge bases are what librarians do best.

The core concept of health informatics and librarianship, including health sciences librarianship, is information. From this it follows that the relationship between health sciences librarianship and health informatics should be symbiotic. Perry (2005) maintains that many of the activities of librarians have migrated into health informatics, such as management of digital rights, network access, and point-of-care delivery of knowledge-based information resources, data mining, information filtering, and a host of nontraditional library work. Libraries are becoming more and more digital and have shifted their emphasis to how to manage information within the context of individual information needs and uses. The advent of the digital age is promoting a movement of health sciences librarianship and health informatics to common areas of operation.

Although the two fields are similar, they are not the same. A major difference is related to the creation of information. Health sciences librarianship does not put much emphasis on the actual creation of information, whereas health informatics, such as imaging informatics, is very much involved in this.

A basic similarity is that both fields supply information for diagnosis, treatment plans, and prognosis; the health informatics professional does this from patient data and the librarian from the literature and other knowledge-based resources. The main barrier for the health sciences librarian in this endeavor at the moment, according to Dalrymple (2002: 5), is the librarian's lack of "domain knowledge." Librarians often lack specific medical knowledge, whereas this comes naturally to the health informatics professional. If librarians want to have a meaningful role in informatics, it is essential that they obtain a more substantial amount of medical knowledge.

Given the similarities and differences between the fields, what does the health sciences librarian have to offer in the informatics environment? The answer is that the librarian has the proven skills and tested knowledge to manage information in whatever form it exists. Health sciences librarians, like the health informatics professionals, are concerned with the organization, storage, transfer, and use of all information related to the healthcare enterprise, and this is the most common intellectual and operational ground between the two fields.

Health sciences librarians should continue to be librarians, modifying their professional missions, roles, knowledge, skills, and research endeavors but not becoming health informatics clones. They should, however, come to understand the principles of health informatics and recognize where and how their librarian skills meld into it.

New Roles and Opportunities

At one time health sciences librarians considered the provision of information to health professionals as their protected domain, but they probably overestimated their perceived importance to the average healthcare professional. To a large extent physicians and other healthcare providers did not give much thought to the mechanics of obtaining information. They read the professional literature, attended conferences, took continuing education courses, and talked to colleagues. Some used health sciences libraries, if they had one closely available, but most healthcare professionals were not highly skilled information retrievers.

Today, new information workers have appeared on the scene and have caught the attention of healthcare providers, primarily as a result of computers and the wide diversity of information technology. The new generations of healthcare professionals are keenly aware of the information revolution and are becoming a part of it, as evidenced by the rise of health informatics. The question is, how deeply involved in and committed to the new changes will librarians be? The opportunities and challenges are there, if librarians are willing to step forward.

Dalrymple (2002) points out that librarians are facing a challenge to their domain of action by other groups that are also regarded as information professionals. Librarians should not resist this challenge but instead should realize that these groups serve complimentary services. Rather than be afraid of these groups, librarians need to "examine and understand the cognate disciplines whose knowledge and functions resemble—even challenge—their own" (Dalrymple, 2002: 2). If librarians do this, a better spirit of cooperation will be possible, and librarians can tout their services and take advantage of new opportunities.

Within health informatics, there is a lack of awareness of just who makes up the workforce. There is no comprehensive quantitative data on the nature and characteristics of the professionals who consider themselves to be in the field (Hersh, 2006). However, the field is beginning to define itself as a profession, and this is opening up real opportunities for health sciences librarians to demonstrate the role they can play in health informatics.

Health informatics is making the healthcare society more aware and more sensitive to the importance of information throughout the entire healthcare infrastructure. Healthcare providers now talk in terms of information in all that they do. This is a chance for health sciences librarians to promote themselves and convince health professionals that the librarians are up to par with the other members of the health team. The reality is that the burden of improving the perception of the viability of the librarian is a tough challenge for health sciences librarians. Both health informatics and librarianship are about *information*. This is an opportunity for health sciences librarians to make the connection.

Some health sciences librarians are uneasy with the rise of nonlibrarians calling themselves information professionals, because they see these new professionals encroaching on their traditional activities to support the healthcare community. Others think of it as an exciting new horizon for health sciences librarians. The following sections examine specific ways in which health sciences librarians might expand their roles.

Health Information Technology Management

Most people involved in healthcare agree that information technology is a major factor in improving the quality and efficiency of healthcare. Hersh (2006) pointed out that much attention is being given to cost and systems problems and technical support but little attention is being give to who will be the leaders and implementers of these systems and how they will be trained. Health sciences librarians have an opportunity in health information technology management because of their proven expertise in information technology and in educating healthcare providers in using the technology.

Hersh and others have also pointed out that there is a lack of knowledge about the personnel who implement and run information technology in health-related organizations. Who are these workers, and what backgrounds, training, skills, and experience do they have? As the technology grows and becomes ubiquitous, these personnel become more and more needed. Three general groups of professionals work full- or part-time in health informatics. The first includes the health practitioners, such as doctors and nurses. Another includes the computer science, professionals, who generally do not have any training specific to health informatics. The third includes medical records management experts and health sciences librarians (Hersh, 2006).

Many healthcare professionals now use technology (sometimes wearing it) to find information themselves, and this will inevitably reduce the librarian's role as information seeker in the traditional sense. Therefore, librarians must modify their role. An obvious modification is to become more involved in information systems design and implementation and in training and mentoring health professionals in the use these information systems.

In 2006, Howse, Bracke, and Keim proposed a concept called *technology mediation*: "The Technology Mediation approach differs from the clinical librarian or informationist model by removing the responsibility for search and critical appraiser." In other words, the librarian (or technology mediator) focuses on having the right technology available and on aiding the healthcare professional in using the technology.

No doubt wireless technology is aiding healthcare providers obtain quick access to accurate information. On the average, it takes about 2 minutes for physicians to find information in a book or journal, but they can find information on a palmtop in about 20 seconds. About 60 percent of family physicians regularly use the Internet for clinical information, and they consider it to be an important tool for their practice (Bennet et al., 2005).

Clearly, the role of the health sciences librarian is changing from being focused on providing "answers" to reference questions to being information technology support personnel. Healthcare professionals increasingly prefer to control the information-seeking process and use online resources, but they still expect technical support. This is where the health sciences librarian can become a *technology mediator*.

Evidence-based Medicine and the Health Sciences Librarian

In most types of libraries, the librarian does not actively evaluate the content of the literature, but health sciences librarians are increasing involved in content evaluation and synthesis. The best example of this is evidence-based medicine (EBM) support, where the librarian is positioned to play a major role.

The development, refinement, and operational implementation of EMB procedures are natural tasks of health informatics. In fact, EBM provides an important opportunity for skilled health sciences librarians to enter health informatics. EBM is founded on the idea of using a systematic approach to optimize methods for identifying and evaluating information, and this makes EBM, health informatics, and medical librarianship natural partners.

The goal of EBM is to find the best information with which to support healthcare. What is the best knowledge about a disease? What is the best treatment? What is best for the patient? The premise is that the healthcare knowledge base holds the best information but that careful, methodological processes must be used to cull out the "best practice" information.

For the healthcare information professional, EBM is an information-based tool, and he or she needs to clearly understand EBM procedures. These procedures can work only if there are people who are skilled in identifying the best available literature on the topic. These professionals may be librarians or other information specialists and, in many cases, are healthcare providers who understand how to search the resources.

EBM is based on a critical appraisal of the medical literature, and working with the medical literature is the core of what health sciences librarians do. What is new to librarians is the element of critical appraisal. Librarians have always been concerned with content analysis in the sense of the "aboutness" of the knowledge record. This is essential to the bibliographic control processes, such as cataloging, classification, indexing, and abstracting. But librarians are seldom called on to analyze and critically evaluate the validity and importance of the content. To become involved in EBM, they must develop this analytical skill (which is a combination of having a certain amount of subject knowledge and highly tuned research skills).

One of the criticisms of EBM is that busy clinicians do not have sufficient time to search, analyze, and synthesize information. Librarians have already demonstrated that they can perform these tasks effectively. For a number of years, health sciences librarians have created systematic reviews, synthesized data and information, and taught classes in EBM to healthcare students and professionals. Finding the best information, formatting it, and presenting it in useable form are what librarians do.

Patient and Consumer Services

The focus of health sciences librarians has traditionally been on providing information only to the healthcare profession. However, health informatics is now bringing in the patient and consumer, creating another rich opportunity for health science librarians. Clearly, in this area health science librarians can draw on the experiences and knowledge of other branches of librarianship such as public librarianship and special librarianship (Dalrymple, 2002).

Health literacy was described in Chapter 4. It is clear that health literacy is a prime area for health sciences librarianship, and health sciences librarians are aware of the need to provide public health information. Promoting literacy, in one way or another, has always been a core function of librarians.

One of the goals of consumer health informatics is to help patients make their own informed decisions about health. Consumers are becoming more sophisticated in understanding and actually searching for health information. Consumers who intelligently make health decisions reduce the need for professional attention and have a sense of empowerment.

The Informationist

Some writers have suggested that a hybrid information professional be created who would be an expert in both information processes and clinical medical informatics. This professional would be called an *informationist* (Davidoff and Florence, 2000; Dalrymple, 2002).

The concept is a modernized version of the idea of the clinical librarian, which arose during the 1970s. The basic idea of the clinical librarian was to place health sciences librarians in the clinical setting and "in context" rather than working from an office in the library. According to Groen (2007), perceptions of the usefulness and success of the clinical librarian are mixed. A number of mostly anecdote-based reports and surveys present a positive picture, but others believe that there is a lack of hard data on the actual impact of this service.

In the early days of the clinical librarian, the technology and the traditional view of the library did not promote much end-user searching for information. The link between the literature and the information professional was the health sciences librarian. With the development of new technologies, the growth of online resources, and the creation of user-friendly searching systems, such as NLM's, the environment changed. These events gave rise to the idea of the *informationist*.

Informationists are not just information searchers but are skilled in both information resources management and medical informatics,. They are a hybrid of both information sciences and clinical work. While their primary services include identifying, retrieving, and synthesizing health information, they must also be skilled in the functioning aspects of clinical work and must work well with the healthcare team (Dalrymple, 2002).

The informationist is an information professional who links clinicians and patients, understands information management, and serves as an information enhancer within the clinical event that is occurring. Some informatics professionals see the informationist as a natural intersection of health informatics and health sciences librarianship, providing an opportunity for the two fields to work together for the common goal of information management (Hersh, 2002).

The term *information specialist in context* (ISIC) is sometimes used to describe those who work with health professionals at the point of care or in a research setting. Those who work at the point of care are called *clinical informationists,* and those who work in research are called *research informationists.* In any case, the informationist is not envisioned as a field worker from a library but as someone based in a healthcare setting and considered a member of that setting. The informationist working in evidence-dependent areas will bring the resources of the digital information age into the real world of healthcare and the research environment. The concept of the ISIC is still evolving. "Considerable work in implementing practices that measure up to the ISIC role in all relevant domains remains however, and the community should guard against equating all advanced practices with ISIC work" (Giuse, Sathe, and Jerome, 2006: 68).

A number of issues must still be addressed. "The informationist's value remains to be demonstrated and measured systematically across multiple settings. A research agenda that focuses on information management, information dissemination, information behaviors, and information economics is essential for the concept to reach maturity" (Rankin, Grefsheim, and Canto, 2008: 203).

Health Sciences Librarians and Bioinformatics

It is quite clear that in the coming years those involved in health information management will need to acquire an understanding of genetics, genomics, and genomic medicine and the basic skills to manage this type of information. According to Lyon et al. (2004: 189), "The rapid advances in the area of bioinformatics and molecular biology create opportunities and challenges for librarians, because maintaining the high level of skills and competences necessary to teach access, retrieval, and use of relevant information is becoming more and more complex."

The specific roles of the health sciences librarians and of the library itself in the bioinformatics revolution are still uncertain, although pathways are beginning to emerge. Bioinformatics is a highly specific, complex, and technical area, and librarians who intend to work in bioinformatics need three basic skills: (1) in-depth understanding of bioinformatics, such as the vocabulary and concepts of genomics and genetics; (2) ability to construct and maintain genetics databases; and (3) retrieval skills related to complex molecular biology information requests. Chapter 12 is devoted to bioinformatics.

Education and Training Roles for Health Sciences Librarians

An old (invalid) cliché says, "Those who can, *do it.* Those who can't do it, *teach it.*" Librarians both do it and teach it as a routine part of their daily activities. Health sciences librarians excel in finding information and delivering it to those who need it, and their skills evolved in parallel with the advances in information technology. They have a unique opportunity to be educators in the evolving health informatics world.

In the late 1800s, librarians began providing library instruction to users. By 1900, library instruction focused on how to use the library, and academic institutions expected librarians to teach students how to use the library (Rice-Lively and Racine, 1997). For many years this continued as a part of the function of the reference department. As computers became integrated into the library, the teaching role of librarians expanded to include computer skills, and it has since expanded again to include how to access the greater sphere of information beyond the walls of a library. Clearly, the types of information skills librarians teach have changed. These skills now include how to use new information structures, new application technologies, and the Internet to find health information and how to evaluate the information.

Information technology has greatly influenced and altered the responsibilities of health sciences librarians, including their role as information educators in the healthcare fields, as they scramble to keep up with the increasing changes. In 2004, King and MacDonald surveyed 26 informatics programs to ascertain the involvement of librarians in the curriculum. The results showed that, in general, librarians do not currently play a central role in instruction, but their involvement and skills are becoming more recognized. The authors believe that opportunities are there, if librarians can find a way to be involved. Some examples of where librarians are involved in informatics programs include (1) searching the Internet, (2) evaluating Internet resources, (3) using search engines, (4) introducing evidence-based medicine, and (5) formulating clinical questions based on literature searches (King and MacDonald, 2004: 211). A major achievement of health sciences librarians is their solid involvement in developing modules and teaching the principles of evidence-based medicine.

HEALTH SCIENCES LIBRARIANS AND A RELEVANT RESEARCH AGENDA

Health sciences librarians interact with research efforts in two ways. First, many health information librarians work in research-rich environments, and those engaged in research activities at these institutions place broad informational demands on the library. Second, many librarians conduct their own research in their fields of interest. These two points of contact are discussed in the following sections.

Health Sciences Librarians and Research

Before 1900, research in librarianship was hardly mentioned. In the first half of the twentieth century, two major events occurred that caused a change, albeit a slow one. The first occurred in 1923 when *The Williamson Report* was issued. This was the first examination of education for librarianship to be published. It did not paint of a very good picture of the state of library education, but its negative conclusions began to stir up the field. Concern grew that if the profession hoped to advance, it needed a meaningful research element.

The second event occurred in 1926 when the University of Chicago received an endowment to create a research-oriented graduate library school. This started a movement toward conducting research in librarianship that has impacted the field to this day.

Pure research aims to enhance the theoretical base of a discipline, and applications research tries to solve local and immediate problems. Understanding research within one's profession is a prerequisite to being a real professional in that discipline. A profession is intellectually framed by its theoretical foundation, and research is key to building that theoretical foundation. Albert Einstein maintained that there is no difference between *practice* and *theory*. All practices are based on a theory. For example, we file things alphabetically in our library because we have a *theory* that this is the most practical way to organize information.

All information professionals who support healthcare professionals need skills in both applications research and pure research. Health sciences librarians must understand the stated needs of users and be able to find the information that best meets those needs. Their ability to do this depends on the level of their research skills and insights gained from research.

Although librarians have always supported research activities in other fields, their research into librarianship itself, for the most part, has not been stellar. Librarians as a group have always seen their role as one of service, not research. They were the "doers." However, there has existed since the 1930s a thread of research that is commendable. A small cadre of librarians understood that a true profession must be undergirded with a strong theoretical base built on accumulated knowledge and fine-tuned with basic research.

Early researchers of librarianship adopted methods from education, such as survey research. Libraries seemed to be ripe for asking questions and tallying the answers, but, beginning in the 1960s, there has been a notable switch to experimental and qualitative research methods. According to Eldredge (2004: 83), "Health sciences librarians and informatics were utilizing a wider array of research methods than in the recent past . . . reflecting the expansion of research methodologies beyond the case study, program evaluation, and survey methods." An example of the move toward quantitative research is bibliometrics analysis, which is a method for studying patterns in subject literatures and, by extension, users of those literatures. In general, modern research in library and information science has become much more sophisticated, moving into management, technology applications, user behavior patterns, and other areas.

Like any profession, librarianship has two overall research needs. One is basic, general research that is common to all areas of the profession, and the other is research related to specific application issues and problems. For example, user information-seeking behavior has common traits in a broad sense, but the information-seeking behavior of primary care physicians has its own peculiarities, specific to the more narrow application area. Librarian research needs reflect the specific community of users that the library serves.

The Medical Library Association (MLA) is very supportive of research as a component of the profession. In 2007, the MLA's Board of Directors published *The Research Imperative,* which is a major update of the 1995 research policy report *Using Scientific Evidence to Improve Information Practice.* The 2007 report is a qualitative assessment of the multitude of views about what the MLA's role is in the profession's research efforts. Several key roles were reviewed:

1. Be a *leader* in encouraging health sciences librarians to integrate research into their practice.
2. Be a strong *advocate* of research in the workplace to funding agencies and library schools.
3. Promote *collaboration* efforts among members, institutions, library schools, and other disciplines.
4. Provide s*ervices,* such as mentors to those involved in research.
5. Provide *education* opportunities, including continuing education and training in grant writing.
6. *Publish* reports, news, and updates on research being conducted.
7. Develop a *research agenda* for the profession.
8. *Recognize the successes* of those who conduct research.

The basic conclusion of the report was that MLA must make it clear that health sciences librarians need "to incorporate evidence into their information practice . . . [envisioning] a future in which it is routine for librarians to provide essential research support, including critical appraise, for health practitioners (Grefsheim et al., 2008: 119). In item number 3, "other disciplines" could most certainly be health informatics.

Research Partnerships with Health Informatics

Collaborations between health sciences librarians and health informatics are natural because both sets of professionals deal with the same domain of applications. The health sciences themselves are interdisciplinary, cutting across the spectrum of physical and social sciences, and so are health informatics and health sciences librarianship. The new roles that health sciences librarians have assumed reflect the changes in the way the health professions access information, and this implies that research in health sciences librarianship also needs to reflect these changes. Common areas where health sciences librarians can collaborate with health informaticists are (1) data mining, (2) knowledge management, and (3) vocabulary design and structuring.

Data mining is developing into a viable information management tool, and librarians increasingly use it, especially in the bioinformatics field where molecular biology has combined with computer science to gather, store, analyze, and integrate biological genetic information. These data are stored in very large databases, which now hold enormous amounts of potential information about the very basics of life. To be meaningful, however, the information has to be "mined" from the data. Librarians are equipped by training and experience to develop mining strategies, protocols, and procedures (Schenke, 2005). Data mining is something librarians understand.

In an earlier chapter the concept of *knowledge management* was discussed. This is another area librarians are familiar with. A primary role of librarians is to manage information. It would be easy for them to enter the realm of knowledge management in the health sciences because information management is the basis for knowledge management. Librarians *are* knowledge managers. There are many other areas where collaboration is viable:

INFORMATICS IN ACTION! 5.1

Mysterious Drug Interaction

Location: Pediatric unit in a large private hospital

Problem: A child who is taking several drugs for a critical condition has an adverse reaction. The pediatrician cannot identify which drugs are interacting to cause the problem. She has consulted numerous standard online drug information tools with no success.

People Involved: The pediatrician, attending medical personnel, and the informationist.

Action Taken: The pediatrician called the informationist in the hospital library, Luis, for assistance. Luis did a search of drug interaction sources to be sure that the pediatrician did not miss relevant information. He verified that there was no overt information readily available. His next step was to use data mining procedures to see if the needed information was reported in the literature but missed by the searches conducted. One of the tools he used was the Science Citation Index system. He started with an article on each individual drug involved, looked for reaction discussions, and then gathered sets of papers that cited the individual articles, looking for connections through citations. After following many cold trails, Luis compiled a set of documents that were internally linked by cross citations and associated information. The information needed about this particular unusual case was found.

Takeaway: The informationist remembered that there are alternate routes to finding information, and data mining association techniques are one of those approaches. His professional training prepared him to effectively use a different path to the clinical information needed.

- Medical ontology, nomenclature, and vocabulary systems
- Information management skills
- Information communication standards and protocols
- Information delivery formats and mechanism
- Information technology interfaces
- Utilization of information
- Global health promotion
- Bioinformatics information management
- Economics of information
- Imaging
- Health literacy
- Disaster preparedness and response

Today healthcare is interdisciplinary and multidisciplinary, and it makes sense that the information management sectors of healthcare also be interdisciplinary and multidisciplinary both in methods and procedures and through meaningful collaborations (Dalrymple, 2003). In 2005, Banks et al. published a paper that drew parallels between competencies in public health informatics and competencies in health sciences librarianship. They identified a number of specific skills that the two fields have in common, including the following:

- Analyzing information and applying it to specific situations
- Planning and developing information policies
- Interpreting information for the community
- Identifying information needs in a community
- Identifying and retrieving the best scientific evidence
- Managing finances
- Providing leadership
- Understanding and working with systems

Banks et al. (2005: 345) concluded that "Exciting correspondence exist between many public health informatics competencies and the skills essential to being a successful health science librarian."

Health sciences librarianship has a proud history of service, and the knowledge and skills of health sciences librarians are very relevant to the changing world of healthcare. The challenge is for health science librarians to become an integral part of this changing environment. As Homan and McGowan (2002: 81) said, there is "the need for health sciences librarians to build on the past and reengineer themselves to meet the information-intensive demands of health care for the future." The time and the environment are right for forging partnerships between the health sciences librarians and the health informatics professionals.

SUMMARY

This chapter reviewed how the evolution of health informatics and its applications have impacted and transformed the way healthcare providers work. These developments offer an excellent platform for health sciences librarians to reengineer old and to discover new avenues to truly integrate into the digital health information environment.

REFERENCES

Banks, Marcus A., Keith W. Cogdill, Catherine R. Selden, and Marjorie A. Cahn. 2005. "Complementary Competencies: Public Health and Health Sciences Librarianship." *Journal of the Medical Library Association* 93, no. 3 (July): 338–347.

Bennet, Nancy L., Linda L. Casebeer, Robert Kristofco, and Blanche C. Collins. 2005. "Family Physicians' Information Seeking Behaviors: A Survey Comparison with Other Specialties." *BMC Medical Informatics and Decision Making* 5, no. 9. Available: www.pubmedcentral.nih.gov/articlerender.fcgi?tool=pubmed&pubmedid=15784135 (accessed October 26, 2008).

Case, Donald. 2002. *Looking for Information.* San Diego: Academic Press.

Cummings, Martin M. and Mary E. Corning. 1971. "The Medical Library Assistance Act: An Analysis of the NLM Extramural Program, 1965–1970." *Bulletin of the Medical Library Association* 59, no. 3 (July): 375–391.

Dalrymple, Prudence W. 2002. "The Impact of Medical Informatics on Librarianship." 68th International Federation of Library Associations Council and General Conference. Glasgow, Scotland, August 18–24, 2002..

Dalrymple, Prudence W. 2003. "Improving Health Care Through Information: Research Challenges for Health Sciences Librarians." *Library Trends* 51, no. 2 (Spring): 525–540.

Davidoff, David, and Valerie Florence. 2000. "The Informationist: A New Health Profession?" [editorial]. *Annals of Internal Medicine* 132, no. 12 (June 20): 996–998.

Eldredge, Jonathan D. 2004. "Inventory of Research Methods for Librarianship and Informatics." *Journal of the Medical Library Association* 92, no. 1 (January): 83–90.

Giuse, Nunzia B., Jeffrey T. Huber, Suzanne R. Kafantaris, Dario A. Giuse, M. Dawn Miller, Dwight E. Giles, Randolph A. Miller, and William W. Stead. 1997. "Preparing Librarians to Meet the Challenges of Today's Health Care Environment." *Journal of the American Medical Informatics Association* 4, no. 1 (January–February): 57–87.

Giuse, Nunzia B., Nila Sathe, and Rebecca Jerome. "Envisioning the Information Specialist in Context (ISIC): A Multi-Center Study to Articulate Roles and Training Models." Chicago: Medical Library Association (2006). Available: www.mlanet.org/members/pdf/isic_final_report_feb06.pdf (accessed November 3, 2008).

Grefsheim, Suzanne F., Jocelyn A. Rankin, Gerald J. Perry, and K. Ann McKibbon. 2008. "Affirming Our Commitment to Research: The Medical Library Association's Research Policy Statement: The Process and Finding." *Journal of the Medical Library Association* 96, no. 2 (April): 114–120.

Groen, Frances. 2007. *Access to Medical Knowledge.* Lanhan, MD: Scarecrow Press.

Hersh, William R. 2002. "Medical Informatics Education: An Alternative Pathway for Training Informationists." *Journal of the Medical Library Association* 90, no. 1 (January): 76–79.

Hersh, William R. 2006. "Who Are the Informaticians? What We Know and Should Know." *Journal of the American Medical Informatics Association* 13, no. 2 (March–April): 166–170.

Homan, Michael J., and Julie J. McGowan. 2002. "The Medical Library Association: Promoting New Roles for Health Information Professionals." *Journal of the Medical Library Association* 90, no. 1 (January): 80–85.

Howse, David, Paul J. Bracke, and Samuel M. Keim. 2006. "Technology Mediator: A New Role for the Reference Librarian?" *Biomedical Digital Libraries* 3, no. 10. Available: www.pubmedcentral.nih.gov/picrender.fcgi?artid=1618854&blobtype= pdf (accessed October 26, 2008).

King, Samuel Bishop and Kate MacDonald. 2004. "Metropolis Redux: The Unique Importance of Library Skills in Informatics." *Journal of the Medical Library Association* 92, no. 2 (April): 209–217.

Lyon, Jennifer, Nuncia B. Giuse, Annette Williams, Taneya Koonce, and Rachel Walden. 2004. "A Model for Training the New Bioinformationist." *Journal of the Medical Library Association* 92, no. 2 (April): 188–195.

McKibbon, K. Ann, Douglas B. Friedman, and Rebecca S. Crowley. 2007. "How Primary Care Physicians' Attitudes Toward Risk and Uncertainty Affect Their Use of Electronic Information Resources." *Journal of the Medical Library Association* 95, no. 2 (April): 138–146.

McKnight, Michelynn. 2005. "Librarians, Informaticists, Informationists, and Other Information Professionals in Biomedicine and the Health Sciences: What Do They Do?" *Journal of Hospital Librarianship* 5, no. 1 (Spring): 13–29.

Medical Library Association. "Librarian's Guide to a JCAHO Accreditation Survey." Chicago: Medical Library Association (July 13, 2007). Available: www.mlanet. org/resources/jcaho.html#Q7 (accessed October 26, 2008).

National Library of Medicine. "Fact Sheet: Opportunities for Training and Education Sponsored by National Library of Medicine." Bethesda, MD: National Library of Medicine (October 10, 2008). Available: www.nlm.nih.gov/pubs/factsheets/ trainedu.html#informatics (accessed October 26, 2008)

National Library of Medicine. "The National Library of Medicine Fact Sheet." Bethesda, MD: National Library of Medicine (January 23, 2007). Available: www.nlm.nih. gov/pubs/factsheets/nlm.html (accessed October 26, 2008).

Perry, Gerald J., Nancy K. Roderer, and Soraya Assar. 2005. "A Current Perspective on Medical Informatics and Health Sciences Librarianship." *Journal of the Medical Library Association* 93, no. 2 (April): 199–205.

Rankin, Jocelyn A., Suzanne F. Grefsheim, and Candace C. Canto. 2008. "The Emerging Informationist Specialty: A Systematic Review of the Literature." *Journal of the Medical Library Association* 96, no. 3 (July): 194–206.

Rice-Lively, Mary Lynn and J. Drew Racine. 1997. "The Role of Academic Librarians in the Era of Information Technology." *The Journal of Academic Librarianship* 23, no. 1 (January): 31–41.

Schenke, Jim. "Librarians, Scientists Enter the 'Data Mine' Together." *News Purdue University.* West Lafayette, IN: Purdue University (May 12, 2005). Available: news.uns.purdue.edu/UNS/html3month/2005/050512.Rein.bioweek.html (accessed November 5, 2008).

Taylor, Paul. 2006. *From Patient Data to Medical Knowledge: The Principles and Practices of Health Informatics.* Malden, MA: BMJ Books.

Williamson, Charles Clarence. 1971. *The Williamson Reports of 1921 and 1923*, including "Training for Library Work" (1921) and "Training for Library Service" (1923). Metuchen, NJ: Scarecrow Press.

Woolf, Steven. H. and Dennis A. Benson. 1989. "The Medical Information Needs of Internists and Pediatricians at an Academic Medical Center." *Bulletin of the Medical Library Association* 77, no. 4 (October): 372.

Part II

Mastering Health Informatics

Chapter 6

The Organization of Medical Knowledge

Medical knowledge is a complex, multidisciplinary accumulation of data, information, and cultural records that have built up over many hundreds of years. Because of its expansiveness and sheer size, plus the complexity of the health enterprise, organizing and structuring this knowledge into forms that are easily accessible and applicable is a formidable task. This chapter introduces the basic concepts related to the organization of medical knowledge.

ORGANIZATION OF KNOWLEDGE

Human societies depend on the collective memories of what has been discovered, thought about, used, and preserved, but to be useful these memories must be organized. It is not enough just to have huge amounts of data, information, and a collection of the knowledge and wisdom of the human race; it is necessary to have this knowledge structured in a way that allows immediate retrieval of the exact information needed at the right time, at the right place, and in an economically viable manner.

Almost everyone organizing information everyday—personal finances, to-do lists, groceries in the pantry. On a higher level, businesses have inventory and accounting systems, computer centers have computer programs and databases, and football coaches put together scouting reports. No aspect of life escapes the task of organizing information. Of course, some people do it better than others.

For the information professional, the task is made more difficult by the vast differences among users and their information needs. Information professionals are not organizing information for themselves but for a multitude of *intended users* who depend on them. Describing the content of information records and determining how this content fits into human-designed knowledge templates is a subjective act, guided by understanding and experience. Librarians and others have done this with bibliographic control tools, such as classification systems, subject heading lists, and indexing. This chapter discusses the very complex and challenging task of organizing information and knowledge in healthcare.

KNOWLEDGE MANAGEMENT AND HEALTH INFORMATION

Healthcare can be grouped into three broad, interrelated categories: (1) the basic sciences, (2), the practice of medicine, and (3) healthcare delivery systems. Healthcare draws from the basic sciences, including biology, chemistry, and physics as well as the interdisciplinary branches of these sciences. The practice of medicine involves the art of combining this scientific knowledge with intuition and judgment to treat patients. Practitioners elicit input from other experts, such as laboratory chemists and technology professionals. Healthcare delivery involves the large-scale management of a myriad of systems and related workers. When all of these aspects are taken into consideration, it can be said that medical knowledge encompasses an enormous domain. Managing this domain of information and knowledge is a challenge.

Knowledge management has been discussed a lot in recent years. Knowledge management evolved out of the traditional idea of information management and from artificial intelligence work with expert systems. Knowledge, as a concept, is on a continuum from data to information to knowledge to wisdom. Data reflect single physical events that happen at concrete points in time. Information is a synthesis of data within a construct of meaning. Knowledge is a subjective concept, representing an interpretation of information, and usually implies a dynamic change in the structure of understanding. Wisdom guides decision making based on the other elements in the continuum. None of this is simply a collection of items. All the parts add up to a sum with its own synergy. Health information and health informatics are about the sum of the parts, which makes the tools of knowledge management central to the activities of health informatics.

Note that databases and knowledge bases are not the same thing. A database contains only facts in the form of numerics, text, or images. A knowledge base incorporates facts and rules for manipulating and integrating new input with stored information to create new knowledge.

The premise of knowledge management is that society does not survive solely on data and information but on the skills and *knowledge* of people applying information to the activities of life. Having information is not the same thing as having knowledge. It is not enough just to store and manipulate data and information; it is the knowledge gleaned from information that is the vital key. Knowledge management structures specific knowledge assets in an organization and develops channels through which this knowledge is made available to personnel in the organization.

Also, a knowledge management system is more than just a historical documentation of events; there is much more to knowledge management than just collecting more data into expanding databases. A true knowledge base contains interpretive experiences of decisions and outcomes, including successes and errors, thus enabling retrospective consultations with experts via the databases in the system. A knowledge base captures the experience and wisdom of the past and integrates it into the current situation. The premise is that because medical decision making includes the recall of similar past situations, knowledge management presents an organized and structured way to do this.

Knowledge management is usually thought of as a support function within an operation. Examples in healthcare could be all the files, procedure manuals, event documentation, financial records, and human resources in a clinic, a hospital, a lab, an imaging center, a research facility, a pharmaceutical company, and any number of other situations. Physically, the knowledge management system might be in a library, in a standalone PC in a physician's office, or within an integrated computer system in a medical center. The major challenges to maintaining a viable knowledge management system are (1) keeping the knowledge up to date and correct, (2) providing knowledge in the right locations, (3) applying knowledge of the most suitable types, and (4) providing knowledge at the time when it is needed (Montani and Bellazzi, 2002).

Health sciences librarians have been leaders in developing and implementing traditional information retrieval systems for many decades, and this continues to be a major facet of their work. These skills remain very relevant to developing knowledge management systems. However, the concept of knowledge management involves more than information storage and retrieval in the traditional sense.

Knowledge system management is about the design of systems that cover the full range of human knowledge and the information sources that feed that vast knowledge base, including the system architecture, taxonomy of language, and content organization and structure. The design of all information/knowledge systems begins with systematic, purposeful organization, tailored to fit the knowledge needs of focused groups of personnel and the specific needs of the members of the group. The following sections in this chapter elaborate on the organization of medical knowledge, including current and potential contributions of health sciences librarians.

MEDICAL TERMINOLOGY

Medical terminology is a critical issue in the health sciences, and it is a major area of interest for healthcare informatics. It has been said that medical terminology is as important to the health sciences as quantitative measuring tools are to the basic sciences (Chute and Cohn, 1998). Approximately 80 percent of clinical records and healthcare communication consist of natural language text (Lincoln and Essin, 2003). Much of this uses a diversity of vocabulary, which changes its meaning as science and technology advance. Managing terminology has always been a concern of both healthcare professionals and health sciences librarians.

First, recorded and transferred information about patients must accurately describe the clinical situation, and it must be clearly understood by all personnel who review the information at a later time or at a different location. In addition, extensive reports are created for regulatory agencies, professional organizations, research funders, accreditation organizations, public health data centers, and many others, and these recipients also must correctly understand the information. Of course, there are always legal issues, and when there is litigation it is necessary that all the parties involved understand the information provided.

Computer informationists expend much effort and resources on standardizing terminology and data formatting, as do information professionals in general, including professional associations, government, and private industry. Within healthcare, numerous national and international agencies and organizations address the issues of standardization and terminology.

Controlling medical terminology has always been important, but it has become even more critical in the electronic information age. Consistent, comprehensive terminology is needed in order to integrate patient information with information technologies. The goal is to maximize speed and accuracy of communication while maintaining the quality and reliability of the data. Clearly, information technology is a powerful tool for doing this. Computers are making the control of health information dynamic and effective, but computers must have information explicitly tagged, with a minimum of ambiguity. In many ways, natural language and computers are incompatible, making it imperative to create a language that both the computer and its human operators understand. Refining medical terminology is a major activity in healthcare and in healthcare informatics.

DEFINITIONS

In medical terminology, a number of concepts are related, but each has its own important meaning. In this section we highlight some of the distinctions.

First, there are *ontologies*. "Ontology [is] a theory of *what exists*, a theory of the kinds and structures of objects, properties, events, processes and relations in every area of reality" (Werner, Smith, Flanangan, 2003: 4). Ontologies present models of what is known in a domain of knowledge, for example, medicine.

Classification is the process of bringing things together on the basis of similarities and differences. It systematically groups and categorizes objects and abstract concepts based on the strength of their similarities and relationships.

While ontologies are concerned with the organization of knowledge, *nomenclatures* and *terminologies* are concerned with the naming problems in a domain of knowledge. *Nomenclature* is a set or system of names or terms used to describe the entities in some domain of knowledge or profession. It is usually implied that the domain being described has been organized and classified, so the nomenclature simply gives names to the aspects of the domain. *Terminologies* usually show more interrelationships.

Whereas nomenclatures are just lists of terms, *vocabularies* are a controlled set of language labels or terms connected to a concept in the domain of knowledge being considered (Bodenreider, 2001). *Coding* is shorthand for representing concepts. It transforms verbal language into a numeric or alphanumeric symbol to represent the concept. *Registries* are databases with data, records, laboratory samples, and so forth, which are kept and made available for research and other healthcare purposes.

MEDICAL ONTOLOGIES

The concept of an ontology, since Classical times, is that it describes reality as it *really is*, not as what one thinks things are from what he or she sees and believes to be true. For centuries the term ontology was a "reality" term, discussed only by philosophers. Today, however, the term is being applied to language processing with computers.

Ontologies are a form of knowledge representation. They define classes and their interrelations and are used to organize information according to the accepted theories in a domain of knowledge. A *medical ontology* attempts to describe the knowledge in the domain of medicine. It attempts to put physical objects and abstract ideas in healthcare into classes and to model logical relationships. Medical ontologies "are being built to perform a job of sharing what we understand about the world of biomedicine" (Bodenreider and Stevens, 2006: 257).

For centuries the healthcare community has recognized the needs for creating knowledge representations, modeling the knowledge domain of healthcare, and developing explicit terminology. Ontologies show structured relationships and the meanings of those relationships. Ontologies facilitate communication among the practitioners within a domain of knowledge. Medical ontologies exist in many forms and have a variety of functions. In the past few years ontologies, for example, Gene Ontology and Microarray Gene Expression Data (MGED) Ontology, have become very important in bioinformatics and molecular biology. The standardization that ontologies bring to a subject domain "facilitates the exchange of information and contributes to semantic interoperability among systems" (Bodenreider, 2008: 68). The next section discusses some of the major medical ontologies.

MEDICAL CLASSIFICATION AND CODING

Classification and coding are the related processes for recording medical information and making the information interoperable between diverse groups of humans and computers, perhaps at different places and points in time. Classification and coding are part of ontology but only implicitly show the logic among objects. Ontology shows both relationships and logic. Medical classification standardizes terminologies and is necessary for effectively and efficiently sharing information, and coding is a mechanism for efficiently transferring that information. Together, classification systems and their codes promote semantic interoperability by preserving meaning and thus enable the understanding, comparison, and integration of data.

Although classification and coding in the medical sciences follow the general principles of information organization, medical classification systems are complex and discipline focused. This is because the medical field is complex and diverse and has a terminology that is equally complex and inconsistent. A common understanding of concepts is necessary if healthcare professionals are going to send and receive understandable information. The purpose of classification and coding is to promote this understanding.

Medical classification together with coding allows the converting of diseases, diagnoses, and healthcare procedures into a convenient, transportable, representative numeric or alphanumeric language. The objective is to have a commonly understood mechanism for exchanging medical information across a diversity of healthcare operations and personnel.

The major challenge to classification efforts has always been to keep the system current with advancing research and the evolution of concepts and terminology. The vocabulary of medicine is nonstatic; therefore, concepts and terms evolve rapidly. A good example is the developments in molecular biological research. In 2006, the U.S. Department of Health and Human Resources (2006: 11) stated, "Ultimately, we may see developed a classification of disease based on molecular characterization rather than traditional empirical and organ classification systems. Such a molecular taxonomy could provide the basis for earlier detection and more effective and less costly treatment." Clearly, medical classification must be flexible and responsive to changing states of knowledge.

Once ontologies, classifications, and vocabularies are established, coding is used to represent verbal, textual, and image naming to numeric or alphanumeric designations. The designations are formal and standardized representations of the natural language concepts of the terminologies. Because the codes are standardized by consensus, they enhance the communication process and reduce the possibilities of misunderstanding. Modern healthcare relies heavily on the exchange of experiences among many individuals. Effectively and efficiently communicating this information depends on standardized ways to code and transfer information. Coding has become especially critical in this age of digital storage and transmission of information, because it allows computers to transfer information in the most effective and standardized way.

The language of healthcare is dynamic, diverse, and often inconsistent, which confounds those who struggle to standardize terminology for computer manipulation and transfer. Coding aims for consistent recording and transferring of healthcare information.

Four general categories of codes are recognized: *Diagnostic codes* represent diseases, including symptoms, medical indications, and morbidity and mortality data. *Procedure codes* record specific health interventions taken by healthcare providers. *Pharmaceutical codes* uniquely identify medications. *Topographical codes* indicate specific locations in the body. Codes are key to (1) analysis of diseases and therapeutic actions, (2) health payer reimbursement information, (3) decision-support systems, (4) surveillance and analysis of epidemic and/or pandemic outbreaks, and (5) medical literature knowledge management systems.

Over the years many medical classification and coding systems have been developed, often overlapping, varying in coverage and completeness, and slow to be accepted. Such systems range from administrative to highly specialized subareas of healthcare. The following few examples illustrate the general nature of these systems.

- International Statistical Classification of Diseases and Related Health Problems (ICD-10). Available: www.who.int/classifications/apps/icd/icd 10online (accessed October 27, 2008). The ICD-10, published by the World Health Organization, is widely used for mortality statistics, reimbursement systems, and automated decision support. Its purpose is to support and promote international comparability of this statistical information. Over the years the ICD has become a major international standard diagnostic classification, used for all general epidemiological classifications and for many health management purposes. The ICD is in its tenth edition, and ICD-11 is planned for 2011. The tenth edition is available online.
- International Classification of Functioning, Disability and Health (ICF). Available: www.cdc.gov/nchs/about/otheract/icd9/icfhome.htm (accessed October 27, 2008). The first edition of the ICF was produced by the World Health Organization in 1980 and was called the *International Classification of Impairments, Disabilities, and Handicaps* (ICIDH). Its purpose is to provide a unifying framework for classifying the consequences of diseases.
- International Classification of Nursing Practice (ICNP). Available: www.icn.ch/matters_ICNP.htm (accessed October 27, 2008). According to the Web site, "The International Classification for Nursing Practice (ICNP®) is a unified nursing language system. ICNP® is a compositional terminology for nursing practice that facilitates cross-mapping of local terms and existing terminologies."
- Healthcare Common Procedure Coding System (HCPCS) Level II. Available: www.cms.hhs.gov/MedHCPCSGenInfo (accessed October 27, 2008). According to the Web site: "Level II of the HCPCS is a standardized coding system that is used primarily to identify products, supplies,

and services . . . such as ambulance services and durable medical equipment, prosthetics, orthotics, and supplies (DMEPOS) when used outside a physician's office."

- Diagnostic and Statistical Manual of Mental Disorders, Fourth Edition (DSM-IV). Available: allpsych.com/disorders/dsm.html (accessed October 27, 2008). According to the Web site, DSM-IV "covers all mental health disorders for both children and adults. It also lists known causes of these disorders, statistics in terms of gender, age at onset, and prognosis as well as some research concerning the optimal treatment approaches."
- Current Dental Terminology (CDT). Available: www.ada.org/ada/prod/catalog/cdt/index.asp (accessed October 27, 2008). The CDT, published by the American Dental Association, includes dental procedure codes, a tooth numbering system, and other components. Its purpose is to promote a standardized coding system to document and communicate dental information related to treatment procedures and services.
- National Drug Codes (NDC). Available: www.fda.gov/cder/ndc (accessed October 27, 2008). The 1972 Drug Listing Act requires that drug manufactures provide the Food and Drug Administration a current list of all drugs manufactured and distributed. The NDC is a universal product identifier for human drugs, as required by this law.
- Current Procedural Terminology (CPT). Available: www.ama-assn.org/ama/pub/category/3113.html (accessed October 27, 2008). The CPT, created by the American Medical Association, is a list of uniform descriptive terms and accompanying identifying codes for reporting medical services and procedures, including medical, surgical, and diagnostic services. CPT is based on widely accepted medical terminology.
- Systematized Nomenclature of Medicine—Clinical Terms® (SNOMED CT®). Available: www.nlm.nih.gov/research/umls/Snomed/snomed_main.html (accessed October 27, 2008). SNOMED CT is a terminology set designed for use in U.S. federal government systems for the electronic exchange of clinical health information. SNOMED CT provides content for clinical documentation and reporting. It strives to be a universal terminology for healthcare, wherever it is needed. The current terminology has more than 350,000 entities, 950,000 terms, and 1.4 million semantic relationships (Hardiker et al., 2006: 320).

REGISTRIES

A different type of medical classification and coding system is the registry. A medical registry is a systematic collection of health and demographic data about patients with specific health characteristics. Registries describe the statistical occurrences and related factors of health events. They are used to determine the incidences of specific diseases, the magnitude of the problems the diseases cause, and trends over time and to identify groups at high risk. Registries began as a method for public health officials to monitor trends in infectious diseases but evolved into, among other uses, tools for following outcomes after disease prevention and treatment programs.

The government (all levels), universities, hospitals and groups of hospitals, nonprofit organizations, and private groups all create registries. There are many hundreds of registries related to healthcare. Perhaps the most common ones are disease registries, but there are a number of other types, such procedural registries, which contain information about patients undergoing a specific medical procedure. Some registries document families with a high tendency for a particular inherited disease. Specific registries include the following:

- Breast and Colon Cancer Family Registries. Available: epi.grants.cancer.gov/CFR/about_breast.html (accessed October 27, 2008). These registries have a comprehensive research infrastructure aimed at assisting collaborative, interdisciplinary research protocols in the genetic epidemiology of cancer. They allow the identity, characterization, and follow-up study of individuals and their family members, spanning the spectrum of cancer risk. The registries are also used to identify genetically susceptible populations that could benefit from enrollment in preventive and therapeutic interventions and help develop an adaptive and evolving informatics model to support ongoing and future research consortia.
- The National Exposure Registry (NER). Available: www.atsdr.cdc.gov/NER/ (accessed October 27, 2008). NER lists persons exposed to hazardous substances. It contains subregistries for specific substances. There are currently four active subregistries—trichloroethylene, trichloroethane, benzene, and dioxin. An important purpose of the NER is to help scientists understand how long-term exposure to hazardous substances affects human health.
- The United States Eye Injury Registry. Available: www.filemaker.com/solutions/customers/stories/41.html (accessed October 27, 2008). This registry collects and documents information on serious eye injuries, particularly, how they occur and how they are treated.
- Immunization Information Systems (IIS). Available: www.cdc.gov/vaccines/programs/iis/default.htm (accessed October 27, 2008). This registry system consolidates immunization information from around the country into one source. In the mobile U.S. society, this registry helps increase the efficiency of accessing immunization records, thus ensuring that children get only the vaccines they need.

- Surveillance, Epidemiology, and End Results (SEER). Available: www. seer.cancer.gov/about/ (accessed October 27, 2008). SEER is a comprehensive set of registries from the National Cancer Institute, focusing on cancer incidence and survival in the United States.

Without doubt, registries contribute substantially to the healthcare endeavor. Slowly, but steadily, healthcare providers are using computer-based systems for documenting clinical encounters and related activities. Computer-based management systems have become an essential part of healthcare facilities. As these systems become ubiquitous, it is critical that efficient and effective knowledge structures be developed and utilized.

In summary, medical terminology is complex. It has always been a challenge to healthcare and is constantly under discussion and revision. The usefulness of a vocabulary depends on how well it meets its intended purpose, on the methods used to update new knowledge and word meanings, and on the ability to change the structure to incorporate new developments. Maintaining a useable vocabulary "is not a trivial undertaking, and there is not a single vocabulary that is accepted as a universal standard for the representation of clinical concepts" (Feng, 2008: 36).

THE MEDICAL LITERATURE

There are three general kinds of medical knowledge: (1) the personal knowledge and skills of the healthcare provider; (2) the operative knowledge collected during daily practice from patient records, laboratory tests, and other immediate events; and (3) the knowledge recorded in the medical literature. Quality healthcare depends on the integration of these three types of knowledge into the daily processes of healthcare. This section focuses on the medical literature.

A subject is defined by its literature. Subject disciplines, such as healthcare in general and its subareas and specialties in particular, generate their own related bodies of literature that represent states of knowledge at a specific point in time. Subject areas overlap and change and therefore are not absolute. The evolutions are reflected in the literatures. A literature is composed of all knowledge records related to the subject area, including published and unpublished materials. These records are paper, digital, audio, and visual—any format that contains information related to the subject.

Medical literature has a long and distinguished history, dating back thousands of years BC. Some of the oldest writings relate to health. By the twentieth century the medical literature had become primarily a journal literature of basic research, discoveries, and new methods. Books still formed an important component, but they were generally textbooks, reference works, or highly specialized monographs. Essentially, the twentieth century was "the century of the medical journal and the proliferation and variety of these publications has been remarkable" (Beatty, 2003: 1851).

Medical Textbooks and Reference Tools

Textbooks and reference tools contain synthesized knowledge, generally agreed on by mainstream experts as being the state of the field at a particular point in time. Here is where the knowledge and opinions of experts on general and specific topics are synthesized and placed in context. There are numerous such textbooks and reference tools in the health sciences, both general and topic specific, reflecting the wide diversity of the health sciences. Textbooks are secondary information sources, which means that they can be outdated, biased, and have errors; so these sources, as necessary and critical as they are, cannot be used exclusively for sources of information. Current and ongoing research must be consulted, and this is primarily recorded in medical journals.

In the past decade there has been a steady movement to put medical textbooks online. Since 1997, MD Consult (an Elsevier service) has been a leading provider of online medical textbooks. Printed medical textbooks may become obsolete, as the trend toward electronic books continues. Electronic books can be downloaded to a PC or a handheld device, or they can be accessed online from any electronic device connected to the Internet. Electronic books can also be constantly updated online, reducing the problem of obsoleteness.

A few of the well-known and authoritative books available online are the *Merck Manual of Diagnosis and Therapy, Gray's Anatomy of the Human Body, Harrison's Principles of Internal Medicine*, and *Griffith's 5 Minute Clinical Consult*. The list continues to grow.

Medical Journals

In the seventeenth century, the journal was created and rapidly developed into a highly effective information tool. Medical journals have since their creation made up a significant portion of the scientific and scholarly literature; they are a major conduit for reporting research and communicating with members of the health sciences professions.

The first journals primarily contained letters and proceedings of professional societies and were distributed to members of the society. Research and professional activities grew so rapidly that this purpose was soon too limited. Journals evolved into collections of approved papers and research reports.

Medical journals provide more than just the latest research. Journals "provide a fascinating potpourri of opinion, philosophy, arguments, gossip, history, theory, and advice" (Gehlback, 2002: 3). They contain suggestions for running a practice, retirement plan opportunities, employment notices, book reviews, professional meetings, and a host of other things. Journals are a means to make social connections, which play an important role in the activities of professionals. Now a lot of these connections are being made via the Internet.

In the past several decades, journals have moved steadily to online status. Hundreds of full-text medical journals can be accessed via the Internet with such searching systems as PubMed Central.

Trends and Prognosis for Medical Journals

The scholarly medical journal has for centuries been the premier medium for the dissemination of research results. Both clinicians and researchers rely on journals for up-to-date information on developments in medical research and applications. However, there are indications that the twentieth-first century is bringing major changes to the concept and role of the medical journal in terms of the publication and distribution process. The accessibility of the new electronic resources and the extraordinarily high cost of manufacturing printed journals have brought a paradigm shift in scholarly journal publishing, namely, the move to computers, the Internet, networking, and open access.

For a century or more, the goal of scholarly and research libraries, including health sciences libraries, was to acquire a large, definitive journal collection, preferably with unbroken, complete sets of paper copies of individual titles. This was always a challenge, but it became a serious problem when the price of journals started to rise, eventually at four times the consumer price index rate of inflation (Groen, 2007). The goal of maintaining extensive sets of journals became daunting and eventually unrealistic.

By the late 1990s it was clear that a new paradigm was needed. According to Groen (2007: 106), "Simply put, librarians want to provide everything to everyone, scientists would like to be right, and publishers want to make money." Many libraries attempted to handle the problem by tightening management controls in terms of selection criteria and acquisition budget allocations, but "by the end of the decade [1990s] a full-blown crises existed" (Groen, 2007: 167).

A partial solution came with the digitalization of scholarly and scientific journals and the development and rapid expansion of the Internet. The digital age opened new commercial opportunities for the publishers and some financial relief to libraries when publishers began to offer packaged and bundled journals sets on CD-ROM. These sets came with licensing agreements, and librarians had to adjust to the idea of licensing rather than purchasing information. Clearly, digitalized journals had advantages, but there were also downsides. If the licensing was discontinued, then the libraries no longer had access to archived materials, unlike the traditional model of owning forever what was purchased. Also, in general, the libraries could no longer select individual titles; rather, they had to accept whatever journals came with individual packages, including titles that the library had limited or no use for. Also, the costs began to grow again. When the Internet came into full bloom, publishers shifted their packages to the Internet, but still with the same licensing model. The debate about how best to provide and to access medical journals continues, especially with the rising concept of e-journals and open access.

E-JOURNALS

As the Internet developed, it quickly became an avenue for providing full-text electronic journals (e-journals), often free to the user. One early e-journal was *Online Journal of Current Clinical Trials*, a joint venture between Online Computer Library Center and the American Association for the Advancement of Science. Another early e-journal was *Journal of Biological Chemistry* (Wineburgh-Freed, 2007).

There is no universally accepted definition of the term *e-journal*, but the most common one, and the one we use in this book, is that an e-journal is a digital artifact that exists only in cyberspace. In general, e-journal are formatted similar to printed journals, and the content is structured the same.

Curran (2002) points out a number of advantages to medical e-journals, such as rapid turnaround from manuscript to publication, reduced cost, and multimedia linking from the paper to external resources. A paper can be available the day after it is written, with few intermediate steps. This not only speeds up the process but also eliminates expensive in-between steps, thereby reducing the costs for all concerned—author, publisher, and consumer. The capability to link the papers to other resources, including other text documents, X-ray scans and other images, audio, and videos, makes the e-journal a powerful tool. A physician reading the paper can immediately find corollary materials and link to related studies and/or individuals he or she might want to communicate with concerning the topic of interest (Curran, 2002).

There is no doubt that the growth of e-journals (and online versions of printed journals) is transforming scholarly communication. Information in a discipline can be quickly and easily accessed and hyperlinked. Web 2.0 is enhancing these capabilities immensely, offering new platforms for scholarly collaboration around the globe.

There are some suboptimal issues related to e-journals. One is the continuing concern for quality control. e-Journals are being subjected to peer review, as printed journals are, but new forms of reviewing have been developed in addition to the traditional reviewing process. One new form is the iterative reviewing process. A manuscript is posted electronically and is openly critiqued online, resulting in changes and revisions, and then the cycle is repeated. Supposedly, this will produce a refined paper of higher quality. Like all review processes, this method is far from perfect, and the research at this point is unclear on its effectiveness.

An issue of greater concern is the preservation of the "online only" digital artifacts. Traditionally, libraries bought the printed journals and archived them in house for future scholarly research. In the digital age, however, the journals are only licensed and few guarantees are in place to ensure that the digital forms will be available indefinitely. In the case of free-access e-journals, it is often unclear how long the journals will be available. This issue is being addressed by librarians, scholars, publishers, and the information technology industry in hopes of developing models that will effectively archive the best e-journals for future scholars.

OPEN ACCESS

The idea of "open access" is constantly debated by both proponents and opponents. *Open access* is an Internet age concept, meaning free, full-text, unfettered access by any user to digital scientific and scholarly information. Everyone concerned with information—publishers, government, librarians, the business world—are involved in the debate.

A major aspect in accessing the medical literature has always been how to obtain a copy once its existence has been identified. Many health sciences libraries made laudable and successful efforts through journal acquisitions and interlibrary loan cooperatives, but the proliferation and rising costs of journals made this very challenging. In the past ten years, the advent of a scholarly communication crisis—the "loss of access to the scholarly research literature, as the rising cost of journal subscriptions far out-strip institutional library budgets" (University of Connecticut Libraries, 2008)—has been discussed. The steep rise in prices was caused partly by inflation and partly by commercial publishing conglomerates maximizing their profit margins through domination of the scholarly communication infrastructure.

More and more, the Internet is providing access to full texts, often for free. A few years ago, very few medical journals were available free on the Internet, but user frustrations with rising costs and access barriers helped fuel the movement for open access. Since the late 1990s, the Internet has strongly impacted scholarly communication by enabling "large-scale, barrier-free access to research and scholarly writings, without necessity of utilizing commercial publishers. The Internet has enabled scholars . . . to communicate worldwide the fruits of their intellectual work" (Bergman, 2006: 108).

Publishers are the major critics of open access. They maintain that a pay-for-access model is necessary for them to stay in business, and with the peer review system they use, they are the best gatekeepers for quality. Some scholars and others also want to protect the peer review process for quality control. Proponents of open access maintain that inappropriate or poor-quality items get published all the time, with or without peer reviews. They also point out the user editing, which is implied in open access, serves, over time, as a quality adjustor.

In 1997, the National Library of Medicine enhanced the movement to open access by making MEDLINE available through PubMed, followed by PubMed

Central, In 2005, the National Institutes of Health's (NIH) Public Access Policy furthered the movement by establishing a voluntary policy that authors of peer-reviewed publications resulting from NIH-funded research provide manuscripts to PubMed Central. In 2008, the policy became a statutory requirement (U.S. Department of Health and Human Services, 2008a). Of course, some publishers and vendors have protested the policy, anticipating that it will cut into their profits.

The attitudes, uses, and economic impact of open access journals are the subjects of numerous studies. Eysenback (2006) performed a longitudinal bibliometric analysis of a cohort of open access and nonopen access health sciences articles and found that open access articles are three times more likely to be cited than nonopen access articles in the first 10–16 months after publication. "This is clear evidence of the fact that OA [open access] accelerates the speed with which new findings are taken up by peers. It ultimately speeds up the pace of progress and knowledge translation" (Eysenback, 2006: 1).

PubMed, PubMed Central, and BioMed Central

PubMed is a biomedical literature citation database, searchable with the National Library of Medicine's Entrez Retrieval System. Entrez is a text-based search system designed for a number of diverse biomedical databases. Publishers submit citations electronically at or before time of publication. If the provider permits full-text access, then a link is added to PubMed. PubMed also links to other databases searched by Entrez. Some publishers charge for access.

The central component of PubMed is the MEDLINE database. According to the U.S. Department of Health and Human Services (2006), MEDLINE is

> the freely accessible online database of biomedical journal citations and abstracts created by the U.S. National Library of Medicine (NLM®). Approximately 5,000 journals published in the United States and more than 80 other countries have been selected and are currently indexed for MEDLINE. A distinctive feature of MEDLINE is that the records are indexed with NLM's controlled vocabulary, the Medical Subject Headings.

Although fees are charged for some items in PubMed, the use of this open database has increased immensely in the past few years. Clearly, users, both healthcare providers and health consumers, want open access.

PubMed Central (PMC) is a free digital archive of full-text biomedical and life sciences journal articles. It is managed by NIH's National Center for Biotechnology Information (NCBI) in the National Library of Medicine, and publishers participate by submitting their texts to PMC. In 2008, MedlinePlus had almost a billion page views (U.S. National Library of Medicine, 2009). Also, in 2008, the computer systems at the National Library of Medicine answered almost 2 billion inquiries related to biomedical knowledge from around the world. The phenomenal development of globally linked communication infrastructures has created a high level of expectation with regard to accessing biomedical information. "People expect up-to-date, easy, fast, reliable, and affordable access to a wide spectrum of information from scientific data to published literature to health information written for the general public" (Lindberg and Humphries, 2008: 1).

Another open access resource is BioMed Central, a British independent service for open access to peer-reviewed biomedical research. The articles in BioMed Central become part of PubMed Central.

Health sciences librarians are using new approaches to find literature relevant to specific healthcare situations. See Informatics in Action! 6.1.

BIBLIOGRAPHIC CONTROL

Information records need to be preserved (stored in an organized way) if they are to remain useful. The method for such organization is called *bibliographic control*. Bibliographic control is a means for providing intellectual access to knowledge. More specifically, it is a set of processes that effectively organizes a body of literature for storage and retrieval. Traditional methods are descriptive cataloging, subject cataloging, classification, indexing, and abstracting. Although these basic methods are still used, they have been modified and applied

---

INFORMATICS IN ACTION! 6.1

Patient/Consumer Access to Health Records

Location: Large managed care company

Problem: The chief executive officer (CEO) of the company wants a consensus from the literature on best practices for allowing patients full online access to their health records.

People Involved: The CEO of the company and the knowledge manager of the company library.

Action Taken: Geoff, the knowledge manager, conducted a literature search and identified several hundred articles on the topic. From them he compiled a list of advantages and disadvantages, attitudes, costs, legal and ethical issues, problems in security and confidentiality, and other pertinent information. He organized the data into tables, created charts, and wrote a comprehensive report. Although the CEO did not request a synthesis of studies on how patients access and use the information in their health records, Geoff included this information too.

Takeaway: The knowledge manager used his searching expertise to identify a set of documents. He used sound analytical and writing skills to generate a high-quality report. Finally, he recognized that certain nonrequested information would also be useful to the CEO, so he supplied that as well.

to new forms of technology, including digitization, networking, integrated library systems, and the Internet.

Key to successful bibliographic control are cognitively friendly structures and ease of use. Maintaining bibliographic control of the health sciences literature is a formable task because of its size, complexity, and diversity. In the remainder of this chapter, we do not attempt to cover the full range of bibliographic control of the health sciences literature but highlight aspects that are important to health sciences librarians working in the realm of health informatics.

Cataloging and Classification

The purpose of cataloging and classification is to organize information artifacts and make the information in those artifacts easily accessible. Descriptive cataloging describes the artifacts, classification arranges the artifacts according to their similarity, and subject cataloging provides a subject approach to retrieving the artifacts.

Over the centuries, numerous medical classification schemes have been developed, often for specific situations. The two most commonly used in medicine today are the Library of Congress Classification (LCC) system and the National Library of Medicine (NLM) classification system. The NLM system was specifically created for health sciences libraries and is popular for a number of reasons. First, it is the only medical classification system that is updated continuously. Any classification system that is static degenerates rather quickly. In addition, the NLM system was designed to meld with the LCC system.

The basic resources used for subject headings in health science books are the Library of Congress Subject Headings (LCSH) and the NLM's Medical Subject Headings (MeSH). MeSH is the subject index to the NLM classification. It is a very comprehensive tool with which to access clinical and research medicine and is particularly appropriate for medical collections (Womack, 2006). Also, MeSH is used for subject indexing in many medical databases.

Little original cataloging is done in house now; rather bibliographic services such as Online Computer Library Center (OCLC) provide cataloging information online. The NLM and Library of Congress create most of the medically related records cataloged by such services (Womack, 2006).

Subject Vocabularies

The traditional principles of information storage and retrieval are deceptively simple. Information that a user might need is collected. From an established vocabulary of terms that describe information, surrogate terms are assigned to each specific information item. The resulting list of surrogates is arranged into a useable format to create records. The records are stored, and a file of index terms is created to access the records. Users retrieve information by expressing their information need in the same vocabulary that was used to organize the information. The system searches the stored information files (paper or electronic), matches requests with stored records, retrieves the records, and presents the results.

So why is the process "deceptively simple"? Problems arise when deciding what a specific document is about. *Aboutness* is not a trivial concept. A knowledge record (e.g., book, article, document, image) is more complex than its surface content. A record's true "aboutness" is informed by the creator of the item, the intended user, and the expected use. Clear expressions of all these facets depend on the vagaries and complexities of human language, such as varied meanings and cultural differences. Subject representation has always been a basic intellectual problem and probably always will be, although a number of workable methods have been developed. There are ways and means.

Every discipline has its own unique vocabulary. Because the field of healthcare is complex and diverse, its nomenclature is complex and diverse. It is therefore critical that the vocabulary of the healthcare field be organized and controlled.

Vocabulary control systems reduce the variations of ways information may be conveyed. The basic problem of information storage and retrieval has always been semantic. If information is coded is a specific, agreed upon way, then subsequent users will not face ambiguity and confusion. Vocabulary control allows controlled levels of detail, standardized synonymous and homonymous possibilities, spelling, and structures.

The Indexing Function

An index is a device that presents in one place information that is scattered throughout a book, periodical, document, computer file, or Internet site. It provides a starting point for the user to find what he or she is looking for. Successful retrieval of useful medical documents from the literature depends on the quality of the document's information representation in the indexing systems. When documents are poorly represented, the quality of the search results will likewise be poor. The mechanics of an index seem straightforward to most users. They don't think much about an index until it fails.

The necessity of indexes became apparent when the number of periodicals published began to proliferate. At first, indexes to individual titles were adequate. By the nineteenth century, however, scholars needed access to information across the journal literature. The answer was to develop indexes providing broader coverage. In the 1850s, W.F. Poole published an index to the contents of many journals, thus establishing the modern practice of publishing a single index for numerous periodicals.

The function of the index has not changed: they link authors with readers. As we entered the electronic age, however, it became clear that new methods and forms of indexes were needed. There are now thousands of indexes and many types, variations, formats, and ways to organize them, reflecting all the changes in modern information delivery mechanisms.

Medical indexing is a major enterprise. The medical literature comprises topics ranging from the social sciences to all the basic sciences, and new topics are added regularly (e.g., genomic medicine, nanotechnology, and fractal geometry in imaging). A number of types of data are indexed in medicine. One type is clinical information, such as the patient and demographic data that are often accessed by public health agencies for analysis. Another type is textual data, such as patient records, lab reports, discharge summaries, research reports, hospital reports to regulatory agencies, and the general medical literature. A third type is multimedia data, such as images, videos, and podcasts.

All indexes are created according to the same basic principles, but clearly specific subjects have specific characteristics. This is certainly true in medical indexing. One of the goals of medical indexing is to serve multiple groups of users. At one end of the spectrum are the healthcare practitioners, who have a highly technical vocabulary. At the other end is the general public (consumers and patients), who have a normative, vernacular vocabulary. Each group has a distinct vocabulary, and it is often difficult to reconcile the two to create an effective medical index.

The explosive rate at which medical knowledge is discovered creates another challenge to medical indexing—the constant and sometimes urgent need to revise the indexing terminology. Terminology is constantly changing as new discoveries are made, new procedures are created, and new medical technologies becomes operational. Terms that once accurately described an area of healthcare suddenly become obsolete as new subspecialties and subtopics erode the boundaries of that area.

Medical indexes usually have a large number of descriptors, and these descriptors represent a high number of precisely defined concepts. Medical concepts can unfortunately be expressed ambiguously because the terminology is a complex combination of thousands of terms. Because of the complex and sometimes ambiguous nature of medical terminology, controlled vocabulary indexing systems, such as MeSH and the UMLS, are still prominent. The free-text style of indexing medical literature spurred by the Web has not caused the demise of controlled vocabulary. According to McGregor (2002: 345), "Contrary to the feeling that indexing has become obsolete or dysfunctional, disillusionment with the haphazard indexing of Websites and intranets has spurred a renewed interest in controlled vocabulary indexing, both in commercial and research settings."

Since its inception, the NLM has focused on medical literature indexing and over the years has engaged many indexers in the phenomenal task of providing bibliographic access to the ever-expanding medical literature. The NLM supports both creating indexes and researching basic indexing methods, including automatic indexing. A prime example of the latter is the Indexing Initiative. According to the U.S. Department of Health and Human Services (2008a), the objective of the Indexing Initiative is:

to investigate methods whereby automated indexing methods partially or completely substitute for current indexing practices. The project will be considered a success if methods can be designed and implemented that result in retrieval performance that is equal to or better than the retrieval performance of systems based principally on humanly assigned index terms.

The continuing involvement of the NLM in indexing underscores the vital importance that indexing plays in the bibliographic control of the medical literature.

Medical indexing is complex and often costly. It is also intellectually challenging and indispensable to effectively manage healthcare information.

THE UNIFIED MEDICAL LANGUAGE SYSTEM

As mentioned, the NLM has always been at the forefront of medical literature indexing and basic research related to indexing. Its development of the Unified Medical Language Systems (UMLS) is a good example. The primary objective of the UMLS is to map different terminologies across many databases.

The heart of the UMLS is the Metathesaurus, a large database of concepts about biomedical and health-related vocabularies. It is multilingual, linking concepts and showing relationships among the concepts. The Metathesaurus incorporates a wide range of vocabularies, including the following:

- The Systematized Nomenclature of Medicine
- The World Health Organization Adverse Drug Reaction Terminology
- The Classification of Nursing Diagnosis
- The Physician's Current Procedural Terminology
- The Medical Subject Headings

The Semantic Network assigns types to the concepts in the Metathesaurus. The major function of the Semantic Network is to consistently categorize all concepts represented in the Metathesaurus.

The Specialist Lexicon is a general English lexicon of biomedical terms used in the SPECIALIST Natural Language Processing (NLP) System, which is a tool for facilitating natural language processing by helping application developers with lexical variation and text analysis tasks in the biomedical domain. The lexicon entry of each term includes the syntactic, morphologic, and orthographic information needed by the SPECIALIST NLP System. The Specialist Lexicon covers both biomedical words and common words. The Information Sources Map contains information about the scope, location, vocabulary, syntax rules, and access parameters of a wide range of biomedical databases.

The UMLS is a powerful resource for retrieving biomedical information from a variety of resources by linking disparate information systems. It is composed of numerous information formats and types, including the medical and general scientific literature, patient records, public health data banks, and practice guidelines and standards.

SUMMARY

This chapter dealt with the major aspects of organizing healthcare information. Information management, in whatever form it exists, begins with the organization of information. In fact, information organization is the heart of health sciences librarianship, medical information science, and health informatics.

REFERENCES

Beatty, William K. 2003. "Medical Literature." In *Encyclopedia of Library and Information Science* (pp. 818–1829), vol. 6. New York: Marcel Dekker.

Bergman, Sherrie. 2006. "The Scholarly Communication Movement: Highlights and Recent Developments." *Collection Building* 25, no. 4: 108–128.

Bodenreider, Oliver. 2008. "Biomedical Ontologies in Action: Role in Knowledge Management, Data Integration and Decision Support." In *IMIA Yearbook of Medical Informatics* (pp. 67–79). Edmonton, Alberta, Canada: International Medical Informatics Association.

Bodenreider, Olivier. "Medical Ontology Research." A Report to the Board of Scientific Counselors of the Lister Hill National Center for Biomedical Communications. Washington, DC: National Library of Medicine (May 17, 2001). Available: http://mor.nlm.nih.gov/pubs/pdf/2001-MOR-BoSC.pdf (accessed October 27, 2008).

Bodenreider, Olivier and Robert Stevens. 2006. "Bio-ontologies: Current Trends and Future Directions." *Briefings in Bioinformatics* 7, no. 3: 256–274.

Chute, Christopher G. and Simon P. Cohn. 1998. "A Frame Work for Comprehensive Health Terminology Systems in the United States." *Journal of the American Medical Informatics Association* 5, no. 66 (November–December): 503–510.

Cleveland, Donald and Ana D. Cleveland. 2000. *Introduction to Indexing and Abstracting*, 3rd ed. Englewood, CO: Libraries Unlimited.

Curran, Charles. "The Medical Journal Meets the Internet." *First Monday: Peer-Review Journal on the Internet* 7, no. 6 (June 2002): Available: http://firstmonday.org/issues/issue7_6/curran/index.html#c1 (accessed October 29, 2008).

Eysenback, Gunther. "Open-access Journals: An Expert Interview with Gunther Eysenback." Medscape Today (2006). Available: www.medscape.com/viewarticle/523727 (accessed October 27, 2008) [requires free registration].

Feng, David D., ed. 2008. *Biomedical Information Technology*. Boston: Elsevier/Academic Press.

Gehlback, Stephen. 2002. *Interpreting the Medical Literature,* 4th ed. New York: McGraw-Hill.

Groen, Frances. 2007. *Access to Medical Knowledge*. Lanham, MD: Scarecrow Press.

Hardiker, Nicholas R., Anne Casey, Amy Coenen, and Debra Konicek. 2006. "Mutual Enhancement of Diverse Terminologies." In *AMIA 2006 Symposium Proceedings*. Bethesda, MD: American Medical Informatics Association.

Lincoln, Thomas and Daniel Essin. 2003. "Medical Informatics." In *Encyclopedia of Library and Information Science* (pp. 1818–1829), vol. 3. New York: Marcel Dekker.

Lindberg, Donald A.B. and Betsy L. Humphreys. 2008. "Rising Expectations: Access to Biomedical Information." *Yearbook of Medical Informatics* 3, no. 1: 165–172.

McGregor, Bruce. 2002. "Medical Indexing Outside the National Library of Medicine." *Journal of the Medical Library Association* 90, no. 3 (July): 339–341.

Montani, Stefania and Riccardo Bellazzi. 2002. "Supporting Decisions in Medical Applications: The Knowledge Management Perspective." *International Journal of Medical Informatics* 68, nos. 1–3: 79–90.

University of Connecticut Libraries. "What Is the Scholarly Communication Crisis?" In *Mandatory Open Access: Friend or Foe? Coming to Terms with NIH and FRPAA Legislation.* UConn Libraries Spring Forum. Storrs: University of Connecticut (March 2008). Available: http://www.lib.uconn.edu/about/publications/scholarly communication.html#Whatis (accessed October 27, 2008).

U.S. Department of Health and Human Services. National Institutes of Health. National Library of Medicine. "The Indexing Initiative." Bethesda, MD: National Library of Medicine (2008a). Available: http://ii.nlm.nih.gov (accessed October 29, 2008).

U.S. Department of Health and Human Services. National Institutes of Health. National Library of Medicine. "Overview." Bethesda, MD: National Institutes of Health Public Access, National Institutes of Health (October 2008b). Available: http://publicaccess.nih.gov/FAQ.htm#2 (accessed October 24, 2008).

U.S. Department of Health and Human Services. National Institutes of Health. National Library of Medicine. "Fact Sheet: What's the Difference Between MEDLINE® and PubMed®?" Bethesda, MD: National Library of Medicine (December 11, 2006). Available: www.nlm.nih.gov/pubs/factsheets/dif_med_pub.html (accessed October 27, 2008).

U.S. Department of Health and Human Services. National Institutes of Health. National Library of Medicine. 2006. *Charting a Course for the 21st Century: NLM's Long Range Plan 2006–2016.* Bethesda, MD: National Library of Medicine.

U.S. National Library of Medicine. "MedlinePlus Statistics." Bethesda, MD: National Library of Medicine (February 19, 2009). Available: www.nlm.nih.gov/medlineplus/usestatistics.html (accessed March 21, 2009).

Werner, Ceusters, Barry Smith, and Jim Flanangan. "Ontology and Medical Terminology: Why Description Logics Are Not Enough." In: *Towards an Electronic Patient Record* (TEPR 2003). Boston: Medical Records Institute (2003). Available: http://ontology.buffalo.edu/medo/TEPR2003.pdf (accessed October 27, 2008).

Wineburgh-Freed, Maggie. 2007. "Scholarly E-Journal Pricing Models and Open Access Publishing." *Journal of Electronic Resources in Medical Libraries* 4, no. 1–2:15–24.

Womack, Kristina R. 2006. "Conformity for Conformity's Sake? The Choice of a Classification System and a Subject Heading System in Academic Health Sciences Libraries." *Cataloging & Classification Quarterly* 42, no. 1: 93–115.

Chapter 7

Health Information Technology

Information technology has been a driving force in the development of health informatics. This chapter describes the role of information technology in healthcare and discusses the current issues and initiatives in the application of information technology to healthcare.

MANAGING HEALTHCARE INFORMATION WITH TECHNOLOGY

Healthcare has evolved from the traditional model of one patient and one doctor into a team approach, with many individuals involved. Sharing data and information in healthcare services is the *modus operandi* today. The team approach requires the exchange of patient information and the need for many people to discuss the care of the patient. Doctors, patients, family, supporting healthcare providers, laboratory personnel, imaging personnel, and representatives of many organizations, institutions, auxiliary services (such as the pharmaceutical operations), libraries, government agencies, and third party payers may all need access to the patient's information at some level. As a consequence, there is increasing interest in, and use of, information and communication technologies to support health services (Coiera, 2006).

According to the Commission on Systemic Interoperability (U.S. Department of Health and Human Services, 2005: vi), problems in healthcare services are usually instigated by problems in information:

> The problems of healthcare have many causes but they share a single characteristic—they result from a lack of information. Clinicians make mistakes not because they are careless, but most often because they lack information necessary to make better decisions. Critical information may exist somewhere in the system, but healthcare information isn't connected and can't move where it is needed to deliver safer and better care, or to reduce inefficiency and improve effectiveness.

Healthcare providers have turned to information technology to help improve the efficiency, effectiveness, quality, safety, and cost-effectiveness of healthcare delivery. Without doubt, such assistance is needed. According to another government report, there have been "five years of consecutive annual double-digit increases in healthcare costs and increases in the numbers of adverse health events. At the same time, reports have suggested that 50 percent of all healthcare dollars are wasted on inefficient processes" (U.S. Department of Health and Human Services, 2006).

Incorporating information technology into the healthcare enterprise is a major endeavor, effecting changes and costing many millions of dollars. Technologies gather information on patient conditions, aid in diagnosis, maintain patient records, control patient practice and hospital systems, implement sophisticated medical imaging devices, drive robotic surgery, provide care over long distances, search knowledge bases, and so on. No area of healthcare has been untouched by information technology.

A number of obstacles must be overcome. They can be classified as situational barriers (including time and financial concerns), cognitive and/or physical barriers (including users' physical disabilities and insufficient computer skills), liability barriers (including confidentiality concerns), and knowledge and attitudinal barriers. Cutting across all of these categories, however, may be the need for a major structural and ideological reorganization of clinical medicine as it is now practiced in the majority of settings (U.S. Department of Health and Human Services, 2006: 5).

THE EXPECTATIONS OF HEALTH INFORMATION TECHNOLOGY

When implementing new technologies, organizations and individuals will have expectations that are both realistic and unrealistic and, of course, some fears and anxieties as well. This is certainly true in the healthcare industry. The general expectations for health information technology are to increase efficiency, reduce costs, create greater patient safety, ensure high-quality care, promote the sharing of data within and across sites of care and among healthcare providers, and improve business processes in health organizations. Table 7.1 summarizes the diverse benefits of health information technology as reported by the Healthcare Leadership Council in 2004.

Information technology is becoming a powerful tool in all areas of healthcare by aggregating information from a wide spectrum of points. Systems are linking patient information, knowledge-based tools, local and external information resources, and automated decision-making aids. The data are merged into larger healthcare information systems, providing a platform for improved decision making and a better sharing of information at every level. Healthcare managers hope that information technology will improve their organization's operational efficiency and financial health.

Table 7.1 Summary of Cited Health Information Technology Benefits

Clinical	Administrative and Organizational	Financial
Reduced medication and other medical errors	Increased staff productivity	More accurate capture of codes and charges
Fewer and avoided adverse events	Increased access to data	Fewer rejected claims
Better communication between patients and clinicians	Increased job satisfaction	More efficient recruitment of qualified clinicians
Better communication with referring physicians	Enhanced recruitment of qualified nurses and other clinicians	Fewer duplicative tests
More timely and comprehensive infection control processes	Easier and more efficient data collection	Decreased operating costs
Increased time for hands-on patient care	Improved work flow	Reduced storage and transcription costs
Improved patient confidence in care	More efficient data flow to payers	Reduced per claim processing costs
Better information for clinical decisions and treatment options	More accurate, legible, and timely clinical documentation	Reduced supply costs
Fewer inpatient hospitalizations	Better compliance with regulatory requirements	
Reduced practice variation	Significant skill enhancement for nurses	
Improved patient satisfaction	Less redundant data entry	
Decreased patient waiting times	More timely public health reporting	
Better patient compliance with treatment plans	Improved data quality for research and clinical trials	
Streamlined disease and case management	Streamlined administrative processes	
	Improved data capture for use in national quality of care, clinical outcomes, and benchmarking efforts	
	Enhanced physician recruiting via electronic health records (EHRs)	

From: Healthcare Leadership Council (2004: iv). Reprinted with permission.

Expectations must be kept in perspective. Better communication does not fix a fragmented system, and better information does not ensure that the right thing is done. Healthcare still involves people (Chang, 2004).

Healthcare professionals hope that information technology will help reduce medical error by monitoring and recording factors that might cause error. Such monitoring is most transparent to the personnel involved in the healthcare activities. Burstin (2008: 503) stated, "Transparency in performance measurement is an important cultural change in the health care landscape that may serve as an additional driver toward greater use of health IT [information technology] in practice."

Some tools of information technology deliver basic information to healthcare professionals, and others support diagnostic and treatment efforts. The major categories of tools that help collect, manage, use, and share healthcare data are outlined in the rest of this chapter.

NETWORKING WITH TELECOMMUNICATIONS

Networking and telecommunication systems are major advances of the information age. Networking "has replaced the desktop as the dominant focus of information systems" (Lincoln and Essin, 2003: 1820). Connecting information technologies over local and remote networks has tremendously empowered some healthcare services. It allows information sharing and collaboration locally and globally on a scale hardly envisioned 25 years ago.

An information system network is basically an interconnected set of computers. The two types of networking systems of interest to healthcare are the local area network (LAN) and the wide area network (WAN). LANs connect a relatively small geographic area, for example, a set of offices or an academic health sciences center. WANs connect a much larger geographic area and can bring LANs into a larger operation. WANs require a much more complex telecommunication infrastructure.

Networks are either wired or wireless. Direct connections are made with wires or with optical fibers. Wireless connections are made via radio transmission and reception.

Finally, it should be pointed out that technology alone does not solve problems. Humans solve problems using information technology as enabling tools. Many problems with healthcare information technology are not caused by a lack of certain tools. The technology continues to develop at an amazingly rapid rate. Rather, a number of problems stem from a lack in the education of healthcare professionals; other organizational problems stem from not knowing how to take advantage of the technology. The healthcare industry was slow to implement networking technologies until it became obvious that networking is a powerful and ubiquitous tool.

MEDICAL DATABASE MANAGEMENT

Databases are organized files for storing information The heart of any information system is its databases, and information systems function by interacting with databases. These databases may be stored on a local computer or externally at remote sites.

In the past two decades databases of all kinds have proliferated. Databases have been created by universities, private industry, government at all levels, scholarly and professional organizations, and individuals. Data repositories are collections of databases, data tables, images, text, bibliographic databases, and mechanisms that organize, store, and provide access to the data for decision support, knowledge management systems, and data mining. Understanding the nature and functions of databases and the principles of database management is essential for all health information professionals, including computer personnel, health informaticians, and health sciences librarians.

Database data are typically organized into fields, records, and files, starting with fields and building upward into files and finally into databases. The fields, for example, a patient's name or an identification number, are used to access records.

In general, databases are organized either hierarchically or relationally. A hierarchical database looks like a tree, with a repeating parent–child relationship in which a parent can have many children but a child can have only one parent. For example, a personnel file has a name and then branches to address, occupation, and so forth.

A relational database is nonlinear, permitting each record to have multiple parent–child relationships, forming a lattice. This allows more natural relationships to be shown among entities. The data are in a table format, and the cells attached to the main entry branch off into related information. For example, a basic record may have a name, and the accompanying cells may branch off into personal data and professional duties; these branches, in turn, may branch of into other related subcategories. The relational database design is currently the most popular of the two because it is a prime tenet of the evolving Web 2.0.

There are two general approaches to using databases, with numerous nuances to each. The first approach is to look at specific databases as standalone sources of information. A user inputs keywords, which are usually subject terms or document authors or titles. The computer searches through a specific database or a set of related databases and returns results. The second approach is the meta approach in which the software looks at broad sets of database collections and sends the query across multiple databases. A well-known example of this is the Internet. The Internet is a very large set of databases of every form and description.

Database Management Systems

Moving health data and information from their creation points to a storage database is a primary concern of health informatics. Over time, the amount of data becomes voluminous, and sound management of these databases is critical. Numerous users access the databases simultaneously, they all have different information needs, and each one has a different search strategy. Database management systems must accommodate these users effectively and at unpredictable times of peak access.

Database management systems (DBMS) manage databases. DBMSs are concerned with the intellectual principles and practical mechanics of structuring data so that they can be accessed according to established protocols. DBMSs consist of computer programs or sets of programs that structure, store, update, and retrieve information from databases. In fact, databases are also created by DBMSs. These systems range in complexity from ones that run on small PCs all the way up to large mainframe computing systems. Anytime there is an application system, there is a DBMS of some type. For example, ATM machines are run by a DBMS, as are airline reservation systems, health sciences library functions, grocery store inventories, clinic electronic health records, and, of course, the mammoth bibliographic and full-text archives of the medical literature.

Multimedia database management has emerged since the advent of the multimedia revolution. Traditionally, database management dealt with text and numeric data, but now imaging, sound, and other types of media generate data in the health sciences. These data too must be stored and retrieved successfully. Imaging databases are discussed in detail in Chapter 10.

In the healthcare field, some DBMSs are aimed at specific medical applications, and others are general, integrated systems. A number of these systems are discussed through this book. Two examples are the following:

- MySOL. Available: www.mysql.com/why-mysql/isv-oem-corner/healthcare. (accessed November 10, 2008). MySOL is a general DBMS that crosses several areas of healthcare information management and promotes the integration of data, including information related to practice management and EMR/EHR documentation (e.g., demographics, medication lists, and patient allergies). It can also monitor medical equipment, such as cardiac machines, and manage digital imaging systems.
- Medstar. Available: www.medstarsystems.com (accessed November 11, 2008). The Medstar DBMS is an integrated healthcare practice management system for, among other things, handling medical billing, medical records, and digital images.

Biomedical Databases

The literature database is the most widely recognized type of biomedical database, but its use goes well beyond providing access to the published literature. In addition to literature retrieval, they are used for factual retrieval, diagnosis support, organization management, laboratory procedures and data, patient records, education and research, and many other medical situations in which current and accurate information is needed.

Once the Internet became sophisticated enough to handle large databases, medical databases migrated there like an avalanche. "The most important reason for the adoption of Internet technologies within the biomedical community has been the development of publicly available databases containing biological information" (National Academy of Sciences, 2000: 109). Modern Web technology and connectivity make the creation and accessibility of databases a simple matter. For little money and a minimum of effort, a Web page gateway can be created to an existing database. As result, thousands of medical databases are now accessible worldwide. Clinical databases exist for almost every disease and clinical situation encountered in the healthcare world: cancer, cardiovascular disease, congenital anomalies, diabetes, general practice research, infectious diseases, mental health, respiratory disease, surgical procedures, trauma and intensive care, and so on.

Searching the medical literature is a complex and often conflicting endeavor because of the volume and variety of databases, inconsistencies among vocabularies, and varying indexing procedures. Fortunately, online tutorials accompany most individual databases and explain the necessary searching method. An excellent example of a database-focused tutorial is the one at the Health Sciences Library at the University of Buffalo (2007). The National Library of Medicine also has outstanding tutorials on how to use their databases.

THE INTERNET

One of the most powerful information technology tools adapted to healthcare is the Internet. Without doubt, the Internet has had an explosive impact on the way society creates, stores, and communicates information, and this phenomenon brought a major new component to healthcare. A bonanza of information is now available from healthcare providers, governments, professional organizations, academic institutions, pharmaceutical companies, health products manufacturers, and private individuals. Internet users can get the latest news on health, current research, and products for sale; they can participate in blogs and wikis; and they can join support groups and other social networks. In fact, the Internet enables access to all aspects of healthcare, including biomedical research, electronic health records, and healthcare finance and administration. The Internet is changing the entire culture of health information and in many ways is changing the practice of healthcare itself.

Health Consumers and the Internet

The Internet is an accessible health information technology tool for the consumer. The Pew Internet & American Life Project (2006) found that over 70 million Americans have used the Internet to find health related information, and over 100,000 active health information Web sites are known. Four out of five American Internet users have searched for medical information. The 2006

Pew survey showed that the top two categories that consumers search on are information on a specific disease or medical problem and information on a particular treatment or procedure.

As more health information flooded the Internet, the inevitable debates began over the perceived harm and benefits this information could have for patients, particularly as consumers of healthcare services and products. On the positive side is the opportunity for patient empowerment. That is, the informed patient, armed with knowledge, can become an active participant in the healthcare process. Many studies in the past decade have assessed the impact on consumers of having health information accessible on the Internet. Potts and Wyatt (2002: 1) concluded that "Overall, this survey suggests that patients are deriving considerable benefits from using the Internet and that some of the claimed risks seem to have been exaggerated."

Potts and Wyatt also pointed out that increased information can improve patients' understanding of their situation and thus improve their state of mind. In addition, doctors also find the Internet helpful in keeping current with new information.

Of course, health information on the Internet is about more than just diagnosis and treatment of disease. It is also a source for identifying services and a social platform for advice, support, and exchange of information. Clearly, the Internet is enabling patients to manage their own health information, improve their communication with healthcare providers, and thus be actively and intelligently involved in the decision-making process.

INFORMATICS IN ACTION! 7.1

Applying Web 2.0 Technology

Location: Cancer clinic

Problem: A social worker in the clinic wants to start an online cancer patient support group using Web 2.0 technology but does not know where to start. She is concerned that the patients are not familiar with the medical terminology used by their oncologist and other healthcare providers.

People Involved: The social worker and the hospital librarian.

Action Taken: The social worker approached Wanda, the clinic librarian. Wanda began by analyzing and synthesizing the literature to find out how Web 2.0 technology is being used for online support groups. She found that blogs were a popular tool, and she instructed the social worker on how to start a blog, blogging practices, and case studies on the use of blogging tools to assist patients. Wanda prepared a plan of action for the social worker, with the recommendation that the blog have health goal-oriented objectives and operational procedures and be a social network for the patients.

Takeaway: The librarian knew Web 2.0 technology, and she saw the opportunity to assist in the implementation of a new service for cancer patients.

On greatest concern expressed on the negative side of the debate is about the quality of the information put on the Internet. Some healthcare professionals are alarmed about the accuracy and timeliness of the information. Hersh (2003) cites numerous examples of out-dated information on the Internet. For example, hundreds of pages promote unproven treatments for cancer, AIDS, heart disease, arthritis, and many other conditions. He also pointed that, in 1999, four of the eight Web sites he found that enumerated cardiovascular risk predictors provided invalid information. Validity and timeliness are clearly real problems.

Another concern is that nonprofessionals may misunderstand the health information on the Internet or be intentionally misled by fraudulent advertisements and cyberspace quacks pushing updated versions of snake oil and other false remedies. Also, some fear that the Internet is giving rise to widespread do-it-yourself medicine. Even when information is of the highest quality, it can be misunderstood, leading to misdiagnosis and wrong self-treatment.

Whether good or bad, the fact is that people are getting more and more of their health information from the Internet. Over half of the United States population is online, and they are turning in great numbers to the Internet for health-related information (Ball, 2003: 20). There is no doubt that the Internet is a major resource for health information. The reference desk at the library is no longer the primary information portal.

Web-based Healthcare Information Systems

The latest frontier of healthcare information on the Internet is the Web-based healthcare information system. This concept continues to evolve, with seemingly endless new innovations and services offering more options for connectivity and integration of every kind. Any healthcare information system planning must aim to maximize the Internet's existing power and ever-growing potential (Felkey, Fox, and Thrower 2006: 127). Web-enabled healthcare information systems utilize Web browsers in combination with software applications and other information sources to deliver information and provide healthcare. These systems are usually based in a health facility and are connected to the Internet, creating a transparent, integrated system. The advantages of these systems are that disparate subsystems in an organization are integrated, bringing about more efficient and effective communication. This expedites information exchange and operations, reducing effort and duplication and usually lowering costs.

Early applications included the delivery of telemedicine, access to data repositories, and development of shareable electronic medical records. Now fully integrated systems are being put in place, enhancing the potential for lower costs and more global access. The trend seems to indicate that Web-based models will eventually prevail over most traditional models.

MOBILE, WIRELESS, AND WEARABLE TECHNOLOGIES

Mobile, wireless, and wearable technologies are three interrelated yet distinct tools. *Mobile technology* is a broad term, meaning portability. It can be used to support a standalone device, such as a laptop computer, an electrocardiographic machine on a cart, a mobile phone, or a portable credit card reader. *Wireless technology* is just what it says: technology that supports communication, both short and long distance, without using connecting wires. *Wearable technology* supports devices that are worn on the body—attached either to clothing or to the body.

Mobile technology, especially when combined with wireless technology, is primarily used at points of care: doctors' offices, hospital rooms, and patients' workplaces and homes. Point-of-care technology (as in transportable and portable devices and handheld instruments) brings needed information immediately to the healthcare provider and patient situation and increases the potential for patients to receive medical results in a real-time manner.

Wireless technology applications have dramatically and dynamically accelerated in the past few years, and their full potential is still to be reached. Riha (2006) estimates that by 2010, $7 billion will be spent on wireless applications in the United States, including the healthcare industry. The wireless healthcare market passed the $600 million mark in 2007. Riha (2006) further estimates that almost 50 percent of physicians use wireless technology in their practices to access patient data and decision-making tools, track processes and operations, monitor patients, respond to emergency situations, and help reduce errors in patient data gathering and recording.

Mobile, wireless, and wearable technologies are becoming both commonplace and very sophisticated. These devices allow users to go directly to specific data with a minimal amount of clicking through hierarchal menus. They enable healthcare personnel to connect immediately with both local and distant colleagues and other resources, including records, lab results, and the Internet. A particularly valuable application is for immediate communications between emergency medical services crews and the hospitals they transport patients to.

Experiences with the Internet enticed healthcare practitioners to expand their use of computers and eventually to use wireless technology. It seems clear that wireless technology will continue to enhance communication in the healthcare industry for years to come (Chen et al., 2004). Wireless devices are easy to install, provide immediate access to network information, and usually increase productivity and convenience. Some of the most common uses include the following:

- *Capture and code information at point of care,* especially collecting and documenting patient data
- *Quickly enter data into and retrieve data from health records* at the healthcare provider's location

- *Support clinical decisions* immediately at the point of care
- *Order lab tests and receive lab results* at the point of care
- *Maintain electronic pharmacopoeias* (drug information databases) for ordering drugs and researching drug interactions
- *Send patient alert messages* to remind patients about medications, self-administered tests, doctors' appointments, and so forth
- *Access medical literature* via the Internet
- *Support medical education* in the areas of evaluating medical students, tracking the procedural experiences of residents, evaluating teaching interactions, and delivering continuing medical education courses
- *Support research projects*, such as collecting on the spot data

Radio frequency identification (RFID) technology was first applied to business activities. It was used to control manufacturing procedures and inventories as well as dozens of other industrial and business operations and processes. In healthcare, it was first used for inventory control. It was then incorporated into monitoring medical devices and tracking patients (Riha, 2003).

Many healthcare providers attaching personal digital assistants (PDAs), wired and wireless recorders, and a host of other devices to their clothes, like electronic apparel accessories, which provides immediate access to personal notes, phones, paging systems, electronic patient records, the Internet, databases, and other computer-based resources. The full potential of these devices has not yet been reached.

Handheld devices are increasingly being used to obtain online information at the point of care in clinical environments. Recent studies show the effectiveness of this application. Hauser (2007: 815) concluded that "handheld computers with wireless Internet connection are effective platforms for online information delivery to mobile clinicians. Evidence-based practice is encouraged by the quick access to the latest available information, including articles in the primary literature" accessible by MEDLINE.

Another application is *biosignal monitoring*, monitoring of patients over time. In the usual case, a doctor orders tests, takes blood pressure and temperature measurements, and so forth at one point in time and then uses these results to diagnose and treat the patient. Biosignal monitoring allows the repetition of this data gathering process over multiple points in time. This technique is used in cases of uncertainty and when a diagnosis cannot be made until a condition has been evaluated over time. This allows the doctor to see the dynamic properties of the situation. The most obvious example of the use of biosignal monitoring is in intensive care units.

Technological advances have reduced the size and increased the power of the mobile devices, making it easy for healthcare providers and patients to take the technology with them wherever they go and giving rise to a new moniker for this type of technology: *wearable*. Another new term that recently appeared in the healthcare vocabulary is *M-Health.* The general concept of M-Health refers to collecting and managing patient vital signs in ambulatory services via mobile technology. M-Health "is a step beyond electronic health-care as it enhances ubiquitous health provisions regardless of the patient's geo-graphic location" (Angelidis, 2006: 239). Wireless, mobile technologies are a trend of the times, and advances in hardware and in procedures continue. These technologies are becoming common in the delivery of healthcare ser-vices and in patient self-management. The *wired physician* is a major develop-ment on the technology horizon.

ARTIFICIAL INTELLIGENCE IN THE HEALTH SCIENCES

The primary objective of information technology is to aid humans in their in-formation processing activities, and since the beginning this has included sup-port for cognitive processes. As a matter of fact, early computers were referred to as "electronic" or "giant" brains, leading to the coinage of the term *artificial intelligence* (AI), the use of which has persisted.

At the most fundamental level, AI is the attempt to create computer-based technologies that exhibit responses that we recognize as being intelligent. Practi-cal AI applications have long been a dream, but, with a few important excep-tions, the dreams have remained elusive. At present, computers can follow algorithms to fly airplanes, run multitudes of devices, and even tell us exactly where we are with global positioning systems. Computer programs can play chess—learning from mistakes even beating expert human players. These sys-tems make decisions, correct mistakes, and learn from feedback experiences. However, computers are not very good at subtle, subjective human mental ac-tivities such as judgment, intuition, and common sense.

The journey to develop true AI has been over a rough road, wrought with many potholes. The problem is that because we still have a long way to go in understanding how the brain works, and we do not know a lot about what human intelligence really is, we don't know exactly how to make computers act intelligently. Our brain does complex things so easily that we are surprised at the difficulty we have trying to program computers to do the same things.

We don't know if we will fully understand how humans think any time soon, but research is producing very interesting simulations of human thought or par-ticular aspects of it. Furthermore, many experts in the field do believe that there are clear indications that our subjective mental processes are no more than very complex brain neuron computations. Once these patterns are mapped, we can create computer algorithms to mimic these brain computations, and this will mark the true beginning of AI. Even if we never reach such a full understand-ing, we can still create more complex practical applications.

AI has been slow to produce viable applications and to be embraced by the healthcare industry, but progress is being made, and the new healthcare technologies may enhance it more. For example, the procedures of evidence-based medicine are compatible with knowledge base processing techniques in AI.

According to Ramesh (2004), many different AI techniques are already capable of solving a variety of clinical problems. However, despite earlier optimism, medical AI technology has not been embraced with enthusiasm. The possible uses of AI in medicine have been contemplated for at least 35 years. Some of the best known AI applications in medicine have been in these fields:

- Expert systems
- Robotics
- Natural language processing

Expert Systems

An expert is an individual who surpasses competency in a domain of knowledge. Simply put, an expert system mimics the decision-making ability of a human expert. We can also define an expert as a person who has special skills or in-depth knowledge of a subject that most of us don't have. Successful computerized expert systems concentrate on specialized areas, usually in narrowly defined domains of knowledge. An expert system acts like a human expert. Typically, a user opens a dialogue with the computer and describes the problem. After a period of processing, the expert system offers solutions to the problem. The user and the computer go back and forth until the problem is properly structured and hopefully solved.

In medicine, expert systems are generally used in the areas of diagnosis, treatment, planning, and management. They offer a number of advantages. In terms of costs, once operational, an expert system can be run on a computer at far less expense than would be required for a high-priced human expert. Also, an expert system might be thought of as a clone of a human expert, and, as such, productivity can be increased. Computers do not take vacations or call in sick.

Critics of clinical expert systems claim that there is not a lot of evidence that these systems can improve patient care in typical practice settings at an acceptable cost in time and money. According to Goodman and Miller (2006: 381), "humans are still superior to electronic systems in understanding patients and their problems, in efficient collection of pertinent data across the spectrum of clinical practice, in the interpretation and representation of data, and in clinical synthesis. Goodman and Miller (2006: 383) also list criteria for using these systems:

- A computer program should be used in clinical practice only after appropriate evaluation of its efficacy.
- Users of most clinical systems should be health professionals who are qualified to address the question at hand on the basis of their licensure, clinical training, and experience. Software systems should be used to augment or supplement, rather than to replace or supplant, such individuals' decision making.

- All uses of informatics tools, especially in patient care, should be preceded by adequate training and instruction, which should include review of all available forms of previous product evaluations.

Robotics

Robots are built by complex information-driven technology that mimics intelligent behavior in order to carry out physical tasks, and they are becoming a success story in the field of AI. Expectations of AI systems continue to go through cycles, but slowly useful and workable systems are being implemented. Robotics is a case in point, and many workable devices are commercially available.

Robots fascinate us. We marvel when we see factory robots and humans engaged together to do things. Robots are finding their way into healthcare through many avenues, where they perform many routines activities, freeing healthcare personnel to focus on higher level activities. They can be used in contagious areas, make deliveries, assist in basic physical exams, and perform a host of other activities.

In some hospitals, robots chug around, moving patient records from one point to another. They stand in front of a patient, processing information and allowing a doctor who is at another site to interview the patient. Robots also serve as scrub nurses, handing surgical instruments to the surgeons.

One interesting application has been in surgery, where robots can enter the body and do the work, guided by the hands of the surgeon. The machines cut, tie, and do all the surgical procedures without the surgeon actually inserting his hands into the patient's body. For example, kidneys can be removed by a process known as *laparoscopic surgery*. The surgeon makes a number of small incisions about a half-inch long; a miniature video camera is inserted into one of the incisions, and the surgeon can study the images of the internal organs that the camera projects on a video monitor. The surgeon then uses miniaturized instruments inserted through the other incisions to perform the procedures. These instruments are small cameras, cutting and tying devices, and other miniaturized surgical tools attached to thin, flexible cables.

In another variation of laparoscopic surgery, a larger incision is made at the belly button, a miniature vacuum cleaner is inserted, and the vacuum cleaner removes the disconnected kidney once it has been cut loose from a multitude of connected blood vessels, other organs, and tissue. In traditional surgery, the surgeon would have had to cut through three muscle groups and break a few ribs to get to the kidney, and the patient would have to stay in bed for at least six weeks to recover. Robotic surgery is a less invasive procedure, resulting in patients returning to normal life much sooner.

An interesting example of the use of medical robots is the da Vinci surgical robotic surgery system, designed by the University of California—Los Angeles and currently maintained by the Center for Advanced Surgical and Interventional

Technology. The da Vinci system is a human patient simulator, with a laparoscopic surgical simulator and accompanying tools. It is a three-dimensional, high-definition system that integrates endoscopy and state-of-the-art robotic technology. This example shows the fascinating current application and potential of robotics (Center for Advanced Surgical and Interventional Technology, 2007). Robotic informatics is primed to be a major area of health informatics in the years just ahead.

Natural Language Processing

Natural language processing is concerned with the problems and applications of creating computers and software that can understand and process natural human language. Of particular interest are the possibilities of human–computer interactions. Application areas of primary interest to healthcare include information extraction, natural language generation, optical character recognition, data mining, and speech recognition.

A major part of a patient's health record is recorded in free text, and recent advances are requiring these data to be coded. Natural language processing is being tested as a method to extract data from the free text and correctly code it for the electronic medical record. Related to this is information extraction. Natural language processing may be able to search a patient's record and reformat the information into summary format for the busy healthcare provider.

Another area where natural language processing is being applied is abstracting and indexing medical documents and published research papers. This is known as *automatic* indexing, extracting, and abstracting and has a long history in the field of information retrieval. The National Library of Medicine has been one of the leaders in developing these systems.

Speech recognition is another application area of natural language processing of vital interest to the healthcare field, particularly for data input, data playback, and directing a variety of instruments and devices related to healthcare. Data input, information searches, and form filling often can be performed more easily when used with a speech-recognition device.

VIRTUAL REALITY

The development of the information technology called *virtual reality* has opened up new opportunities in healthcare. Virtual reality is the technology that lets a user interact with a computer-simulated situation, which may be an actual situation or one imagined. It draws together many elements of informatics, such as computer hardware and software, robotics, telecommunications systems, imaging, and animation. These elements are combined, enabling individuals to experience three-dimensional visualization, usually with manipulability components and auditory capabilities.

Virtual reality has been used for years in such applications as flight simulation training, but only in the past decade has it become operational in healthcare. Virtual reality was first applied to healthcare in the 1990s when it was used to plan surgery, give preoperative training, and guide imaging during surgery (Arvantis, 2006). It is rapidly being adapted for other purposes, such as virtual endoscopy, telediagnostics, telesurgery, diagnostics, education, and rehabilitation. Numerous virtual reality applications in medical diagnostics have been based on anatomical data sets from the Human Visible Project. In education, students can develop understanding and skills in a simulated realistic situation before dealing with patients. In research, virtual reality technologies offer avenues for experimentation and testing theories.

Major advancements in both basic medical research and in clinical applications have been made in the past 15 years. Informatics tools have become valid tools for education, research, and patient care.

CONNECTIVITY AND INTEROPERABILITY

As the health information infrastructure became more complex and ubiquitous, concerns arose about connectivity and interoperability. Connectivity is concerned with implementing networks to transport healthcare information seamlessly through multiple levels and across widely diverse points of healthcare. Interoperability means making information compatible and accessible where and when it is needed. Despite the prevalence of information technology today, obtaining needed information, when and where it is needed, is still a problem. According to the Commission on Systemic Interoperability (U.S. Department of Health and Human Services, 2005: vi):

> The problems of healthcare have many causes but they share a single characteristic—they result from a lack of information. Clinicians make mistakes not because they are careless, but most often because they lack information necessary to make better decisions. Critical information may exist somewhere in the system, but healthcare information isn't connected and can't move where it is needed to deliver safer and better care, or to reduce inefficiency and improve effectiveness.

To be compatible and interoperable, information must be governed by agreed upon rules as to how it is created and transported among computer systems. This will allow health providers to share health information, such as medical history, lab results, and drug information with each other in a real-time environment. The quality of our healthcare, on both societal and individual levels, is suffering from the lack of a connected system of healthcare information. The cost comes in injury, wasted resources, and lost lives. The problems of the lack of connectivity and interoperability remain, despite the enormous investment in technology. The technology exists and the expertise is available, but it is generally being applied to infinitely less critical concerns such as making travel plans online and checking bank balances at any ATM (U.S. Department of Health and Human Services, 2005: 14). We need to take the steps to make connectivity and interoperability a reality in healthcare.

Connectivity and interoperability are obtained with a combination of technology, standards for transmitting data, and agreement among communication partners on rules and processes. The purpose is to connect users to information, knowledge, and each other. New forces, both political and economic, are pressuring the healthcare industry to improve its delivery structures, and one of the top priorities is to ensure connectivity and interoperability.

Many involved with the problems of connectivity and interoperability envision solutions being achieved with creation of a national health information infrastructure (NHII). Americans spend $1.7 trillion on healthcare every year, $5,670 per capita, leading the world in expenditures, but the general consensus is that the United States lags in information technology infrastructure in healthcare (U.S. Department of Health and Human Services, 2005).

The idea of an NHII began to be discussed at least two decades ago, and in the intervening time the concepts have started to become a reality. Despite the steady progress in the use of information technology, and its obvious potential to strengthen the healthcare system, however, there remain too many instances of problems in getting quality data to healthcare providers. According to Detmer (2003: 1), "When fully implemented, the NHII would also enable automation of routine tasks, simplification of complex tasks, democratization of functions, customization of services, management of the knowledge base, and greater collaboration across the domains of the health sector." Early discussions of an NHII focused on personal health, healthcare delivery, and public health, but in recent years this has expanded to envision it as a platform for aggregating data, information, and knowledge and making them universally accessible for medical decision-making and promoting a robust research effort.

The question naturally arises as to who should lead the development of this infrastructure. As in any other undertaking, it probably should be a combination of both public and private efforts, but the consensus is that the federal government must provide the backbone of the structure by passing laws, setting standards, and creating a communication network. The government should also work with the private sector in developing mechanisms, structures, and policies and in obtaining funding. Without doubt, a robust and sustainable national health information infrastructure is crucial to the future of healthcare in this country, and it is equally important globally.

SUMMARY

This chapter presented a broad overview of health information technology, including its scope and general applications. Healthcare professionals envision a time when its full potential will be realized. Hopefully, says Mike Leavitt, Secretary of the Department of Health and Human Services: "The day is not far off when we can walk into a medical clinic and not be handed a clipboard to enter the same information you've filled out a hundred times" (U.S. Department of Health and Human Services, 2005: 18). Health information technology will make this a reality.

Over time and through new generations of healthcare personnel, health information technology has become ubiquitous. It is rare to find a doctor who does not use information technology in his or her daily activities. Even U.S. presidents (Bill Clinton and George W. Bush) have called for the implementation of electronic medical records, and the U.S. Congress is active in promoting a healthcare information technology infrastructure for the country. It is no longer a matter of accepting the technology. Clearly, health information technology in healthcare is no longer just a promising possibility. It is an integral part of the total enterprise. Both healthcare professionals and the general public now expect information technology to be used in healthcare.

Finally, we note that effective use health information technology requires robust health information management systems. Chapter 9 discusses these systems.

REFERENCES

Angelidis, Pantelis. 2006. "Mobile Telemonitoring Insights." In *Handbook of Research on Informatics in Healthcare and Biomedicine* (pp. 234–239), edited by Athina A. Lazakidou. Hershey, PA: Idea Group Reference.

Arvantis, Theodore N. 2006. "Virtual Realty in Medicine." In *Handbook of Research on Informatics in Healthcare and Biomedicine* (pp. 59-67), edited by Athina A. Lazakidou. Hershey, PA: Idea Group Reference.

Ball, Marion J. 2003. *Consumer Informatics: Applications and Strategies in Cyber Healthcare*. New York: Springer-Verlag.

Burstin, Helen R. 2008. "Achieving the Potential of Health Information Technology." *Journal of General Internal Medicine* 23, no. 4: 502–504.

Center for Advanced Surgical and Interventional Technology. 2007. "What Is CASIT." Los Angeles: UCLA David Geffen School of Medicine. Available: www.casit. ucla.edu (accessed October 29, 2008).

Chang, Sophia. "The Challenge: Chronic Disease Care and the Promise of HIT." In *Health Care Information Technology 2004: Improving Chronic Care in California*. San Francisco: California HealthCare Foundation (November 18, 2004). Available: www.ehcca.com/presentations/cahealthit2/chang.ppt (accessed October 28, 2008).

Chen, Dongquan, Sing-jaw Soong, Gary J. Grimes, and Helmuth F Orthner. 2004. "Wireless Local Area Network in a Prehospital Environment." *BMC Medical Information Decision Making* 4 (August 31): 12.

Coiera, Enrico. 2006. "Communication Systems in Healthcare." Clinical Biochemist Reviews 27, no. 2 (May): 89–98.

Detmer, Don E. 2003. "Building the National Health Information Infrastructure for Personal Health, Health Care Services, Public Health, and Research." BMC Medical Information Decision Making 3 (January 6): 1.

Felkey, Bill B., Brent I. Fox, and Margaret R. Thrower. 2006. *Health Care Informatics: A Skills-based Resource*. Washington, DC: American Pharmacists Association.

Goodman, Kenneth W. and Randolph A. Miller. 2006. "Ethics and Health Informatics: Users, Standards and Outcomes." In *Biomedical Informatics: Computer Applications in Health Care and Biomedicine* (pp. 379–402), 3rd ed., edited by Edward H. Shortliffe and James J. Cimino. New York: Springer.

Hauser, Susan E., Dina Hemner-Fushman, Joshua L. Jacobs, Susanne M. Humphrey, Glenn Ford, and George R. Thoma. 2007. "Using Wireless Handheld Computers to Seek Information at the Point of Care: An Evaluation by Clinicians." *Journal of the American Medical Informatics Association* 14, no. 6 (November–December): 807–815.

Healthcare Leadership Council. Chief Executive Task Force on Quality and Patient Safety. "Recommendations to Congress to Advance Implementation of Health Information Technology." Washington, DC: Healthcare Leadership Council (June 2004). Available: www.hlc.org/IT_White_paper_FINAL.pdf (accessed October 30, 2008).

Hersh, William R. 2003. *Information Retrieval: A Health and Biomedical Perspective,* 2nd ed. New York: Springer.

Lincoln, Thomas and Daniel Essin. 2003. "Medical Informatics." In *Encyclopedia of Library and Information Science* (pp. 1818–1829), vol. 3. New York: Marcel Dekker.

National Academy of Sciences. Committee on Enhancing the Internet for Health Applications: Technical Requirements and Implementation Strategies, Computer Science and Telecommunications Board, National Research Council. 2000. *Networking Health: Prescriptions for the Internet.* Washington, DC: National Academies Press.

Pew Internet & American Life Project. Online Health Search. Washington, DC: Pew Research Center (October 29, 2006). Available: www.pewinternet.org/pdfs/PIP_Online_Health_2006.pdf (accessed October 30, 2008).

Potts, Henry W. and Jeremy C. Wyatt. 2002. "Survey of Doctors' Experience of Patients Using the Internet." *Journal of Medical Internet Research* 4, no. 1 (January–March): e5. Available: www.jmir.org (accessed October 29, 2008).

Ramesh, A., C. Kambhampati, J.R. Monson, and P.J. Drew. 2004. "Artificial Intelligence in Medicine." *Annals of the Royal College of Surgeons of England* 86, no. 5 (September): 334–338.

Riha, Chris. 2006. "Growth of Wireless Technology in Healthcare Institutions." *IT Horizons,* 43–45. Available: www.aami.org/publications/ITHorizons/toc2006.pdf (accessed October 29, 2008).

University of Buffalo. Health Sciences Library. "Tutorials for PDAs, Biomedical Databases, and Library Research Techniques: A Guide to the Resources." Buffalo: State University of New York (September 25, 2007). Available: http://ublib.buffalo.edu/hsl/resources/guides/tutorials.html (accessed October 30, 2008).

U.S. Department of Health and Human Services. Agency for Healthcare Research and Quality. 2006. *Costs and Benefits of Health Information Technology.* Rockville, MD: AHRQ Publication No. 06-E006 (April).

U.S. Department of Health and Human Services. Commission on Systemic Interoperability. 2005. *Ending the Document Game: Connecting and Transforming Your Healthcare Through Information Technology.* Washington, DC: Government Printing Office.

Chapter 8

The Electronic Health Record

The electronic health record (EHR) is becoming the hub for patient-centered information. A master universal EHR will potentially contain not only specific patient data but also links to imaging sources and Internet-based information resources specific to the patient. This chapter examines the background and current status of the EHR.

THE NATURE OF HEALTH RECORDS

The patient health record has always been a fundamental component of healthcare. Patient health records have been kept since classical times, but the need to have complete, accurate, and up-to-date records has become much more critical in modern times. Traditionally, the health record contained lists of data related to the patient's situation, supplemented by detailed notes scribbled in by the physician.

A patient's health record generally is a conglomeration of paper documents, collected by the physician and nurses, arranged in descending chronological order. Documents include lab tests and results, images, charts, checked forms, and narratives generated during the periods of care of active patient care, showing the progression of a patient's case and describing the services rendered to the patient at those points.

Health records contain three broad categories of information: (1) administrative, (2) insurance, and (3) medical history. Specific data include such things as the patient's address, phone number, family relationships, marital status, health insurance company, billing information, detailed medical history, and sometimes information not specifically related to the present conditions. Data also include lab test results and radiology reports, especially any diagnoses and further testing recommendations from the lab and/or radiology department. All therapeutic interventions, the course of the illness, the responses to treatments, and any complications are recorded (Leiner et al., 2003).

Healthcare records have traditionally been accessible only by physicians, who used the records for making decisions about the individual case at hand. With the trend toward team healthcare delivery, however, the paradigm is changing. Providers "need to share healthcare information with a growing range of professional colleagues, often on multiple sites. Patients are often under the care of more than one team or specialty at the same time: for example a diabetic patient may be under a diabetologist, an ophthalmologist, a nephrologists, a dietician . . . their GP and a District Nurse" (Kalra and Ingram, 2006: 138). The single file patient record is very inefficient for this ubiquitous use. Also, patient data have become complex, and the volume of data continues to increase.

There are three areas of concern related to health records: (1) their accuracy, timeliness, and completeness; (2) the domain of personnel who can access them; and (3) the cost to adequately maintain them. High levels of accuracy, currency, and completeness depend on how the information is obtained and how it is entered into the record, and both processes are susceptible to human error and carelessness. To ensure security and privacy, organizations establish policies regarding who can access the records. Costs depend on how much labor is involved for record creation and management, what kind of storage space is needed, and the technology used to drive the system. These three basic concerns exist with paper-based systems as well as with electronic systems.

Problem-oriented Health Records

As described earlier, health records have traditionally been structured as a list of data. Typically, the data are not cross indexed or aggregated to summarize and explain the interactions. An alternative structure is the problem-oriented health record, which organizes information by clinical concepts, such as diagnosis. Proponents claim that concept organization is more natural for the decision-making process. For example, "a physician may navigate to a page in the chart to satisfy one information need, but spontaneously decide to satisfy additional information needs while they are there" (Post and Harrison, 2006: 646). Concept organization makes this linkage more viable.

The primary purpose of a problem-oriented health record is to provide a platform for communication among the healthcare team working with individual patients. In a sense, this method can be thought of as a scientifically designed problem statement, which is fundamental to the scientific method. This problem could be "a symptom, a sign, an abnormal laboratory or radiological finding, a social burden, or a previously diagnosed disorder" (Savage, 2001: 275). This structure allows the various healthcare providers to understand one another's thinking processes and decision-making rationales rather than relying on an independent examination of a list of data items each time the record is accessed. For this kind of approach to be successful, the data must be well-defined, specific, complete, and structured for ease of electronic handling.

Personal Health Records

A different kind of health record is the personal health record. At present, this is a somewhat ill-defined concept that has been discussed for years but with new interest since the rise of health information on the Internet. The idea of the personal health record is that it belongs exclusively to the patient, who is responsible for building and maintaining it and who has complete control over who can access it. The record is available only to the individual and to those whom the individual designates.

The physical nature of the record can take a variety of forms. For example, the record may be a simple loose-leaf binder or paper file, a document stored on a private computer, or a record accessible through an online service. It can also be stored on a computer chip that individuals have on their person at all time.

Although the concept of personal health records includes paper records, the current thought is that personal health records should be electronic-based applications. Patients would directly enter their own data into secure repositories that could be accessed as needed (Kim and Johnson, 2004). The rationale is that this type of record can be a second level of information to aid in routine medical care, emergency care, and health self-management. Over the years, an individual accumulates many health records from a number of primary care physicians, specialists, and related healthcare professionals. These providers keep their own records, but it is unlikely that the providers communicate with one another. As a matter of fact, what each individual provider *does not know* about what has been done elsewhere might be crucial to a person's health. A personal health record can help alleviate this problem.

When personal health information is needed, it should be immediately accessible. In any health event, the more complete and accurate the health information, the better it serves the patient and the healthcare provider. A personal health record can come into play in many incidents, such as a visit to an out-of-town doctor or a trip to the emergency room. In general, the personal health record promotes a more active role in one's own healthcare.

Personal health records can originate through a variety of portals. The basic platforms are (1) individual Web pages, where patients enter their own information; (2) health provider services; (3) employer-based services; (4) payer-based services, and (5) commercial vendor services (Halamka, Mandl, and Tang, 2008). Data will come from a number of sources, including healthcare providers, pharmacies, healthcare facilities, and Internet resources.

In response to the recent interest in personal health records, many collaborative projects and activities are being developed. Healthcare professional organizations are promoting discussions through public education seminars and Web sites. The American Health Information Management Association provides procedures and forms on its Web site (www.myphr.com) that the public can use to create personal health records. The U.S. Department of Veterans Affairs (www.myhealth.va.gov) offers a powerful gateway to information about veteran health benefits and services. This Web site links to My Health*e*Vet, which offers a Personal Health Journal for recording personal health information.

Vendor services have increased dramatically in recent years. A number of companies have online services for maintaining and managing personal health records. One example is the recently launched service by Google, called *Google Health*. The service gathers medical records from doctors, hospitals, and pharmacies and organizes it all in one place. Personal health records put the patient at the center of the patient's healthcare, allowing security and assurance that needed personal health information will be available at the right time and the right place.

THE EHR

The EHR is an information technology application that has become a major trend in healthcare. It is promoted as a solution to a number of problems related to health records and reflects the broadening concept of the purposes of a health record.

Definition

The term *electronic health record* has many synonyms: medical health record, electronic patient record, computer-based health record, computer-based patient record. Electronic health record is becoming the preferred term.

In EHR systems, the patient's medical information is stored in digital form and can be easily viewed and altered on computers by authorized personnel involved in the patient's care. It is a patient record in electronic form but ideally with more information, accessibility, connectivity, and interoperability than the paper record. It is more than just a computerized version of the papers put into manila folders.

Need for the EHR

In today's information-driven society, the healthcare world is moving toward the EHR. The leaders in healthcare view the EHR as a vehicle to improving patient safety and quality of care. Research shows this to be true, especially in the area of medication errors and following clinical practice guidelines (Crosson, 2005).

As the structure of healthcare delivery becomes more complex, more sophisticated ways of tracking data are needed. Tools are needed to capture both administrative and patient information, to promote the consumer awareness movement, and to encourage patients to become more involve in their healthcare. Many believe the EHR will assist in all of these areas.

The U.S. government promotes the EHR as a way for improving healthcare. President George W. Bush, in 2004, set the goal that every American would have an EHR by the year 2014. This resulted in a number of initiatives to promote the EHR, such as the Office of the National Coordinator for Health Information Technology (ONC) and the American Health Information Community (JAHIC) (Simborg, 2008).

Universality of EHRs

Healthcare is a collaborative effort and successful collaborative work inherently depends on effective interchange of information. Universal and integrated health record systems are envisioned as a main vehicle for information transfer among healthcare providers and healthcare facilities. Numerous organizations, the private sector, and government agencies are engaged in developing universal EHR systems.

The need for universal EHRs became particularly apparent after Hurricane Katrina. One of the recommendations in *The Federal Response to Katrina: Lessons Learned* was to "foster widespread used of interoperable electronic health records (EHR) systems, to achieve development and certification of systems for emergency responders" (The White House, 2006). As a result, the ONC (Department of Human and Health Service, 2006) released *Emergency Responder Electronic Health Record Detailed Use Case* to address the issues and the recommendations in the *Federal Response*. A universal EHR is a key element in the goal for global connectivity of healthcare systems and the exchange of information.

Challenges

EHR systems must be able to accommodate the changing paradigms of healthcare services. The clinical workforce is becoming more distributed and mobile, and healthcare professionals are altering their work patterns and the ways they approach their tasks.

Other challenges include accessing the overwhelming amount of available medical information. Some EHRs include external links to medical information resources, but doing this effectively is major task. The ever-present challenge to maintain confidentiality and privacy of patient records becomes critical when patient information moves to universally accessible electronic formats. From a technical viewpoint, a major challenge is to understand the complex operational environment in which the EHR is used, including common terminologies and specific communication standards.

Finally, there is the challenge of cost. EHR systems are expensive both to implement and to maintain. Proponents of the EHR point out that a way to fully optimize resources is to speed up access and reduce duplication, which in turn will help alleviate the high costs associated with the systems. In general, the healthcare industry is accepting the idea that EHRs are needed, but it remains a challenge to implement the EHR in an effective and cost-efficient way.

Electronic versus Paper Patient Records

What is wrong with paper health records? Anyone who has ever worked in a paper-based office knows the answers to this question. Paper records get misfiled and lost. Paper input can lead to gaps in the information, and in healthcare this can mean the difference between life and death. If the record cannot be found, then the healthcare professional must start from scratch to re-create it. Inconsistent recording standards for lab reports and illegible handwriting can lead to confusion, misunderstandings, and mistakes. Last, but not least, paper systems are static, not capable of providing the dynamic information interactions allowed with electronic systems.

At the most basic level, electronic records allow the management of information with a computer-based device. New data are added, old data are updated, and information is retrieved using a computer interface device. The EHR allows the user to do the same things that the paper record does but more as well.

EHRs take up less physical space, data can be retrieved quickly, and the records are accessible at any place there is an authorized computer interface. EHRs can incorporate multimedia input, both locally and remotely. A major advantage is that EHRs can be effectively and conveniently archived in electronic form. Paper archives have usually been subject to poor care and maintenance; EHR archives can be better organized and maintained. In general, EHR systems have little impact on the amount of time spent with patients, but there is definitely an impact on time spent accessing records.

One of the advantages of the EHR is its accessibility from many locations by many different individuals who perform various tasks. Some EHRs may allow the patient to access the record so that they can be more involved in their own care. EHRs support collaboration, automatic reporting, access to medical databases, and transference of records to different locations. They support management by enhancing the efficiency and effectiveness of healthcare professionals. EHRs document justifications for actions and diagnoses for legal, as well as medical, reasons. Data and statistics for policy and program development can be mined from EHRs. Finally, EHR systems support education and learning by supporting clinical research and medical education (Kalra and Ingram, 2006). Clearly, the EHR is far superior to the traditional paper file.

Despite the appeal of EHR systems, there are disadvantages. The most obvious are that they are expensive and they usually cause major organizational changes. EHRs still rely on humans to collect and input data and to apply the technology to their activities and responsibilities. This involves replacing familiar ways with new ways and new systems. These changes sometimes generate a fearful or uncooperative attitude.

EHR systems can fail for several reasons. At times, the system just does not work for an organization, and making adjustments involves unexpected additional costs. Some systems fail for technical reasons. When an EHR system fails, all records in the system go down, whereas if a paper record is lost or destroyed, then only one patient's record is affected. Unlike paper records, however, EHRs are almost impossible to lose. Server computer crashes that destroy large amounts of data are now uncommon because of secure backup systems.

Basic EHR Functions

EHRs have many functions, and the scope of their capabilities keeps changing. Functional components include detailed, integrated data about the patients, some degree of clinical decision-support capability, automated clinical ordering, external links to knowledge resources, and integrated reporting and communication capability (Tang and McDonald, 2006). Other functions include capturing demographic information for public health purposes and research; creating guidelines, protocols, and patient-specific care plans; managing consents and authorizations; monitoring of drug interactions in prescription orders; supporting accurate specimen collection; sending alerts for preventive services and wellness; supporting clinical task assignments and routing; communicating with pharmacies; providing patient and family education materials; and generating reports. The number of functions being incorporated into EHR systems keeps expanding.

The Ideal EHR

A number of attempts have been made to describe the ideal EHR. In 2007, the Society of General Internal Medicine (Blue Ribbon Panel of the Society of General Internal Medicine, 2007) suggested that EHRs have the following:

- Rapid accessibility and response time
- Intelligent and flexible data presentation
- Consistency
- Contextual sensitivity
- Prioritization
- Promotion of quality improvement
- Electronic communication
- Patient involvement.

The ideal EHR requires being current, complete, flexible, and integrated. It contains complete, up-to-date, and error-free information. Beyond these basics, it will contain advanced functionalities for linking to a variety of information resources, drawing on lab, radiology, registries, and prescription systems, including wireless access from a variety of locations. The ultimate, ideal EHR system will be wireless, with entry and reception available at the point of care or other locations and the ability to send alerts. It will allow single entry points with simultaneous access by many authorized personnel. It will link to other systems, including decision-making software, telemedicine systems, the Internet, and the health sciences literature. It will be effective and cost efficient.

Some long-range goals for EHR systems are to provide the infrastructure of a universal health care information system, which links all health care providers and organizations in the nation and around the world. Also, the EHR will promote the reduction of errors and reduce the time and human resources expended in managing paper files so that more time can be given to patients and their care. EHR systems continue to develop in terms of concept, structure, and supporting information technology. Much potential lies ahead for EHR applications.

Selection of an EHR

Selecting an EHR system can be a difficult, expensive, and time-consuming task. Holbrook et al. (2003) described a systematic, multifaceted, rigorous team approach to EHR selection and determined that there is no perfect system. During the selection process it was felt necessary to revisit the goals and objectives for the system. Each stage of the evaluation raised new issues, and the different team members had a hard time understanding the many features of the system.

Chapter 9 describes in detail the process of selecting and implementing a health information management system that includes EHR functions. It should be noted at this point that robust EHR systems will have automated support for legal compliance, the most obvious one being HIPAA. This is a time-consuming task, and having a built-in function in the EHR system is useful, to say the least. Patient health records are a major place where security locks and privacy protection are critical and should be both effective and efficient.

User Interfaces

The user interface component of the EHR is of paramount importance because the input and output is complex, varied, and of high volume. It is the interface that ensures a smooth operation and control of human error. For this reason, the interface must be addressed throughout the entire process of analysis, design, implementation, and evaluation of the EHR system.

Effective user interfaces are intuitive and logically designed in a way that makes them easy to learn and use. Some vital questions are: What information will be needed, and how does the user go about finding the information? Can the user easily find patient records and the detailed information needed from the record? Can new data be easily entered? The interface should make the entry and retrieval of information intuitive, with a minimum amount of ambiguity for the user. Are the different screens easy to read and understand, with clear-cut menu choices? Does the system allow alternative paths with the ability to return to the previous point in the process? If the user gets lost or does not understand an option, is the help function fast, compressive, and appropriate to the immediate problem? Data will be entered and retrieved by physicians' offices, labs, operating rooms, nursing stations in the hospital, the patient's room, and other locations, and the user interfaces must be of the highest quality.

Implementation of the EHR

After the EHR system has been selected, the next step is implementation. In most cases, implementation failure is not due to the technology or the system selected, if the selection process was done effectively. Failures are caused by poor organizational structures, inaccurate requirement definitions, poorly planned implementation, and, most prominently, by people. The very first thing to understand is that implementing the system should involve more than just one systems person. In today's world of complex systems and advanced technology, there is too much for one person to do alone.

Organizational issues are also present when major changes are undertaken during implementation of the EHR. Structuring and workflow must be re-tooled, and there is a natural resistance to change. Much of the resistance can be overcome by involving those concerned in the implementation process, providing high-quality training, and showing patience. The working environment needs to be collaborative, where people feel they are an important part of a team and no one is marginalized.

After an EHR system has been implemented, there remains the critical step of evaluating its performance. This step must be carefully planned and must involve the users of the system at every level. Chapter 9 discusses further details of evaluating information systems.

Web-based Systems

As discussed in Chapter 7, there is a steady movement toward Web-based, universal health information provision, with the EHR being a center focus. The increasing functionality of the Web is creating new avenues for health information connectivity and resource access. Three major advantages are (1) access to very large stores of information, (2) ubiquitous access at anytime and at any-place where there is computer interface, and (3) cost control.

A number of benefits are being touted for the Web-based health record. First, healthcare providers can have full and immediate access to the patients' records, at any time and in any place, within the scope of an organization or outside it, all on a global scale. The provider can see such things as the patient's medication list, history, and past treatments at the point of care, which speeds up and enhances the quality of treatment.

Another benefit is that patients have access to and better control of their own health information. Insurance companies and other support elements of healthcare can have their own management control and oversight, avoiding duplicate testing and unnecessary treatment, thereby reducing costs. Storage management is also less expensive; there is no need to buy servers and backup media, because they come with the Web service. Estimates range up to a 75 percent cost savings over in-house systems.

Issues and Caveats

Some basic concerns about health records are common to both paper based systems and EHR systems, and some concerns have arisen with implementation of the electronic form. Shortliffe and Blois (2006: 8) highlight four major issues currently facing efforts to implement EHRs.

- Need for standards in clinical terminology
- Data privacy, confidentiality, and security
- Challenges of data entry by physicians
- Difficulties associated with the integration of record systems with other information resources in the health care setting

NEED FOR TERMINOLOGY STANDARDS

The necessity for standards governing terminology is intensified when EHR systems are involved. It is essential to have the proper information technology configurations and a set of common standards for transferring information. Uniformity of data and transfer is vital for system compatibility, connectivity, and interoperability. The standards cover the processes from the way data are coded, entered, and transported to the technological interfaces of the communication equipment.

DATA PRIVACY, CONFIDENTIALITY, AND SECURITY

The explosion of the information technology age has brought many benefits to healthcare, and many exciting potentials are on the horizons. At the same time, there are concerns about the issues of patient privacy, confidentiality, and data security in health records. Accurate, more complete information is being provided to users at incredible speeds, from a widening range of locations and times. The increased numbers of both individuals who are allowed access and points of possible access create vulnerabilities for security and privacy. Proper controls must be in place to protect privacy and confidentiality.

Privacy and security can be jeopardized in two ways: patient information is released inappropriately by authorized personnel and unauthorized people enter the system. In the first case, authorized personnel may intentionally or unintentionally access or disseminate information, and in the second case outside intruders may hack into the system. Some aspects of security and privacy are regulated by law, for example, HIPAA. Maintaining secure, abuse-free EHRs will depend on the system designers, technology people, and rank-and-file users. It will also require the diligent oversight of management.

CHALLENGES OF DATA ENTRY BY PHYSICIANS

Data input presents a challenge because it requires time and careful attention, even with the use of information technology. The two major methods of data entry are manual entry and electronic capture. Manual data entry is labor intensive; therefore, it is costly and susceptible to error. Electronic entry is a preferred option when dealing with data from electronic sources. A number of healthcare personnel input data, but, with the rise of the EHR, more of the duty is being shifted to the physician. One of the hurdles in the implementation of the EHR has been to convince physicians to enter data electronically. In the beginning, some revolted against the idea of a doctor doing "clerical work" and felt it was too time consuming, but training the doctors to enter data electronically has resulted in greater use of the EHR and an understanding of its value. The creation of input software has helped the situation. Some of this software is powerful, allowing such things as image input and manipulation of the databases in the system. Many doctors are choosing handheld computers with pen interface and voice input. They have learned to actually like the input methods, and they are pleased especially with systems that allow them to text input, which they are familiar and comfortable with, and to build databases in styles and forms that suit them.

Computerized physician order entry (CPOE) has decreased error related to handwriting and verbally communicated orders for patient care. Also, doctors are pleased with the ability to enter data at the point of care, thus reducing the delay factor in completion of data entry and ordering. Despite the advances, much research and testing is still needed to improve data entry by physicians.

DIFFICULTIES ASSOCIATED WITH THE INTEGRATION OF RECORD SYSTEMS

The piecemeal fashion in which the healthcare industry began to automate led to a potpourri of local systems of all kinds. Slowly, networking and the advent of the Internet have pulled together many of these disparate systems, but still the reality is that integrating these resources is a formidable task. Because the concept of an ideal EHR envisions this linking, how to achieve this integration in an effective and cost-efficient way remains a critical issue.

Health Record Information Ownership

Health records are primarily composed of personal information about a patient, potentially including private information such as family history, mental status, and sexual preferences. The question is who owns this information and who should have ultimate control over accessing the information (Sharpe, 1999). A growing number of patients believe that they should have control over their health information, and healthcare professionals are increasing agreeing with this stance. On the other hand, other healthcare professionals and professional associations maintain that the information belongs to the health-care provider and that patients have no ownership rights. Sharpe (1999: 36) asks seven basic questions related to ownership of health record information:

1. Who may access data?
2. Who may mine or manipulate data?
3. Who may use data and for what purpose?
4. Who may sell data?
5. Who may disclose or publish data?
6. Who must pay to access, use, publish or sell data?
7. Who is required to disclose data in response to subpoenas or court orders?

Trends and Potentials of the EHR

Large medical organizations (medical centers, clinics, health maintenance orga-nizations) have spent billions of dollars to convert to electronic records, but small healthcare operations don't have the finances to do so. According to Freudenheim (2005), up to 60 percent of Americans receive their primary care at small-scale physicians' offices. Unless these medical practices can find ways to get into the mainstream of information technology, millions of Americans will not have access to the latest and most advanced healthcare.

An example of the powerful potential of the EHR occurred in the aftermath of Hurricane Katrina in 2005. Katrina left approximately 1 million people dis-placed, the great majority without any health records. This created a difficult sit-uation for healthcare providers and the patients. Health officials built electronic databases of prescription drug records for these victims. A universal EHR would have solved the problem. Health and Human Services Secretary Mike Leavitt said the chaos wreaked by Katrina "powerfully demonstrated the need for elec-tronic health records" (Freudenheim, 2005).

On the other hand, the Department of Veterans Affairs' EHR system clearly illustrated the potential usefulness of these systems during hurricanes Katrina and Rita. Health records of their patients were accessible even when disaster struck and patients were displaced from their homes.

Although use of EHR systems is still low, interest in their potential is gaining momentum at the federal level. For example, the Agency for Healthcare Research and Quality is investing millions in health information technology research. The past two U.S. Presidents have made major speeches on healthcare technology in which they urged the move toward the EHR. The Centers for Medicare and Med-icaid Services are planning to launch a 12-city project designed to nudge more small doctors' offices toward computerized systems. The project will include incen-tives, such as giving doctors cash bonuses from Medicare for buying EHRs systems and then reporting quality improvements to the government. The project hopes to overcome the reluctance of some healthcare professionals to adopt the EHR. Ac-cording to Kerry Weems, the acting administrator of the Centers for Medicare and

Medicaid Services, "Many smaller practices have been slow to buy the systems, which can cost between $20,000 and $40,000 per year" (Zwillich, 2007). Also, many doctors are reluctant to buy a system before industry and government groups have settled on a single standard for how the programs operate and communicate with each other. Blue Cross/Blue Shield has also said they will launch an incentive program to encourage doctors to use EHR systems (Zwillich, 2007).

A survey conducted by the National Center for Health Statistics (2005) indicates that "one-quarter of office-based physicians report using fully or partially electronic health record systems (EHR) in 2005, a 31% increase from the 18.2 percent reported in the 2001 survey. Although these estimates show that progress has been made toward the goal of universal electronic health records, there is still a long way to go."

The issue goes beyond just implementing EHR systems; a number of other problems still need to be solved. According to Simborg (2008: 29), "The current policy of promoting adoption of EHR systems requires some re-thinking. Adoption, per se, is not the goal. We must focus, in addition, on correcting the problems in EHRs and more importantly, on the financial environment which underlies those problems."

A National Health Record

Some people envision a national health records network, and efforts toward this goal are being made on several fronts. The idea is to integrate all electronic health information records, across institutions, into a national system. The idea

---

INFORMATICS IN ACTION! 8.1

National Network of EHRs

Location: Renowned health research center

Problem: The research center wants to establish a network of connected EHRs. It needs information on software available for linking EHR systems.

People Involved: The research center's project team and the informationist in the library.

Action Taken: Albert, the informationist, has a graduate degree in information technology and years of experience managing health record systems in a variety of environments. He knew that there were numerous "linking software" packages on the market. He did an extensive literature search for reviews and identified user reports in order to come up with comparison charts depicting the strengths and weaknesses of the different software packages. Albert wrote a report with his analysis and recommendations and submitted it to the research center's project team.

Takeaway: Albert had the experience necessary to evaluate software, but his most important strength was that he knew how health records are structured and used. This gave him critical insight when he analyzed the available linking software systems on the market.

was given a boost in 2004 when President George W. Bush made his proposal regarding all Americans having an EHR. He appointed a National Health Information Technology Coordinator to direct this effort. The ideal system will allow any doctor's office, hospital, or clinic to link to networks, both local and globally.

Creating such a network is a formable task, but promising efforts are under way. In 2008, the Coordinator of Health Information Technology announced plans to make the Nationwide Information Network (NIN) include EHRs from the Department of Defense, the Department of Veterans Affairs, the Indian Health Service, and some independent networks. Also, NIN will integrate their system with the healthcare databases that Google and Microsoft have for storing individual private health records. EHRs systems are a difficult challenge, but at the same time they are an opportunity for providing a major impact on healthcare delivery.

OPPORTUNITY FOR THE HEALTH SCIENCES LIBRARIAN

Librarians certainly have a role to play in the development and implementation of EHRs because of their expertise in organizing, structuring, storing, and retrieving information on demand. One of the areas being developed in EHRs is embedding links in individual patient records to online information resources that have a direct bearing on the particular patients. Health sciences librarians are involved in finding ways to link primary research and the "best medical evidence" to specific patient records. The theoretical and practical problems of building EHRs are about structuring information for effective and efficient retrieval and use, and this is the main domain of librarians.

SUMMARY

Throughout history, societies have recognized that it is essential to keep accurate and easily accessible healthcare records. The current volume and complexity of these records have produced new challenges for doing so. The EHR is a potent tool in keeping robust health records. Steady progress is being made in developing EHR systems, and the healthcare profession is beginning to accept and embrace these systems. This is opening up opportunities for the health sciences librarian to be directly involved in the health informatics enterprise.

REFERENCES

Blue Ribbon Panel of the Society of General Internal Medicine. 2007. "Redesigning the Practice Model for General Internal Medicine: A Proposal for Coordinated Care." *Journal of General Internal Medicine* 22, no. 3 (February 2): 400–409.

Crosson, Jesse C. 2005. "Implementing an Electronic Health Record in a Family Medicine Practice: Communication, Decision Making, and Conflict." *Annals of Family Medicine* 3, no. 4 (July): 307–311.

Department of Human and Health Services USA. Office of the National Coordinator for Health Information Technology (ONC). *Emergency Responder Electronic Health Record Detailed Use Case.* Washington, DC: ONC (December 20, 2006). Available: www.hhs.gov/healthit/usecases/documents/EmergencyRespEHRUseCase.pdf (accessed December 6, 2008)

Freudenheim, Milt. "Doctors Join to Promote Electronic Record Keeping." *New York Times*, September 19, 2005. Available: www.nytimes.com/2005/09/19/technology/19ehealth.html?scp=3&sq=katrina+medical+records&st=nyt (accessed: December 27, 2008).

Halamka, John D., Kenneth D.Mandl, and Paul C. Tang. 2008. "Early Experiences with Personal Health Records." *Journal of the American Medical Informatics Association* 15, no. 1 (January–February): 1–7.

Holbrook, Anne, Karim Keshavjee, Sue Troyan, Mike Pray, and Peter T. Ford. 2003. "Applying Methodology to Electronic Medical Record Selection." *International Journal of Medical Informatics* 71, no. 1 (August): 43–50.

Kalra, Dipak and David Ingram. 2006. "Electronic Health Records." In *Information Technology Solutions for Healthcare*, edited by Krzysztof Zieliński et al. New York: Springer.

Kim, Matthew I. and Kevin B. Johnson. 2004. "Patient Entry of Information: Evaluation of User Interfaces." *Medical Internet Research* 6, no. 2 (April–June): e13.

Leiner, F., W. Gaus, R. Haux, and P. Knuap-Gregori. 2003. *Medical Date Management: A Practical Guide.* New York: Springer.

National Center for Health Statistics. "Electronic Health Record Use by Office-based Physicians: United States, 2005." Washington, DC: National Center for Health Statistics (2005). Available: www.cdc.gov/nchs/products/pubs/pubd/hestats/electronic/electronic.htm (accessed August 27, 2008).

Post, Andrew and James Harrison, Jr. 2006. "Data Acquisition Behaviors During Inpatient Results Review: Implications for Problem-oriented Data Displays." In *AMIA Annual Symposium Proceedings* (pp. 644–648). Bethesda, MD: American Medical Informatics Association.

Savage, Peter. 2001. "A Book That Changed My Practice: Problem Oriented Health Records." *British Medical Journal* 322, no.7281 (February 3): 275.

Sharpe, Charles C. 1999. *Health Records Review and Analysis.* Westport, CT: Auburn House. Citing: Waller, Adele A. and Oscar L. Alcantara. 1998. "Ownership of Health Information in the Information Age." *Journal of the American Health Information Management Association* 69, no. 3 (March): 28–34.

Shortliffe, Edward H. and Marsden S. Blois. 2006. "The Computer Meets Medicine and Biology: Emergence of a Discipline." In *Biomedical Informatics: Computer Applications in Health Care and Biomedicine* (pp. 3–45), 3rd ed., edited by Edward H. Shortliffe and James J. Cimino. New York: Springer.

Simborg, Donald W. 2008. "Promoting Electronic Health Record Adoption. Is It the Correct Focus?" *Journal of the Medical Informatics Association* 15, no. 2 (March–April): 127–129.

Tang, Paul C. and Clement J. McDonald. 2006. "Electronic Health Record Systems." In *Biomedical Informatics: Computer Applications in Health Care and Biomedicine* (pp. 476–510), 3rd ed., edited by Edward H. Shortliffe and James J. Cimino. New York: Springer.

The White House. *The Federal Response to Katrina: Lessons Learned.* Washington, DC: The White House (February 26, 2006). Available: www.whitehouse.gov/reports/katrina-lessons-learned (accessed December 6, 2008).

Zwillich, Todd. "Medicare to Offer Incentives to Persuade Doctors to Use Electronic Health Records Systems." WebMD Medical News (October 30, 2007). Available: www.webmd.com/medicare/news/20071030/doctors-urged-to-get-electronic-records (accessed August 27, 2008).

Chapter 9

Healthcare Information Management Systems

The amount of health-related information is enormous, ranging from information generated by the offices of physicians to global Internet resources. To be useful, this information must be effectively and efficiently managed—acquired, organized, archived, retrieved, and distributed. This can only be done with quality management systems. This chapter describes healthcare information management systems.

INFORMATION MANAGEMENT

An almost universal consensus exists that information technology can improve operations in healthcare organizations, but this will happen only if information systems are successfully defined, developed, implemented, and maintained. Health information management deals with information technology, with the basic principles of information management, and with human users of information. The information manager's primary task is to make decisions related to these factors, especially with regard to how these factors interact.

By virtue of the nature of medicine, information systems always have been a part of the delivery of healthcare services, for centuries in manual paper form and in modern times in electronic form. Traditional paper systems maintained patient records, scheduled treatments and appointments, and handled billing. Electronic systems perform the same basic functions, but they are enhanced with a host of modern technologies, such as physical monitoring devices, information input/output mobility, networking, and advanced communication. These technologies are rapidly being incorporated into the healthcare infrastructure. It is rare nowadays to find a doctor's office, clinic, hospital, or any other healthcare facility without some type of computer-based management system, but the level of complexity and functions varies widely among systems.

There are different ways of looking at information systems in healthcare because of the complex web of relationships among units, staff, and operational functions. Activities exist in a maze of connections among numerous subunits in a healthcare organization, and these relationships must be given careful attention when designing, implementing, and managing a health information management system.

Correct Information at the Right Time

Having the correct information delivered to the right person at the right time at the right place seems both logical and essential, but it has always been a challenge. This is true of both clinical data and management data at all levels. Effective information management systems deliver the fundamental information that enables the care of patients and the smooth functioning of healthcare facilities and institutions.

Complexity of Healthcare Information Systems

Healthcare is a vastly complex enterprise; therefore, the information systems that support it are equally complex. Krabbel and Wetzel (2000: 2–3) pointed out three basic aspects of complexities that need to be considered when implementing information systems in hospitals, but they equally apply to all healthcare organizations:

- First, because of the high amount of existing cooperative work, designers need to understand the relationships and interdependencies among single activities.
- Second, another source of complexity lies in the heterogeneity of the involved user groups and their often competing requirement, while at the same time designing an integrated system to connect the different groups. In today's complex healthcare environment, information needed for specific situations is rarely found in a single computer or particular computer system. Sharing of information through networks is the new paradigm.
- A third reason for complexity is that implementing a hospital information system certainly causes changes in the entire work organization.

Understanding Information Needs and Opportunities

When designing and implementing an information management system, the first concern is the information needs of the people who will use the system. A wide variety of groups will use the healthcare information systems for reasons related to their specific tasks. Therefore, when designing a system, each group's needs must be equally addressed and included in the design of the system.

Although it is important to keep up with the latest hardware and software advances, understanding user needs is the highest of priorities. The system must support the needs of the users, as defined by the users themselves. Everybody who will use the new system should be involved in the system analysis and design processes, not only to be sure their needs are met, but also to win their acceptance and support early on. Perhaps the hardest lesson that system analysts have to learn is to listen to what people *mean*, not just what they *say*.

Information Resources Management

Information resources management (IRM) is the overseeing of the acquisition, installation, and operation of information resources in an organization. It is usually an executive level position, with the manager reporting to a deputy executive or sometimes directly to the organization's chief executive office. IRM is a set of principles, plans, and practices for managing information resources. It is involved with the planning and operation of information resources, including technology, humans, and related financial resources. The widespread use of information technology and the increasing complexity of the information infrastructure in healthcare have created the need for qualified information resources managers. This manager is often called the Chief Information Officer (CIO).

In healthcare, the concept of the CIO often evolved into the position of Chief Medical Information Officer (CMIO) in order to ensure the input of medical professionals. Medical personnel felt that information management systems were being designed without adequate input for the actual users of the systems and saw a need for clinicians to have informed input to the planning and implementation of these systems. In the early years of the development of health information systems for health organizations, the CMIO was not likely to be a technology person, per se, but rather a physician who was savvy in health information technology. However, the CMIO position has evolved to a management position for the oversight of all aspects of information management. According to Leviss, Kremsdorf, and Mohaideen (2006: 573), "interviews with those individuals indicate that executive leadership skills are more valuable to a CMIO than formally trained informatics expertise." It appears that CMIOs use their leadership and informatics expertise to instigate health system changes and accomplish institution goals and objectives rather than just using their technical knowledge to build information systems.

The duties of the CMIO usually include, among other things, serving as a liaison between the medical staff of the organization and the senior administrators of the information unit. The CMIO participates in the planning and implementation and performance assessment of clinical information technology and is involved in the long-range strategic planning regarding the information technology. As part of this, the CMIO elicits input about user needs for information technology and helps plan and direct training of the healthcare personnel who will be using the technology.

MAJOR TYPES OF HEALTH INFORMATION SYSTEMS

Because of the diversity of healthcare and the complex infrastructures involved, it is difficult to categorize all types of information systems. These systems are in various states of merging, integrating, interconnecting, and centralizing, particularly with the migration to Internet-based systems. The following are some general categories of modern healthcare systems.

Clinical Information Systems

A clinical information system provides a database of information related to patient care, handles the business processes of health providers, and often includes decision-making functions to aid the physician in diagnosis and treatment. The practical goals of clinical information systems include improvement and enhancement of the quality of patient care, support of clinical management and research, increase in productivity, and reduction of operating costs.

Clinical information systems are patient centered, providing immediate information at the point of care at the time needed. Point of care can include physicians' offices, hospitals, telemedicine distribution centers, and any other place where care is being provided.

These systems provide integrated access to electronic medical records, clinical guidelines, drug interaction alerts, electronic messaging capabilities, and decision-support systems. They link and integrate pharmacy systems, laboratory systems, radiology systems, and other ancillary systems. These systems can accept provider orders and deliver results back to the provider and can generate on-demand status reports. Input devices to these systems include PC terminals, intranet connections to supportive systems, and mobile devices for caregivers for collecting data and viewing reports and archival information.

Some additional functions of clinical information systems may include the capability to go online and access the medical literature. Also, it is useful when the system responds with advice regarding proposed therapies or diagnostic tests and issues automatic alerts when something in the patient's data needs attention. In addition, some systems check activities against standard guidelines of care and earmark any possible deviations (Sittig et al., 2002).

A clinical decision-support function in a clinical information system assists in patient care decisions. Data are gathered from numerous information systems, such as patient records, laboratory systems, pharmacies, diagnostic imaging systems, and nursing information systems.

EXAMPLES OF CLINICAL INFORMATION SYSTEMS

The following are examples of the wide range of available services and systems for managing clinical information:

- EMRitus. Available: www.ergopartners.com (accessed December 27, 2008). EMRitus includes patient management, clinical documentation, order processing, outcome tracking, and more. It is a functionally flexible module that adapts to clinical documentation needs. Examples of functions include recording patient encounters, assigning diagnoses, submitting orders for lab tests, and creating treatment plans. It includes clinical vocabularies.

- INTERACTANT. Available: www.hcsinteractant.com (accessed December 27, 2008). INTERACTANT is a fully integrated clinical and financial information system.
- Site of Care Systems. Available: www.siteofcare.com (accessed December 27, 2008). Site of Care Systems is an example of a narrowly focused, specific system dealing with perinatal and neonatal information.
- AccuStat EMR. Available: www.accustatemr.com (accessed December 27, 2008). AccuStat is a company that focuses on electronic medical records.
- Clinical Information Systems Consultants, Inc. Available: www.ciscon.com/Products.html (accessed December 27, 2008). This consulting firm works with clients in order to focus on specific needs. It specializes in the implementation of clinical information systems.

Hospital Information Systems

The purpose of a hospital information system is to manage the information that hospital personnel need to do their jobs. Hospital information systems are integrated systems that handle the administrative, financial, and clinical operations in a hospital. They assist in carrying out the daily activities of a hospital, including such things as patient tracking and coordination of clinical functions.

Administrative procedures were the first functions automated in healthcare, following the pattern of societal computer applications in general. The functions were most often financial operations, because that was the primary state of the art at the time. These systems were standalone operations in individual units, usually duplicated in other units and not integrated. Over time, hospitals realized the inefficiency of not being able to share and integrate information, and slowly, as enabling technology developed, the movement was toward integrated and networked systems. Hospital information management systems have many subsystems and access to information by the subsystems is frequently different, but they generally fall into three application areas: patient care, administrative and regulatory process, and decision making and quality improvement (Wickramasighe, Gupta, and Sharma, 2005).

Patient Admission, Transfer, Discharge, and Billing

Typically, a patient arrives and is checked into the hospital. At the admission point, demographic information is collected and identification codes are assigned to the patient. Records are checked to see if the patient has been admitted before, and new information is inputted. Once the patient arrives at the treatment points or wards, examinations, lab results, diagnoses, therapies, and nursing orders become part of the record. Traditionally, this record was a growing file of paper forms and charts, but computer workstations, run by management software, are taking over much of the drudgery involved.

Patient admission, transfer, tracking, and discharge systems are management systems that follow patients from the time they are admitted into a facility until they are discharged. It has been estimated that in the United States it costs $250 billion a year for checking in, verifying eligibility for insurance, billing, updating events, and eventually discharging. Surely, one answer to reducing cost lies in effective and efficient automation of the total process. Internet-based transactions might drop this cost by tenfold (Wickramasinghe, Gupta, and Sharma, 2005).

DOCUMENTATION, REPORTING, AND PLANNING

A hospital has many documentation obligations. The primary one is to record all clinical information related to individual patients, including diagnosis, treatment, ongoing responses of the patients, orders, and other such data. Another documentation need is external legal reports, such as epidemiological registries and legal compliance. Also, complete and accurate documenting is required for administrative control and billing. In addition, hospitals need to gather operational information in order to plan ahead. Many of the commercial hospital information management systems contain functions for aiding in these activities.

ADMINISTRATIVE SUPPORT SYSTEMS

Administrative support systems assist administrators and managers in making decisions based on current information. Clinicians need information that is patient specific, but hospital administrators need a broader range of information in order to run their complex organizations. Information is needed for daily operation, planning, communication among disparate groups in the organization, and documentation and reporting requirements. This information is gathered from a variety of sources, such as accounting and marketing, and is used for many purposes. Some major examples of administrative information needs include the following:

- Inventory and supplies: Hospitals need to track, order, and pay for supplies. A typical hospital has many hundreds of supply items. Electronic health management systems have incorporated techniques developed in the business world to monitor and control these activities.
- Human resource management: A large percentage of hospital budgets are expended in human resource management, including hiring, personnel record keeping, payroll, and work assignments.
- Strategic planning: Planning in hospitals has been aided by computer systems since the beginning of automated information systems in healthcare. Effective systems are used to aid in understanding the needs and opportu-

nities in the future of the hospital and to aid in good decision making for planners.

- Facilities management: Facilities management is always a major activity in healthcare organizations, and in hospitals this involves many people and substantial amounts of money. Efficient information systems can streamline procedures and promote cost effectiveness.

NETWORKS

Many hospital administrators and health information technology professionals are seeing a movement toward Internet-enhanced hospital procedures and operations: "Many chief information officers (CIOs) believe that the Internet makes provider organizations an offer they cannot refuse—lower costs, widespread access, and interface engines for in-place hardware and software" (Coile, 2001: xv). More than 80 percent of all U.S. hospitals are members or affiliates of integrated systems and networks (Coile, 2001).

It appears that Web-based connectivity is going to eventually replace most traditional models. Common examples of benefits for Web-based systems include online purchasing and time and cost reduction in insurance management and billing. Also, there is reduced time in obtaining laboratory results. Delivery of lab reports can be reduced to hours rather than days. In additions, these Web systems allow instantaneous global linking of healthcare professionals, along with many other applications.

Related to this are hospital intranets. An intranet is a network *within* an organization, technically similar to the Internet. Intranets are usually in the top ten lists of priorities for healthcare executives. Hospitals see intranet systems as a way to connect internal resources, people, and procedures in order to produce more effective and cost-efficient services. Hospital-sponsored intranets, which connect physicians for minimal up-front or subscription fees, are proving highly popular (Coile, 2001). These intranet capabilities are providing clinicians the means to access and share data with each other at different locations and synthesize information regarding individual patients.

EXAMPLES OF HOSPITAL INFORMATION MANAGEMENT SYSTEMS

One of the pioneer hospital information systems was Medinet at General Electric Company in the 1960s. There were also early systems at Massachusetts General Hospital in Boston, Latter Day Saints Hospital in Salt Lake City, Kaiser Permanente in Oakland, and at Stanford University (Felkey, Fox, and Thrower, 2005). Currently there are numerous hospital systems on the market. Here are a few examples:

- HospitalPortal™NET. Available: www.hospitalportal.net/HospitalPortal/Main.aspx (accessed December 27, 2008). The system builds intranet and extranet sites. According to the homepage, it is "a turn-key solution that

comes with . . . tools to address all of the common needs of a typical Intranet or Extranet environment in healthcare organizations."
- PRO/Scheduler™. Available: www.programmingresources.com/solutions.jsp (accessed December 27, 2008). This is an example of hospital patient scheduling software. Also, it includes an inventory management component.
- HealthQuest®. Available: www.mckesson.com/en_us/McKesson.com/For%2BHealthcare%2BProviders/Hospitals/Hospital%2BInformation%2BSystems/HealthQuest.html (accessed January 9, 2009). This system provides a number of integrated functions, including a financial management system and a receivables management system for accounting collections.

Professional and administrative staffs in hospital spend at least 25 percent of their time handling information (Haux et al., 2004). High-quality hospital information management systems are needed to increase the quality of care and to maintain an economically viable operation through better management.

Supportive Health Information Systems

Throughout the healthcare system, numerous information subsystems support the primary activities of healthcare. The following are typical support systems, although the list is not exhaustive.

LABORATORY MANAGEMENT SYSTEMS

Laboratory information management systems are software programs that organize and track the processes that occur in the laboratory. These systems keep track of data about individual patients, organize the tests results, and route the information to appropriate points. The system may also help manage personnel and operations in the lab. Ideally, the system is networked and integrated, allowing the access and transfer of secure data to and from other systems electronically.

A medical laboratory tests clinical specimens for information about the health situation of patients and thus constitutes a major factor in diagnosis and treatment plans. According to Cowan (2005: 2), "about 70% of the information used in the management of patients comes from the clinical and anatomical pathology laboratories. . . . [I]n one large medical center in which information flow is tracked, about 94% of requests to the EMR are for laboratory results." The three major types of medical laboratories are hospital labs, which are a part of a hospital system; in-house clinical labs; and private labs (usually for-profit operations). There are other variations, such as public health labs and those labs affiliated with research operations.

RADIOLOGY INFORMATION SYSTEMS

Radiology information systems organize, process, and distribute radiological data and images related to patient care. These systems receive orders from health providers, schedule patients, manipulate and distribute test results and images, and provide diagnosis to the personnel who requested the information. They also manage workflow in the unit and do inventory control, purchasing, and billing. Modern systems are often networked and send results rapidly and effectively to the points of care. Medical imaging is discussed in Chapter 10.

PHARMACEUTICAL MANAGEMENT SYSTEMS

Pharmaceutical information systems are used to manage the full range of activities involved in the provision of patient medication. There are two major facets of these systems: filling of prescriptions and managing the pharmacy operation.

Automated pharmaceutical systems fill over one third of the more than three billion prescriptions dispensed each year in the United States (Felkey, Fox, and Thrower, 2006). These systems keep patient records, check on the validity of prescriptions, scan drug interaction information, verify insurance information, and update patient records as the prescriptions are filled. Often these systems are linked to medication information systems, which are database systems containing information about medications. The information from these databases can be used by pharmacists in their duties and can also provide educational information for the patient.

From a management viewpoint, pharmaceutical information management systems help organize the pharmacy unit, control workflow, chart personnel assignments, handle inventory control, and manage billings and payments for the patients and the pharmacy. Pharmacy information management systems save the time of pharmacy personnel, increase productivity, reduce costs, help improve accuracy, and reduce medication errors.

EXAMPLES OF SUPPORTIVE INFORMATION SYSTEMS

Many supportive information systems are available commercially. The following are examples:

- Cerner PathNet®. Available: www.cerner.com/public/Cerner_3.asp?id= 199 (accessed January 10, 2009). This is a laboratory information system. It integrates operational and managerial processes of laboratories. It addresses four key components: clinical, anatomical pathology, genetic information, and laboratory outreach.
- Centricity® Pharmacy. Available: www.gehealthcare.com/usen/img_info_ systems/centricity_clin_info/products/pharmacy.html (accessed January 10, 2009). This GE Healthcare product is a complete pharmaceutical system that maintains all the functions expected from a high-end pharmaceutical information system. It is also an example of an integrated pharmacy system that allows sharing of information directly with other caregivers.
- Siemens Pharmacy. Available: www.medical.siemens.com/webapp/wcs/ stores/servlet/StoreCatalogDisplay~q_catalogId~e_-1~a_langId~e_-1~

a_storeId-e_10001.htm (accessed January 10, 2009). This supports the clinical, operational, and management functions of a pharmacy. It is an example of a medication order processing system. It begins with order entry and maintains check points throughout the process, such as validation and clinical conflict screening. It includes clinical decision support and automatic notifications.

- MedStar RIS. Available: www.medstarsystems.com/ris_system.html (accessed January 10, 2009). This service computerizes patient scheduling, demographics, billings, claims preparation, and imaging. It interfaces with external vendor imaging systems. It is also an example of a radiology information system with speech-recognition capabilities.

HEALTHCARE INFORMATION SYSTEM ANALYSIS

The acquisition and implementation of a healthcare information management system requires a careful and professional analysis of the existing system and the design of the new system. System analysis and design is an art and a science, and it could be described as the orchestrating of change. Like any activity that involves change, planning and keeping it on target are not simple tasks. An analyst can receive valuable assistance in planning and implementing a system from a few key individuals in an organization, but consultation within a wider group is critical. The planning team should include officials from top management, middle management, and the rank-and-file operational personnel. When appropriate, nonstaff persons may be involved, such as advisory board members, patients, and community members. Many viewpoints are needed, but at the same time the team should not be so large as to become unwieldy.

The systems analyst is generally only a "middle person" between the user of the system being analyzed and the technical experts, vendors, or some other people who implement the recommended design. For example, the systems analyst gathers data from the users of a system, analyzes it, documents the analysis and findings from the data collected, and then develops a design document. To ensure that the system analyst has accurately described the current system, the documentation is given to the users for their concurrence. The design document subsequently forms the basis for either the in-house programming and development of the system or the purchase of a commercial turnkey system design. It should be clear that the systems analyst communicates the existing system (from information supplied by the end users) to the technical personnel, or vendor, generally followed by a description of the new, improved system that is envisioned.

Careful, detailed planning is the only way to successfully implement a complex health information management system. A good information system cannot be designed without a clear analysis of the problems and the outcomes desired. There is a growing literature that supports the idea that a large

INFORMATICS IN ACTION! 9.1

An Integrated Hospital Information Management System

Location: Metropolitan hospital affiliated with a medical school

Problem: The hospital recognizes that its patchwork, decentralized information systems are archaic, ineffective, and wasting resources. The various units have individual systems, with their own information technology (IT) staff, unevenly qualified. The hospital needs a modern integrated system.

People Involved: The hospital chief executive officer (CEO), the vice president for information resources in the medical school, the systems librarian in the medical school center library, and a task force with representatives from throughout the hospital.

Action Taken: The hospital CEO knew that Jodie, the systems librarian, has a state-of-the-art information management system in the library and is very knowledgeable in the area of IT. The CEO appointed her to co-chair a task force with the head of IT for the hospital. The task force had the charge to study the implementation of a new information management system for the hospital. Jodie went to the heart of the matter by telling the CEO that the main problem was organizational. The hospital needed a centralized IT unit with a chief information officer. Once this infrastructure is in place, then the task is to acquire information systems for the hospital. The CEO agreed and redirected the task force to develop a plan to establish an information technology unit for the hospital.

Takeaway: The systems librarian at the medical school center library identified the organizational problems. Her insight was based on her years of experience in the area of IT implementations. She had experience in working in interdisciplinary teams.

number of medical errors are the result of systems problems. There are many major and minor systems in healthcare that need careful analysis, for example, scheduling, operations, billing, correct handling of lab tests, making sure patients get the correct medication, double checking for drug interactions, and so on, where system problems can cause malfunction. A new system does not just implement old routines; it enhances the operation and opens new doors of opportunity.

Basic Rules for Acquiring an Information Management System

The design and implementation of any information system has three basic, easy-to-understand rules. Often these rules are violated, usually with unhappy results. The rules are:

1. Determine what needs to be done.
2. Decide what the new system will encompass.
3. Install the best technology to meet the system requirements.

Each of these rules involves a number of steps and processes, consisting of complex analysis, creative designing, and the marshalling of human resources.

DETERMINE WHAT NEEDS TO BE DONE

Selecting a computer-based system does not begin with hardware. The starting point is a clear identification of your application needs and an understanding of the processes of the operations. If the processes are poorly understood, the new system will be poorly designed and will simply allow the same old mistakes to be made at an incredibly faster rate.

Understanding the variety and complexity of the healthcare information system needs comes from a careful analysis of processes, outcomes, and the perceptions of the users. Also, regardless of the type of healthcare facility and the institutional information architecture, organizational and external factors always influence the information needs. Such factors include the cultural, technical, structural, psychosocial, temporal, and managerial aspects (Tan, 2001), and they must be investigated. Other factors that affect the selection include governmental initiatives and laws, economics factors beyond the control of the institution, mergers, sociological factors, and current technology advances and trends.

DECIDE WHAT THE NEW SYSTEM WILL ENCOMPASS

Will the new system replace a paper-based system? If it replaces an existing computer-based system, will it be a total replacement or a partial replacement and update (Wiederhold and Shortliffe, 2006)?

There is a natural tendency among systems analysts to want to design the "perfect system," one that has every feature even remotely desired by the users. Such a system is simply not achievable: no one ever has the financial resources or time necessary to achieve it. User requirements change during the system design process, so you're always shooting at a moving target. The best scenario that you can hope for is to write functional specifications that meet most of the requirements of most of the users most of the time.

INSTALL THE BEST TECHNOLOGY TO MEET THE SYSTEM REQUIREMENTS

Do you purchase a commercial system (a turnkey system), or do you develop the software in-house? In the ideal situation, you can buy a commercial system that will meet the needs of the organization, and this is often the case. Despite the numerous systems commercially available, however, the specific, local needs often cannot be adequately covered, and an internal self-developed system is necessary. Some commercial systems are easily adapted, and some are inflexible—"what you see is what you get."

Generally, commercial systems are less expensive than self-developed systems, but flexibility and adaptability are often compromised. Turnkey systems rarely exactly fit an institution's needs, lacking some necessary functions and including some other superfluous functions, but building your own system is a challenging task (Wiederhold and Shortliffe, 2006). It requires a highly knowledgeable and experienced technical staff and the dedication of all individuals involved.

Few organizations have the resources needed to be able to rely entirely on in-house development.

Whether the system is purchased or designed in-house, high priority should be given to making the system integrated. Health information management systems were traditionally developed as add-on structures. Single function systems were first implemented and then additional functions were attached, somewhat like adding additional rooms to a house. When these systems worked, they were usually complex, with slow interfacing. Gradually, this approach gave way to multifunctional systems, built with increasingly sophisticated interrelated structures. On a broad level, these systems could be accessed from many points because of their numerous options. These systems are loosely related but essentially are independent subsystems. In such cases, duplication of activities is usually unavoidable and costly. This is one of the reasons that modern information technology focuses on integrated, networked systems.

There are many reasons for having integrated systems, but probably the most compelling one is that various groups, at diverse locations, need the same information. For example, a patient record may be part of clinical information system, and at the same time the record may be a part of the administrative system in a hospital. Surgeons need patient information to prepare for surgery. Nursing stations need instructions and reports from the surgeon. Referring doctors need to be updated, and administration needs information for billing (Haux et al., 2004). In the past few years, managers have been turning to integrated information systems as the best solution. Unnecessary expenses often arise when the same data are acquired repeatedly for different tasks instead of using the information in multiple ways (Leiner et al., 2003). Modern times demand integrated systems.

Once you have identified your application requirements in specific, concrete terms, then identify software that will meet your requirements. A wide variety of resources will help, for example, *software directories*, which are collections of review materials and/or manufacturers' product descriptions. Keep in mind that most of these write ups are descriptions, *not* evaluations; they provide only basic information, such as application features, memory requirements, price, and services included.

Another important resource is the in-depth product *review*. Although there are many avenues to finding reviews, popular magazines and professional journals are the most common sources. Reviews often show screen shots, which give a quick look at the program. One word of caution: popular computer magazines rarely will have reviews by healthcare professionals.

Trade and professional associations are good sources because the software recommendations come from knowledgeable professionals in specific fields. Identify the state, regional, national, and international associations that are appropriate to your tasks. They often have publications related to software.

You can also directly contact software companies that might have appropriate software, and they can give you specific technical details and costs. Look for ads in the professional journals or talk to exhibitors at meetings and conventions. When you attend professional meetings, visit the exhibits and ask hard questions about the software and its compatibility with your needs.

There are a number of *software databases* that describe software and are especially useful for obtaining full technical details. A good example is DataPro (www.data-pro.com/). Many systems analysts have relied on DataPro for years. It is very detailed and includes reviews by individuals using particular software.

Searching for information about software on the *Internet* is another approach. The Internet's search tools will retrieve articles, reviews, and other information about many types of software. Searches will often identify the Internet sites of commercial vendors as well as sites offering shareware and firmware packages. Some sites will allow you to download demonstration or examination copies of the software. One of the best ways to evaluate software is to obtain a demo copy and test it out.

Engaging a *consultant* is also a good option. Advice from experienced consultants who are knowledgeable about healthcare software can save you many hours studying and pondering over what you are doing. After identifying a group of potential software packages that may work, compare the specific features of each package to the specifications of your needs. For example, will the software handle 100,000 records or more? Many software packages are under constant revision—*make sure you are buying the latest version.* Also, note that many companies advertise that they provide HIPAA compliance, but "compliance" can be interpreted in many ways.

Making a sound decision requires a good grasp of the capabilities of computers, how software is designed, and how to match needed specifications with software features. While it helps to have quite a bit of experience in the field of information technology to make the right choice, even neophytes can generally do an adequate job of selecting appropriate hardware and software from the myriad of choices available today.

The quality of support vendors give their customers after purchase varies. Some vendors provide "hotline" technical support, bulletin boards, support groups, blogs, or e-mail service. Others provide no technical support at all. Know what type of service the vendor provides before you make a purchase, and be sure to read carefully any disclaimer at the bottom of the contract.

Once you have identified the appropriate software package, prepare a request for proposal (RFP). An RFP is a formal document you send to vendors and suppliers inviting them to submit a proposal to provide the product or service. RFPs are usually distributed based on a bidding process, which has the advantage of several potential companies competing to offer the best deal. The RFP briefly describes the hardware, software, and services needed. It does not get into exact details, leaving this to be suggested by the companies in their proposals. Proposals are negotiated before accepted.

Once you choose a vendor, prepare a detailed contract. The contract addresses many specific items. The following list of questions that your contract should answer is adapted from Cowan (2005: 35):

- What is being bought?
- How much will it cost, and what are the terms of payment?
- How will it be installed, and who will install it?
- What are the installation costs, and how much time will installation require?
- What are the physical requirements for the computer room?
- What electrical services are required?
- Who will do the training, where and how will training occur, how much does training cost, and who pays for it?
- Who will operate the system?
- How should the system perform?
- What is the definition of system acceptance?
- Who maintains the system, and who repairs it?
- Who upgrades the system?
- What are the rights and obligations of the organization?
- What are the rights and obligations of the vendor?
- What are the penalties for failure of the system to perform to specification?

Contracts are legal documents. If you are part of a larger organization (i.e., a hospital within a health system within a university), there will be personnel designated to handle the legal issues, along with attorneys. Also, vendors like to require that any litigation be handled in the state of the vendor; you should require that it be handled locally.

Successful Information System Implementation

When a new system is implemented, the way operations are performed, the tasks of the staff, and the relationships among units will change. The installation of a new system or changeover from one system to another requires skillful management and sensitivity to people. Departmental structures may change and some jobs may be eliminated, while new structures may come into place and new jobs are created. This is naturally a stressful situation for the staff.

The project manager must oversee both the development of the system and the changing perceptions of the system. Leicht and Sauter (2003) maintain that the project manager needs to keep the users aware of developments: "Keeping users abreast of developments means they will rest easier, they will not be surprised by outcomes, and they will be more convinced that the project is being well managed; as a result, users' attitudes toward the project will be better."

Systems fail when users' needs are not met or when their expectations of the system don't become a reality. Sometimes their expectations are unrealistic, but in many cases the problem is that they were not truly involved in the process.

HUMAN–COMPUTER INTERFACES

An information system is only as good as the quality of its interfaces. When a user has difficulty interfacing with a system, he or she considers it to be a system failure. A typical computer system has multiple interfaces—human– computer, computer–computer, computer–noncomputer devices, robots, printers, and graphic producers. System failures are often caused by poor computer–user interfaces. The structure of the system and its informational intent may be excellent, but if an interface breaks down and frustrates the users, they may very well reject the entire system.

Good user–computer interfaces are intuitive, fast, efficient, and easy to use. The physical devices for human–computer interfacing are straightforward and include keyboards, the mouse, display screens, and audio devices. Some psychological and environmental problems involved with user interfaces, however, often cause problems when implementing a system. A great deal of attention has been given to these problems over the years.

Healthcare professionals have long agreed that entering patient data into computers is tedious and time consuming (McKenna, 2003). Nowadays data are often captured with a minimum of human intervention, and wearable technology is changing the negative attitudes of physicians and other healthcare personnel toward self-input of data. They understand that the computer allows fast and effective retrieval and analysis of the information; however, the interfaces between humans and computers and between computers and computers remain a concern. Information must be presented in ways that users quickly understand. There should be a minimum of puzzlement time. The effective presentation of information is related to visual format, generic organization, and compatibility of vocabulary.

QUALITY CHECKLIST

Wiederhold and Shortliffe (2006: 259–260) list some basic parameters for a successful computer information system implementation:

1. Quality and style of interface
2. Convenience
3. Speed and response
4. Reliability
5. Security
6. Integration

The implementation project was successful if it was:

1. On *time*: The system is up and running by the date as projected in the timeline.
2. On *budget*: The cost was as forecasted and given a reasonable leeway.
3. Of high *quality*: The system functions as intended, and the performance is smooth and acceptable to the users.

Finally, always remember this difficult fact of life: the actual implementation usually does not go exactly as planned. Careful planning and good lines of communication can minimize the likelihood that total disaster occurs.

Managing Change

The deployment of information technology is not always totally successful in any industry, including healthcare. All too often in the history of information technology, there has been a lack of a true understanding of the human factors when systems were planned and implemented. This understanding is critical, especially when it comes to healthcare system implementation, because the decision-making of the clinician is intrinsically interwoven with how the technology is used and how the results are interpreted (Goldstein et al., 2007).

It is to be expected that people will resist change. People will automatically be sensitive about their job responsibilities and any apparent threat to their well-being. Change must be carefully planned. Implementing change involves more than technology. It involves politics and human sociological factors. People have their own agendas, conflicting priorities, and needs, and most are uneasy about change. Research suggests that "a failure to discover, describe, and address both technical and social problems during health information systems design is likely to result in poor system performance and low acceptance" (Irestig and Timpka, 2008: 12).

The system's team must always be sensitive to the importance of user acceptance of the system. According to Anderson and Aydin (2005: 2), "Despite the fact that they are technologically sound, more than half of medical information systems fail due to user and staff resistance." Complex information systems are used by humans, who also are complex and often filled initially with uneasiness. Several general types of resistance to change can occur when new information systems are implemented. One is resistance to the environment. People want to just keep doing what they are comfortable with. Related to this is resistance to organizational change, which might mean being shifted to another department or to a new supervisor. Sometimes personnel don't like the "changers" themselves, for various reasons, and this is reflected in their resistance to proposed changes. Finally, resistance can be very specific, for example, not wanting to change from one type of computer to another (Lorenzi, Riley, and Dewan, 2001).

Environmental changes are related to the general ambiance of the situation and the associated infrastructure of the organization and its general functions. New systems, manual or automated, change work routines and often change relationships among personnel. Perceived radical change makes people worry about their roles and even about their own viability in a new environment. Sometimes proposed changes bring to the surface personal conflicts, and individuals or groups may oppose simply because they object to any suggestions made by certain other individuals or groups. Also, some individuals may believe a specific change is "just the wrong way to go" and will resist on a perceived sense of right or wrong.

Automated systems require users to standardize their actions, and often healthcare professionals resist this because they feel it infringes on their reliance on their professional judgments in decision making. Lorenzi, Riley, and Dewan (2001: 1304) list a number of reasons why physicians resist information technology changes:

1. Perceived low personal benefits
2. Fear of loss of status
3. Fear of revealing ignorance
4. Fear of an imposed discipline
5. Fear of wasted time
6. Fear of unwanted accountability
7. Fear of new demands

Technology is only one element of implementing a new system. Systems involve people, who can make or break the success of the new system. Never be surprised when there is resistance. "Experience tells us that motivated, involved people can make bad systems work. After all, they have done it for years. In the same way, unmotivated—or, even worse, negative motivated—people can bring the best system to its knees" (Lorenzi, Riley, and Dewan, 2001: 1304).

Evaluation of an Information System

The purpose of system evaluation is to determine the effectiveness, efficiency, and value of the new system by careful study and appraisal. Evaluation is done in order to determine how good the new system is, and the informatics professional's work is not complete until such evaluations are made. A good or bad system is not the result of a single component but of many factors, including hardware, software, human judgment, and economic constraints.

The system will go through various stages of quality assurance. Whether a system is designed within the organization or purchased, it must be implemented on a trial basis to test that it meets the objectives and the design specifications established before the final implementation. The testing process can be informal or extremely rigorous, depending on the time and money available and on the demands of the organization. Once the system is installed and has been operating for a reasonable period of time, inferences can be made about its performance, reliability, and capacity to deliver the benefits anticipated. Testing is something that is done before, during, and after implementation.

Evaluation starts at the beginning when you decide what the system should do and list the functions and benefits expected from the system. For each functional subdivision and component at a given level of analysis, quantitative characteristics can be identified, such as the volume of work, the amount of time, the cost, and the number of errors. Statistics on utilization give a quantitative picture of how the system is being utilized.

And after the immediate postimplementation testing has been completed, it is necessary to follow up and continually review the operation with all operating personnel involved. Particular attention should be paid to the problems they have experienced and to the corrective measures they recommend.

One of the functions of follow-up evaluation is to isolate the causes of system malfunctions. A world of caution: if things go wrong, the staff will quickly blame the new system rather than admit to any mistakes on their part. Experience shows that only gradually, as operating personnel become more familiar with the system, do they begin to observe that system malfunctions may be the result of their own mistakes.

Throughout the life of a system, it requires routine management and maintenance. From the moment the new system is implemented, obsoleteness sets in. This is why we speak of systems as having a finite life cycle. If the system is designed well, however, it will be optimal for its destined lifetime.

THE ROLE OF THE LIBRARY

Health sciences libraries play a vital role throughout the healthcare industry, including the application of information technology. This manifests itself in two basic ways. First, health sciences libraries are a portal to the research literature, providing fast access to current information on developments in the healthcare field. Second, health science librarians are effective information technology consultants in the acquisition and implementation of information technology.

Health sciences libraries are full of knowledgeable and expert advisors, yet the healthcare information systems literature reveals a deficiency of discussion of the role of the library. This should be seen as a challenge. Health science librarians are well equipped to address questions such as: Do we need to integrate knowledge resources in healthcare information management systems? When and where are knowledge resources needed? What types of interfaces are required? The quality of patient care depends on the effectiveness of the information systems and on the professionals who manage these systems, and this includes health sciences librarians.

SUMMARY

Health information management systems play a key role in healthcare. It is the most sensible approach for today's complex health enterprise. Selecting and implementing a healthcare information management system requires a combination of technological knowledge, the ability to manage people, and an understanding of the objectives and the outcomes expected. It is essential to consult experienced professionals in similar healthcare organizations, and to study current industry and technology trends. Above all, throughout the process, base decisions on user information needs.

REFERENCES

Anderson, James G. and Carolyn E. Aydin, eds. 2005. *Evaluating the Organizational Impact of Healthcare Information Systems,* 2nd ed. New York: Springer Science Business Media.

Coile, Russell C., Jr. 2001. *The Paperless Hospital: Healthcare in a Digital Age.* Chicago: Health Administration Press.

Cowan, Daniel F., ed. 2005. *Informatics for the Clinical Laboratory: A Practical Guide.* New York: Springer-Verlag.

Felkey, Bill G., Brent I. Fox, and Margaret R. Thrower. 2006. *Health Care Informatics: A Skills-Based Resource.* Washington, DC: American Pharmacists Association.

Goldstein, Douglas E., Peter J. Groen, Suniti Ponkshe, and Marc Wine. 2007. *Medical Informatics 20/20.* Sudbury, MA: Jones and Bartlett Publishers.

Haux, Reinhold, Alfred Winter, Elske Ammenwerth, and Birgit Brigl. 2004. *Strategic Information Management in Hospitals: An Introduction to Hospital Information Systems.* New York: Springer-Verlag.

Irestig, Magnus and Toomas Timpka. 2008. "Politics and Technology in Health Information Systems Development: A Discourse and Analysis of Conflicts Addressed in a Systems Design Group." *Journal of Biomedical Informatics* 44, no. 1 (February): 82–94.

Krabbel, Anita and Ingrid Wetzel. 2000. *Hospital Information Systems.* Hershey, PA: Idea Group Publishing. Available: www.idea-group.com/downloads/excerpts/armoni. pdf (accessed December 27, 2008).

Leicht, Michael and Vicki Sauter. "Managing User Expectations." St. Louis: University of Missouri St. Louis (1999). Available: www.umsl.edu/~sauterv/analysis/user_ expectations.html (accessed December 27, 2008).

Leiner, Florian, Wilhelm Gaus, Reinhold Haux, and Petra Knaup-Gregori. 2003. *Medical Data Management: A Practical Guide.* New York: Springer-Verlag.

Leviss, Jonathan, Richard Kremsdorf, and Mariam Mohaideen. 2006. "The CMIO— A New Leader for Health Systems." *Journal of the American Medical Informatics Association* 13, no. 5 (September–October): 573–578.

Lorenzi, Nancy M., Robert T. Riley, and Naakesh A Dewan. 2001. "Barriers and Resistance to Informatics in Behavioral Health." In *MEDINFO.* Amsterdam: IOS Press.

McKenna, Mindi K. 2003. *High Tech Medicine: Building Your Medical Practice with Computers and the Internet.* Kansas City, MO: Fordham University Press.

Sittig, Dean, Brian L. Hazlehurst, Ted Palen, John Hsu, Holly Jimison, and Marc C. Hornbrook. 2002. "A Clinical Information System Research Landscape." *Permanente Journal* 6, no. 2 (Spring). Available: http://xnet.kp.org/permanentejournal/spring02/landscape.html (accessed December 27, 2008).

Tan, Joseph K.H. 2001. *Health Management Information Systems. Methods and Practical Applications*, 2nd ed. Gaithersburg, MD: Aspen Publishers.

Wickramasinghe, Nilmini, Jatinder N.D.Gupta, and Sushil K. Sharma. 2005. *Creating Knowledge-based Healthcare Organizations.* Hershey, PA: Idea Group Publishing.

Wiederhold, Gio and Edward H. Shortliffe. 2006. "System Design and Engineering in Health Care." In *Biomedical Informatics: Computer Applications in Health Care and Biomedicine* (pp. 233–264), 3rd ed., edited by Edward H. Shortliffe and James J. Cimino. New York: Springer.

Chapter 10

Medical Imaging

Imaging is one of the fastest growing segments of healthcare. In a few decades the field has evolved from various applications of basic X-rays to an enormous range of devices, techniques, and applications. One of the intriguing developments is *digital* imaging, which has revolutionized the storage and transport of images. This chapter describes the background and current status of medical imaging.

INTRODUCTION

Imaging is the application of information technologies and bodies of techniques to manage visual images. It is the processes by which visual images are captured, edited, enhanced, stored, retrieved and transformed, and today they are appearing more and more in digital form. Imaging is widely used throughout modern society, including surveillance cameras, satellites, Mars land rovers, bar codes, bank checks, and X-rays. It can be simple when it is a bar code but complex when it is a pilot training with a virtual reality simulator (Cleveland and Cleveland, 2001). Hardly any sector of society is exempt from image processing. We encounter it throughout the day, and seemingly we are becoming an image-based information society. A floodgate of imaging is opening, brought on by new multimedia technologies and global networking. Text, voice, audio, graphics, images, and animation are being integrated into heterogeneous packages, and this has presented new challenges to find a way to organize these packages in an effective way.

The information technology advances in the past decade have brought many changes, including a rapid rise in visual databases and digitized imaging. With the Web helping to usher in a new age for visual information, the rapid increase of digitized resources is changing our concepts of information storage and retrieval.

The new digital technologies and applications have also become a part of the healthcare world. The move to digitization is one of the most significant technological breakthroughs in the history of the healthcare profession. Of course, images have always been a part of healthcare, going back to classical anatomical drawings related to the human body and to disease. Many of these drawings were masterpieces of illustration, albeit not always totally accurate.

Medical imaging deals with complex sets of tools, technology, and procedures to manage images for healthcare services, education, and research. It supports all healthcare services, regardless of the specialty or setting of health provision, including doctors' offices, clinics, hospitals, and telemedicine sites. It is closely related to a number of other modalities and technologies, both inside and outside of the healthcare area. It has borrowed from other fields, such as mining, seismology, and cartoon animation (Moe, 2003). It overlaps with related fields, such as biological imaging, biomedical engineering, medical physics, and radiology.

Medical imaging provides a method for finding, identifying, and diagnosing disease and in some instances provides interventional treatment. Medical imaging allows healthcare professionals to see into the living body, with a minimum of physical invasive procedures. Details about the inner structures and real-time functions of the body can help provide specific diagnoses, leading to appropriate treatment plans and patient monitoring. When it comes to medical imaging, the cliché that a picture is worth a thousand words is certainly true.

Most of the time, imaging procedures are easy and painless for the patient, although the patient has to be very still. The exposure to radiation varies greatly based on types of equipment and imaging modalities.

Imaging techniques and procedures continue to advance at a rapid rate. Many new technologies, procedures, and research involving imaging have occurred in the past ten years, and they are of major interest in health informatics.

MEDICAL IMAGING BASICS

Medical imaging as a specialty incorporates technologies developed by numerous sciences to harness the forces of magnetic fields, high-frequency sound waves, X-rays, gamma rays, and others to capture, store, and present images of the organs and other internal structures of the body. It is used to detect and diagnose disease. When used as treatment, it is called *interventional radiology*. According to Sorantin (2008: 1276), medical imaging "consists of the following steps: (1) data acquisition, (2) data (image) processing, (3) further data processing by the computer graphic system, (4) image display, and finally (5) visual perception and interpretation."

Two basic types of medical imaging are structural imaging and functional imaging. Structural imaging deals with the physical structures of the body, and functional imaging deals with metabolic processes. Structural imaging provides information about the physical organization of the body, showing abnormalities, which allows the physician to extrapolate to an explanation of the situation.

Until recently, most functional conclusions were inferred from viewing structural images and correlating with other tests and observations.

In the past few years molecular imaging has allowed real-time observation of metabolic processes as they occur. For example, functional magnetic resonance imaging (discussed later) allows observation of metabolic changes in the brain as a subject performs specific cognitive activities.

Most images are two dimensional, but advances are being made in three-dimensional imaging. Three-dimensional images present an illusion of depth and provide a more realistic view of the structures and functions of the body.

Most medical imaging is structural imaging, and advancements are made as we try to obtain better views of the body's structures. However, no single modality satisfies all of the diagnostics needs. Various situations require different kinds of imaging modalities. In the past few years, two of the important changes have been the shift of images from static pictures of anatomy and functions to real-time views, sometimes with movement, and the generation of graphs, maps, and details extracted from digital images and synthesized for the healthcare provider.

DIGITAL IMAGING

An increasing number of imaging modalities are digital. Traditional film modalities are still widespread, but there is a steady movement toward the digital format.

In basic terms, a digital image is usually a bit-map in a computer. The bit-map is an array of numbers that represent the intensity in an image in a small area of a picture, which is called a *pixel.* The pixels may also indicate color. These condensed pixels are scanned on a metalevel by the human eye and are interpreted by the brain as an image. This is similar to the multidots that convey an image in print formats, such as a newspaper.

Digital images can be created directly when the image is captured, or they can be created by converting existing analog images. The advantage is that images in digital format can be manipulated just like any computer data. To the computer, an image is just numbers to be manipulated; it is immaterial if the numbers represent text or images.

Digital imaging is the preferred tool for many reasons. Digital processes (1) allow noise-free and therefore better quality data; (2) capture data over time, which allows patient monitoring; and (3) store and manipulate data more efficiently and effectively. Digital imaging has reduced the cost and physical space needed for storage and has cut down on the time needed to process traditional film-based images. Even more important, because the digital format allows computer management of the images, the images can be accessed and transmitted globally with great speed (Greenes and Brinkley, 2006).

Digital images are durable and do not deteriorate over time because of chemical or other environmental factors. They are much easier to manipulate in terms of reshaping, cropping, enhancing color, reducing/magnifying, compressing for electronic transmission, and so forth. They can be copied without affecting the original. Digital images can be linked to other records such as textual resources and database repositories of image catalogs. These catalogs generally contain collections of similar images, allowing the healthcare provider to make comparisons. Digital images can be transmitted via the Internet, over local area networks and wireless networks, and by cell phones (Indrajit and Verma, 2007).

The number of digitally produced medical images is steadily growing. Some images are still being converted from analog items, but many more are being initially created in digital form.

IMAGING AND MEDICAL PRACTICE

Medical imaging plays a pivotal role in modern healthcare and is ubiquitous throughout the healthcare structure. Over 380 million radiological examinations are performed each year in the United States (Gunderman, 2005). Medical imaging has become an indispensable tool in clinical diagnosis and therapy, health sciences classrooms, and research labs. New hospital and clinical information system designs now usually integrate digital radiology systems into the electronic health record. This allows image viewing at distributed computer workstations, both locally and remotely.

In the daily practice of medicine, healthcare providers want to see the images themselves, often expecting to do their own verification of the interpretations accompanying the images. They want the images to be of the highest quality and, when appropriate, to be integrated into the electronic health records.

Imaging Acquisition Modalities

Modalities are the different medical imaging techniques that are used to acquire images. Most modalities produce two-dimensional images, particularly in the clinical environment, but the use of three-dimensional imaging is increasing and is opening new avenues for research and applications. Virtual reality systems are an obvious example, but three-dimensional methods are being applied to other important applications, such as modeling and simulation.

X-RAYS

Internal body imaging began with X-rays over a century ago and revolutionized surgery and medical practice in general. An X-ray machine works by sending electromagnetic radiation to a targeted region of the body. The radiation passes through to an X-ray film on the other side. Denser objects, such as bones and tumors, absorb more radiation, and as a result these appear as white objects on the developed film. The less dense material appears as black or gray areas, thus highlighting the desired target for observation. Now these images can be converted into digital form for storage, viewing, and transporting.

COMPUTED TOMOGRAPHY

Computed tomography (CT), or computed axial tomography (CAT), was developed in the 1970s. The CAT scan, as it is commonly called, uses an X-ray beam to take a cross-sectional picture of the body, including the soft tissues and blood vessels. These pictures are called *tomographs*, derived from the Greek word that means "slices," like a slice of bread. The X-ray beam is mounted on a wheel that rotates around the subject. Because it is taking pictures from all angles, bones and soft tissues do not block the view. A contrast media may be injected into the bloodstream to produce better images of the areas of concern. The computer combines a number of these cross-sectional images into a multi-dimensional view of the internal organs. CAT scans contain more subtle contrasts than simple X-ray images because of the computer-based algorithmic processing.

NUCLEAR MEDICINE MODALITIES

Nuclear medicine has emerged as an important component of healthcare and has major applications in imaging. Nuclear medicine utilizes radioactive isotopes to locate, diagnose, and treat diseases. Nuclear medicine is based on the principle that a radioactive element has energy that is unstable, and, in its effort to reach a more stable state, its nucleus emits excess energy in the form of radiation (Moe, 2003). The radiation then allows images to be created and captured. Examples of applications are magnetic resonance imaging (MRI), functional magnetic resonance imaging (fMRI), and positron emission tomography (PET).

MRI technology involves a mixture of magnets, atoms, radiofrequency, imaging techniques, and computers (Moe, 2003). In 1976, Dr. Raymond Damadian developed the first MRI scanner. MRI creates detailed images of the structures and functions of the visual subject from any plane or viewpoint. MRI scanners create a strong magnetic field around the subject, and forces spin hydrogen atoms in the body's tissues to align themselves with the magnetic field. Pulses of radio waves at a special frequency then add energy to those hydrogen atoms, which are forced to spin in a slightly different direction. When the hydrogen atoms realign themselves with the magnetic field, they give off the extra energy, which is detected and transformed into an image. These images have greater soft tissue contrast than CTs, allowing more in-depth analysis, and can actually be used to measure various metabolisms in body tissues.

An advanced model of MRI, called fMRI, can do such things as recognize blood flow and thus capture functions in real time. The "f" stands for *functional,* because it shows living tissues in action, not just as static pictures. For example, a scan of the brain can show which part of the brain is active when something is going on, and this opens up a world of possibilities for research and diagnosis (Cleveland, 2005).

PET works by injecting isotopes into the subject, creating three-dimensional color pictures. The radioactive isotopes give off a positron, a tiny piece of antimatter. When this positron collides with an electron in the tissues, the two particles annihilate each other and give off a gamma ray, a very powerful electromagnetic pulse that can be detected by the scanner. An important advantage of a PET scan is that it reveals metabolic activities inside organs in real time, for example, blood flow or glucose metabolism. An even higher diagnostic accuracy can be achieved by combining PET scans with CT images.

Ultrasound

Ultrasound uses sound waves and their echoes to create images. It is acoustic energy with a frequency above human hearing. Diagnostic ultrasound scanners operate hundreds of times beyond the limit of human hearing, in a range of 2 to 18 megahertz. The scanners create images of muscles and internal organs in real time by bouncing high-frequency sound waves off the body structures being targeted for examination. No radiation is used in the ultrasound process, and the skill of the technician is vital to obtain an accurate image. Modern ultrasonic scanners can create three-dimensional images, and real-time body functions can be recorded for later computer-based observation. Ultrasound allows imaging of tissue structures on a large scale and is better at differentiating the boundaries between organs. The system works by picking up changes in the velocity of ultrasound as it moves from one tissue type to another, being highly sensitive to the macroscopic biological structures within tissues.

Fluoroscopy

Fluoroscopy is an X-ray–based technique that allows the health provider to view real-time images. The patient is placed between an X-ray source and a fluorescent screen. An X-ray beam moves through the patient and strikes the fluorescent plate, producing and image that is amplified for on-the-spot viewing. Contrast agents that are given to the patients help delineate anatomical structures and body functions. Fluoroscopy allows healthcare providers to see the body functioning in real time. Modern fluoroscopy systems record and save images for storage and later viewing.

Digital Angiography

Angiography is a radiological technique for studying blood vessels. When the technique is applied to the arteries, it produces an *arteriogram*. When applied to the veins, it produces a *venogram*. The basic procedure is to inject the patient with an iodinated compound and then to use X-rays to study the blood vessels. Conventional X-rays usually does not show the blood vessels very well. Angiography is commonly used to detect arteriosclerosis.

MAMMOGRAPHY

Mammography is a low-dose X-ray procedure for creating images of the human breast. Currently, mammography is the first choice of image screening for the early detection of breast cancer. It uses conventional film techniques, but there is a movement toward digital methods.

Digital mammography and film-screening mammography basically use the same techniques; the difference is that with digital imaging the results are sent directly to a computer where they can be enlarged, highlighted, and manipulated in other ways. Whether or not digital screening is more effective than film has been debated. Most studies in the past few years report that there is little difference in diagnostic abilities. A recent study concluded that "No statistical significance in sensitivity and specificity was observed between digitized images and mammograms for each breast composition. Original screen-film mammograms were observed to perform better than digitized images" (Liang et al., 2008).

ENDOSCOPY

Endoscopy is a visual light procedure that uses a tube—either flexible or rigid—and fiber optics to observe patients internally through the body's passageways. The light is reflected back to viewing lenses for real-time observation. The endoscope is also used to obtain tissue samples for biopsy tests, administer drugs, and perform irrigation. The tube may have a tiny camera for taking picture for later study or archiving.

Major Uses of Imaging in Healthcare

Images are used in a number of ways in healthcare. Major areas are diagnosis, assessment and treatment planning, and education and research.

DIAGNOSIS

Diagnosis is a fundamental objective in healthcare, and modern imaging is a powerful aid. Images are used in diagnosis primarily to identify abnormalities. If an image shows a suspicious abnormality, then other diagnostic methods are used to pinpoint a diagnosis. For example, an image may suggest a tumor, but then a biopsy will clarify the situation.

ASSESSMENT AND TREATMENT PLANNING

After diagnosis, images are used to track changes, benchmark treatments, and help revise prognosis. Real-time imaging is playing an increasingly important role in medical procedures, such as endoscopy and minimally invasive surgery.

One of the exciting developments in imaging is the capability for assessment and treatment planning through electronic communication and networking. Imaging and long distance eHealth are natural companions.

EDUCATION AND RESEARCH

Imaging is a major tool in education and research. Medical students utilize a wide range of image databases, online tutorials, case studies, three-dimensional models, and virtual reality programs. Images are used as visual aids in teaching anatomy and physiology. More and more health sciences students are accessing image databases to supplement their classroom studies. In research, MRI, fMRI, and PET allow real-time examination of bodily processes. For example, PET scans of the brain are allowing researchers to track the early development of Alzheimer's and other dementia diseases. Imaging is also being used to study pulmonary functions and disease and hearing disorders. Researchers are finding imaging a powerful tool for direct observations in medical research. Imaging is especially useful when combined with three-dimensional visualization and virtual reality systems.

MANAGING IMAGING INFORMATION

The combination of modern information technology and communication networks is allowing healthcare providers to connect with a variety of information systems in order to carry out all of the routines and procedures related to medical radiology. Clinicians can order imaging work from their desktops and/or wearable devices. The images can be processed and integrated with other information systems to enhance, store, and retrieve the images. Finally, the images, with accompanying interpretation, can be returned to the ordering clinician.

Image management is the processes, procedures, and policies related to organizing, storing, transmitting, displaying, and retrieving images. Such imaging management systems are called *picture archiving and communication systems* (PACS) and are discussed later in this chapter.

Image Manipulation

Since the beginning of photography, users have been interested in manipulating the images. Usually, images are manipulated, or altered, in an attempt to improve their quality. However, manipulated images can also be used to perpetrate fraud, for example, by placing an alternative head on a body. Before computer imaging software became available, retouching was done with ink, patching parts together, or, as in the case of Polaroids, scratching things out.

Medical images are manipulated to make them clearer and more revealing of a medical situation. Manipulations are made to increase sharpness and focus, enhance contrast, and alter colors to highlight abnormalities and relationships among the structures and functions being studied. Also, images can be resized, flipped, rotated, mirrored, and converted into different formats as needed for viewing, transporting, or archiving.

Color and texture are key elements of medical images. These two aspects can be related to the overall, global-level image or can be related to specific points in the graphic. Other elements include image segmentation and semantic interpretation. The latter deals with how users perceive the names of the items in the image and the relationships among the images.

The basic steps in imaging processing are the following:

1. Acquisition: Images are captured by some device, such as a CT or MRI scan.
2. Enhancement: Images are edited to improve their quality. This may include manipulating sharpness, contrast, and coloring.
3. Compression: Images are compressed, using computer algorithms and procedures, in order to reduce storage requirements.
4. Representation: Images are indexed and tagged to indicate content in order to integrate the images into information archiving and retrieval systems.

Image Transport

Images need to be transported from point of creation to point of use, often to multiple sites of use. Traditionally, X-rays were put into an envelope and delivered by courier or in hand by the patient. Today's technology allows instant electronic transport from creation point to the appropriate healthcare professional, and this requires standardized methods for formatting and transporting.

Medical standards, in general, deal with the procedures used to diagnose and treat diseases and health problems and to provide healthcare. Information transport standards deal with formatting and protocols for electronically exchanging information, including images.

There are many information standards, and the two most widely known health standards are Health Level Seven (HL7) and Digital Imaging and Communications in Medicine (DICOM). HL7 is a standard for exchanging electronic information among disparate health systems. It focuses on the exchange of clinical as well as administrative data and information. This is a transmission standard and is not concerned with the nature of the content of the message. The "Level Seven" indicates the application level of the International Organization for Standardization (ISO) procedures for establishing standards.

The standard's original purpose was to establish a common data exchange standard among diversified hospital computer applications in order to improve the efficiency and costs of programming activities needed to maintain these operations. The mission of HL7 (Health Level 7, 1997) is described as follows:

HL7 provides standards for interoperability that improve care delivery, optimize workflow, reduce ambiguity and enhance knowledge transfer among all of our stakeholders, including healthcare providers, government agencies, the vendor community, fellow SDOs and patients.

HL7 is maintained by an international group of healthcare experts, informatics professionals, and related persons who collaborate in creating protocols and formats for the exchange of electronic healthcare information. HL7 aims to create flexible and cost-effective interoperability among healthcare systems. This standard has evolved through numerous versions, each one adjusting to the changes in technology and established information protocols.

The DICOM standard is the most common format for managing and transporting images, and it addresses technical interoperability issues in medical imaging. The DICOM standard was created by the National Electrical Manufacturers Association (NEMA), based in part on earlier imaging standards from the Association. Its purpose is to have a consistent format for distributing and viewing medical images.

Basically, the standard addresses file formatting and network communication protocols. DICOM allows full network capabilities, including the transfer of images, graphics, and textual reports. A simple DICOM image has a header with information about the patient, such as name, the type of scan, image dimension, and other basic information describing the particular image.

DICOM is having a major impact on communication management of digital medical imaging. "While the digital imaging revolution in radiology can be attributed to a number of factors, there is little doubt that the standards put forth by the Digital Imaging and Communications Standards in Medicine Committee serve as a major 'technology enabler' " (Oosterwijk, 2005: iii).

Image Organization, Storage, and Retrieval

The rapid and extensive growth of imaging in recent years was accompanied by the need for effective methods to store and retrieve images from archives. O'Sullivan et al. (2005) described it this way: "Recent advances in digital image capture and storage technologies have increased the problem of information overload in imagery task domains. As a consequence, intelligent application support is needed to help manage imagery tasks."

Image Indexing

Image indexing is based on the old adage that a picture is worth a thousand words—that even a great amount of descriptive text cannot convey as much understanding as actually viewing the image. Image indexing is a difficult task. Efficient retrieval of biomedical images requires robust and effective indexing procedures. The nature of the wide-ranging image material in medicine is complex and requires specialized adoption of general indexing procedures to the process.

The problem is how to choose the relevant information content from a multitude of possible facets for representation. The larger problem is how to select images with the needed information from a large, heterogeneous collection of images, often numbering in the thousands for a specific topic. The basic theoretical difficulties in indexing images are "(1) images do not satisfy the requirements of a language whereas textual materials do, (2) images contain layers of meaning that can only be converted into textual language using human indexing, and (3) [because of the]multi-disciplinary nature of the images . . . the terms assigned are the only access points" (Neugebauer, 2005).

Once all the cognitive and environmental attributes have been identified, the next task is to filter the information and turn it into content indicators in the form of an index. The content of medical images is highly specialized requiring adapted indexing procedures. There are three basic approaches to indexing images: textual indexing, content-based indexing, and context-based indexing. In practice, all three approaches may be used at the same time. These three facets are related to *all* domains of imaging, including medical imaging.

TEXTUAL INDEXING

Traditionally, images were indexed largely by adapting textual indexing procedures developed around the idea of concept indexing. Indexing involved human indexers using controlled vocabularies to describe the physical characteristics and information content in the images. Many controlled vocabularies tools were developed, such as the *Art & Architecture Thesaurus*. The thesauri of the Library of Congress and the National Library of Medicine formed the basis of the vocabulary used in the medical sciences. The indexing results were then moved into metadata structures, which placed the images into related physical and intellectual categories for storage and retrieval.

There are many shortcomings to the textual indexing method. A major one is that the uniqueness of individual images is lost. As Jörgensen (2003: 97) stated, we "need to preserve the uniqueness of the object or image . . . while providing access to the object through some type of constrained vocabulary within an information retrieval system." Capturing the *aboutness* and *level of meanings* in the object being indexed has always been a concern in textual indexing, but this concern became acute when applied to indexing images.

Another challenge in using textual indexing procedures is to achieve sufficient depth and specificity. The greater the depth and specificity achieved, the more time, effort, and money will have been spent. These concerns, among others, have resulted in new approaches to indexing images.

Healthcare providers and researchers need to find images based on the features of the images, in other words, on the content of the images. This has led to what is called *content-based image retrieval.*

Content-based image retrieval does not rely on metadata, such as keywords, to find the image. It relies on actual pieces of image content, such as shape or color—any appropriate information that can be derived directly from the image itself. Images involve such things as textural and cognitive attributes that come through several sensorial inputs. In text indexing the source is the printed word, but an image source is richer; therefore, content-based indexing enhances cognitive understanding of the image. This method is being rapidly adopted for digital imaging.

Content-based indexing uses techniques and algorithms adapted from computer visual applications, pattern recognition, and statistics. Automatic content-based indexing of images is done with software written specifically for this task and can be tied to Internet search tools. Most of the work to this point on content-based indexing has concentrated on similarity-based retrieval for constructing search engines to match scientific images. Content-based systems work well when the images are relatively stable in terms of shape, color, and texture but do not work as well when these characteristics are not maintained consistently over time, as in videos and other streaming images.

Although commercial software packages for content-based image retrieval are being developed for general imaging, according to the National Library of Medicine (Antani, Longa, and Thoma, 2008) this has not happened yet for medical images:

> Content-based Image Retrieval (CBIR) for medical images has received a significant research interest over the past decade as a promising approach to address the data management challenges posed by the rapidly increasing volume of medical image data in use. Articles published in the literature detail the benefits and present impressive results to substantiate potential impact of the technology. However, the benefits have yet to make it to mainstream clinical, biomedical research, or educational use. No major commercial software tools are available for use in medical imaging products.

For the image databases now coming online to be used to their fullest potential, it is necessary to develop effective and efficient database management techniques, especially in the retrieval of data and information based on the content of the databases. "To do so, effective techniques for feature representation and data management are required, and images must be suitably organized for rapid retrieval based on their contents" (Leung, 1999: 463).

CONTEXT-BASED INDEXING

An image is more than just its overt content. It was created in a specific environment, including the activities and tasks shown in the image and the reasons why the image was produced. The aim of context-based retrieval is to use this environmental information, or context, to enhance the accuracy of the retrieval results. Context-based image indexing does not replace textual or content-based image indexing; rather, it enhances the meaning of the image by providing further background and source information. For example, knowing the research lab or the medical researcher who created the image would be useful for some users.

Sometimes describing the content of an image can be more complex than describing the content of text. It can be difficult to reach a consensus on what certain images are about and what they represent. Identifying the objects in images is not the major problem. The major problem is how to represent their meanings. Debate continues regarding exactly which image attributes should be emphasized and indexed.

AUTOMATIC EXTRACTION OF IMAGING REPORTS

Methods to automatically extract information from medical reports, including image information, are being actively discussed, researched, and applied. Radiological reports include not only images but also textual information about the medical situation. These reports are usually stored as unstructured free text. Keyword tagging and query formulation are often insufficient to capture the specific information that the healthcare provider needs. This fact, plus the enormous volume of information being searched, often makes retrieval difficult and time consuming when retrospective information is needed.

Automatic extracting and data mining techniques are being developed to address this issue. Current research and development are yielding more sophisticated and effective tools for data mining from images. This is an exciting area of research and possible applications.

Image Access

Images are archived and subsequently retrieved for use. This is a relatively straightforward procedure when images related to a specific patient are needed. The tags assigned for that specific patient are entered, and the images are retrieved. Archiving and retrieving images is much broader and complex than this, however, because most images are not of particular patients. Physicians need to see images related to the case at hand, such as ones showing different diseases when contemplating differential diagnoses. In fact, most medical images are unrelated to specific patients. Therefore, effective image storage and access systems are needed for images in general.

It is natural to attempt to use text retrieval techniques. Two basic principles in information retrieval are that a feature frequent in a document describes that document well and that a feature frequent in the collection is a weak indicator to distinguish documents from each other (Müller et al., 2004). A picture of Abraham Lincoln might be described as a man with a beard wearing a tall black hat. That describes that particular image very well. However, if a general collection of images is searched using "man with a beard and wearing a tall hat," thousands of such pictures will be retrieved, most of which are not of Abraham Lincoln.

In text information retrieval, the basic concept is to cluster objects with similar content in order to satisfy a user's query regarding a certain topic. If the clustering is based on very specific details, it will yield a more closely related set of documents. This is called *retrieval precision*. If the clustering is based on a broad set of concepts, it will bring in more documents. This is called *retrieval recall*. Items are stored and queries are formed with these two principles in mind. Similar principles are applied to the storage and retrieval of medical images. Often, clinicians turn to imaging databases because, for the "clinical decision-making process it can be beneficial or even important to find other images of the same modality [or] the same anatomic region of the same disease" (Müller et al., 2004: 6). In other words, the classical information retrieval model is still valid for images, albeit with some important differences.

Traditionally, techniques commonly used in text database searches have been used to retrieve images. Image records are assigned fields for the artist or photographer, a title, the date produced, and so forth, including one with descriptive text. Keyword and Boolean operators are then used to search. Content-based image indexing is similar to textual based indexing in other ways, too. For example, both normally deal with large databases. Also, there is a high degree of uncertainty on the part of the users of image databases, requiring effective feedback for relevancy.

Most current image searches are based on either similarities of appearances, such as low-level features like color and shape, or natural language textual querying, where similarity is determined by comparing words in a query against words in semantic image metadata tags. The biggest problem arising from these techniques is the so-called semantic gap (Hollink et al., 2004), the mismatch between the capabilities of the retrieval systems and the user's needs (O'Sullivan et al., 2005).

Some systems enter the database via text from the patient record or a research study, while other systems use a set of descriptor terms, either free text or from a controlled thesaurus. Relying on text as the starting point of a database search may not be the best way, because it is quite possible that the text does not necessarily define the image content. The image itself may carry information not explicit in the text. According to Müller, "The combination of textual with visual features or content and context of the images does have the most potential to lead to good results. One can also be used to control the quality of the other or to obtain a better recall of the retrieval results" (Müller et al., 2004: 10). The combination of textual and visual feature descriptions can yield more successful results.

Formulating an effective query is key to successfully accessing information, something that librarians have known for centuries. At the same time, it is not a simple, straightforward procedure because of the vagaries of language and the difficulty some people have when expressing themselves. When query formulation involves images, the problems are magnified.

Image Quality

Producing quality images is a major challenge. To be useful, medical images must allow the healthcare provider to detect very subtle details. He or she often must decide if an anomaly is an actual body pathology or simply a glitch in the image itself. Quality control procedures, including precise measurements and definitions of image quality can help avoid such situations.

Three types of resolution affect image quality. First is the sharpness of the image, which is called *spatial resolution.* Second is the differentiation of small differences in intensity, called *control resolution.* The third is, the amount of time it took to create the image, called *temporal resolution.* Very high temporal resolution images can capture physical events, such as heart beating and blood flow.

PICTURE ARCHIVING AND COMMUNICATION SYSTEMS

A picture archiving and communication system (PACS) is a method of image management. According to Dreyer, Mehta, and Thrall (2002: 4), "This technology encompasses such elements as workstations, archives, networks, and acquisition devices that enable the digital creation, transfer, and storage of medical data."

A PACS is an electronic system that stores, retrieves, distributes, and presents images for healthcare services and research. PACSs are now part of the fundamental technological infrastructure supporting radiology practices. PACSs are composed of technologies, people, and policies. Image capturing modalities, processing hardware and software, and storage devices are networked with one or more computer systems.

Radiologists, hospitals, and other healthcare providers and organizations are moving from analog to digital radiography, albeit somewhat slowly. The transition depends on both the creation of advanced technologies and the financial ability to purchase them. The technologies have come a long way in the past few years, but cost is still a major obstacle. Hoyt, Sutton, and Yoshihashi (2007: 208) highlight a number of basic issues related to PACSs:

- Initially hospitals purchased film digitizers so routine x-ray film could be converted to the digital format.
- Now digital images go from the scanning device *directly* into the PACS.
- PACS usually has a central server that serves as the image repository and multiple client computers linked with a local or wide area network (LAN or WAN).
- Images are stored using the Digital Imaging and Communications in Medicine (DICOM) standard.
- PACS is made possible by faster processors, higher resolution monitors, more robust hospital information systems, better servers and faster Internet connections. PACS is also aided by voice recognition to expedite report turnaround.
- Input into PACS can also be from a teleradiology site via satellite.
- Most monitors are still grayscale as they have better resolution (3–5 megapixels on a standard desktop monitor).
- It is estimated that about 25–30 percent of hospitals now have PACS.

PACSs continue to evolve, with more and more enhancements. According to Valenza, "PACS is not just about image archiving anymore. The latest PACS trends are providing radiologists with more automatic image processing, integrated enterprise workflow, and the ability to seamlessly share images with anyone, anywhere in the world" (Valenza, 2008).

EMERGING IMAGING TECHNOLOGIES

If healthcare professionals 50 years ago had been able to read about medical technology in our time, they would have thought they were reading highly imaginable science fiction, particularly regarding medical imaging, and what is ahead looks even more exciting. Medical imaging is developing into one of the most important areas of healthcare. To many, medical imaging is the most promising and exciting area in healthcare.

The future will bring extensive developments in networking, which will allow a global PACS for immediate medical decision making around the world. Truly integrated clinical information systems will contain transparently structured images driven by retrieval methods based on structured information, free text, and visual content. Future systems will have effective user-friendly communication interfaces for both input and output.

Advances are being made rapidly and are effecting changes in the practice of medicine. Gunderman (2005: 241) believes that "radiology is the medical community's paradigmatically visual discipline. Perhaps more than any other medical field except pathology, it has contributed to the objectification of patients and their diseases."

MEDICAL IMAGES AND THE HEALTH SCIENCES LIBRARIAN

Health sciences librarians are well positioned to be major players in the imaging revolution. To be used effectively images must be tagged, organized, archived, and then searched for and retrieved. Organizing information and developing ways to retrieve information is what librarians have always done and what they are trained to do. In today's imaging environment, they can become experts at developing, managing, and searching image databases. Librarians are thoroughly experienced with digital libraries containing images of millions of information artifacts.

Librarians also excel at database searching. Large repositories of medical images are available through the Internet. These images are used by healthcare providers to make diagnoses and to teach classes, and they are good study aids for students (Müller et al., 2004). Images illustrating practically every area of medicine and healthcare services can be found on the Internet.

Atlases are collections of images that, combined with symbolic representations, help illustrate and explain anatomy. These collections are being digitized, which enhances their quality and expands their usefulness. Atlases are used most extensively in medical education. Health sciences librarians use the following medical imaging databases and atlases to support healthcare providers:

INFORMATICS IN ACTION! 10.1

Training PACS Users

Location: Large medical center hospital

Problem: Hospital officials recently implemented a state-of-the-art PACS, and they are concerned about the way personnel are using the system. They suspect that inadequate training may be the problem.

People Involved: Hospital staff and the medical center library librarian.

Action Taken: Maria, the systems analyst/librarian in the medical center library, has years of experience in information technology applications, particularly in training and evaluation. She is appointed by the hospital officials to evaluate the situation. Maria discovers that personnel training consisted of a couple of hours of explanation by the vendor. She sets up an experiment. Maria divides new users of the PACS into two groups. The first group is given the current two-hour orientation. The second group is given an extensive three-day training course. After a month on the job, the two groups are tested for their level of knowledge and skills with the PACS. Those who took the three-day course have a much higher performance level. As a result, Maria recommends that all new employees be given the three-day course.

Takeaway: The medical center librarian's solution appears self-evident, but her controlled experiment provided documented evidence for the hospital officials.

Anatomy Atlases. Available: www.anatomyatlases.org (accessed January 11, 2009). According to the Web site, this is a "digital library of anatomy information and contains full color digitized books on anatomy and first aid. It is written for and intended primarily for use by Medical Students, Residents, Fellows, or Attending Physicians studying anatomy."

ARTstor. Available: www.artstor.org/index.shtml (accessed January 16, 2009). This collection contains hundreds of thousands of digital images and related data and includes tools for using the images. The images may be used "for noncommercial, educational and scholarly purposes."

Catalog of Clinical Images. Available: http://meded.ucsd.edu/clinicalimg (accessed January 16, 2009). This is a Web-based collection of physical examination findings.

Embryo Images: Normal and Abnormal Mammmalian Development. Available: www.med.unc.edu/embryo_images (accessed January 16, 2009). This database is used primarily to teach mammalian embryology.

Historical Anatomies on the Web. Available: www.nlm.nih.gov/exhibition/ historicalanatomies/home.html (accessed January 16, 2009). This site is "designed to give Internet users access to high quality images from important anatomical atlases in the National Library of Medicine's historical collection. Atlases and images were selected primarily for their historical and artistic significance."

Multi-Dimensional Human Embryo. Available: http://embryo.soad.umich. edu/index.html (accessed January 16, 2009). This database consists of three-dimensional images of the human embryo, created with MRI and is for students, researches, clinicians, and the general public.

Public Health InfoLinks: Medical/Health Image Collections. Available: www.sph.emory.edu/PHIL/PHILimage.php (accessed January 11, 2009). This general directory contains dozens of medical imaging databases of all kinds. The project can be viewed in several formats, including MRI and CT scans and photographs.

The Visible Human Project®. Available: www.nlm.nih.gov/research/visible/ visible_human.html (accessed January 16, 2009). One widely known online medical imaging tool is the Visible Human Project® from the National Library of Medicine (NLM). This tool is built on two- and three-dimensional digitized images of an anatomically complete man and woman. The NLM (2008) describes the project as:

> [T]he creation of complete, anatomically detailed, three-dimensional representations of the normal male and female human bodies. Acquisition of transverse CT, MR and cryosection images of representative male and female cadavers has been completed. The male was sectioned at one millimeter intervals, the female at one-third

of millimeter intervals. The long-term goal of the Visible Human Project® is to produce a system of knowledge structures that will transparently link visual knowledge forms to symbolic knowledge formats such as the names of body parts.

SUMMARY

This chapter summarized the major aspects of medical imaging. No area of the health sciences has been impacted more by information technology in the past few decades than imaging. The technology continues to develop at a fast pace. The challenges are not so much about the technology itself but about developing procedures and management systems for the increasing volume of images being produced and making them more accessible. For example, effective indexing of images is still at a somewhat primitive stage and needs much attention. The future is bright for medical imaging. All areas of health informatics offer windows of opportunities, but probably nowhere is this more obvious and exciting than in the area of imaging.

REFERENCES

Antani, Semeer, L. Rodney Longa, and George R. Thoma. "Bridging the Gap: Enabling CBIR in Medical Applications." Bethesda, MD: U.S. National Library of Medicine, National Institutes of Health (February, 2008). Available: http://archive.nlm.nih.gov/pubs/ceb2008/2008011.pdf (accessed January 16, 2009).

Cleveland, Donald. 2005. *How Do We Know How the Brain Works?* New York: The Rosen Publishing Group.

Cleveland, Donald B. and Ana D. Cleveland. 2001. *Introduction to Indexing and Abstracting,* 3rd ed. Englewood, CO: Libraries Unlimited.

Dreyer, Keith, Ainit Mehta, and James H. Thrall. 2002. *PACS: A Guide to the Digital Revolution.* New York: Springer.

Greenes, Robert A., and James Brinkley. 2006. "Imaging Systems in Radiology." In *Biomedical Informatics: Computer Applications in Health Care and Biomedicine* (pp. 626–659), 3rd ed., edited by Edward H. Shortliffe and James J. Cimino. New York: Springer.

Gunderman, Richard B. 2005. "The Medical Community's Vision of the Patient: The Importance of Radiology." *Radiology* 234, no. 4 (February): 339–342.

Health Level Seven. 1997. "Mission Statement." Washington, DC: Health Level Seven, Inc. Available: www.hl7.org (accessed January 9, 2009).

Hollink, Laura, Guus Schreiber, Bob Wielinga, and Marcel Worring. 2004. "Classification of User Image Descriptions." *International Journal of Human Computer Studies* 61, no. 5 (November): 601–626.

Hoyt, Robert, Melanie Sutton, and Ann Yoshihashi. 2007. *Medical Informatics: Practical Guide for the Healthcare Professional.* Pensacola: University of West Florida.

Indrajit, I.K. and B.S. Verma. 2007. "Digital Imaging in Radiology Practice: An Introduction to a Few Fundamental Concepts." *Indian Journal of Radiology Imaging*
17, no. 4 (November): 230–236.

Jörgensen, Corinne. 2003. *Image Retrieval.* Lanham, MD: The Scarecrow Press.

Leung, Clement. 1999. "Introduction." *Image and Vision Computing* 17, no. 7 (May):
463–464.

Liang, Zhigang, Xiangying Du, Jiabin Liu, Xinyu Yao, Yanhui Yang, and Kuncheng Li.
2008. "Comparison of Diagnostic Accuracy of Breast Masses Using Digitized
Images Versus Screen-film Mammography." *Acta Radiologica* 49, no. 6 (July):
618–622.

Moe, Barbara. 2003. *The Revolution in Medical Imaging.* New York: The Rosen Publishing Group.

Müller, Henning, Nicholas Michiux, David Brandon, and Antoine Geissbuhler. 2004.
"A Review of Content-based Image Retrieval Systems in Medical Applications—
Clinical Benefits and Future Directions." *International Journal of Medical Infor-
matics* 73, no. 1 (February):1–23.

National Library of Medicine. "Visible Human Project®." Bethesda, MD: National Library of Medicine, National Institutes of Health (April 1, 2008). Available:
http://nlm.nih.gov/research/visible/visible_human.html (accessed December 26,
2008).

Neugebauer, Tomasz. 2005. "Imaging Indexing." *Photography Media Journal.* Available:
www.photographymedia.com/article.php?page=All&article=AImageIndexing (accessed January 15, 2009).

Oosterwijk, Herman. 2005. *DICOM Basics,* 3rd ed. Aubrey, TX: OTech.

O'Sullivan, Dympna, Eoin McLoughlin, Michela Bertolotto, and David C. Wilson.
"Capturing and Reusing Case-based Context for Image Retrieval." Nineteenth
International Joint Conference on Artificial Intelligence, Edinburgh, Scotland
(July 30–August 5, 2005). Available: www.ijcai.org/papers/post-0068.pdf (ac-
cessed January 5, 2009).

Sorantin, Erich. 2008. "Soft-copy Display and Reading: What the Radiologist Should
Know in the Digital Era." *Pediatric Radiology* 38, no. 12 (December): 1276–1284.

Valenza, Tor. "PACS: Top Trends for Today and Tomorrow." *Imaging Economics* (May,
2008). Available: www.imagingeconomics.com/issues/articles/MI_2008-05_01.
asp (accessed January 13, 2009).

Chapter 11

Ethical and Legal Issues in Health Informatics

This chapter describes the major ethical and legal concerns related to health-care and health informatics. Professional ethics and legal affairs in medicine have roots that go back to ancient times. In the digital age, these concerns have become complex and compelling. Ethics and law are not synonymous concepts, but clearly they can be interrelated when we address some of the pressing issues facing healthcare.

ETHICS AND MEDICINE

Ethics is concerned with what is right or wrong, appropriate or inappropriate, praiseworthy or blameworthy (Goodman, 1998). Ethics is about what we consider to be societal norms of conduct. It is more than just a strict concept of what is right, wrong, or legal. It includes a sense of what is good for oneself and for others.

There are three general levels of ethics. First, individuals have personal codes of ethics based on their own philosophies of life and on their perceptions of what it means to be a member of a particular profession. Second, organizations and groups have sets of values that management and employees expect everyone to adhere to. These are not "written down" but are societal behavior norms that groups of people expect from one another. At the third level are formally coded, published, and distributed sets of ethical rules and regulation developed by management, professional organizations, associations, and government agencies.

The strong belief that healthcare providers behave ethically dates back to the earliest times. In fact, some societies developed rigid sets of rules for the conduct of healthcare providers, with severe consequences for misconduct or malpractice.

The *Gale Encyclopedia of Nursing and Allied Health* (Wells, 2006: 1623) contains the following definition of medical ethics:

Medical ethics refers to the discussion and application of moral values and responsibilities in the areas of medical practice and research. While questions of medical ethics have been debated since the beginnings of Western medicine in the fifth century B.C., medical ethics as a distinctive field came into prominence only since World War II. This change has come about largely as a result of advances in medical technology, scientific research, and telecommunications. These developments have affected nearly every aspect of clinical practice, from the confidentiality of patient records to end-of-life issues. Moreover, the increased involvement of government in medical research as well as the allocation of health care resources brings with it an additional set of ethical questions.

Stedman's Online Medical Dictionary (2009) defines medical ethics as "the principles of proper professional conduct concerning the rights and duties of the physician, patients, and fellow practitioners, as well as the physician's actions in the care of patients and in relations with their families."

Because healthcare deals with the very core of human existence, it naturally follows that ethical issues are of central importance. Over time, physicians, lawyers, and philosophers have been keenly interested in medical ethics and in the past few decades nurses and other healthcare professionals, clergy, policy makers, and consumers have joined the discussion.

Expectations regarding ethics in the healthcare field evolve as societies change. For example, the publication of the Institute of Medicine's report *To Err Is Human: Building a Safer Health System* in 2000 spurred increasing attention toward medical errors, specifically by addressing such errors in codes of ethics. eHealth is another example of modern influences on medical ethics. *eHealth* describes healthcare practices based on electronic processes and communication, and ethical issues regarding confidentiality and security of electronic records and the global use of patient data for research and health management abound. Other ethical concerns in modern healthcare include end-of-life care and issues related to biotechnology, such as DNA forecasting and genetic engineering.

Concept of Professional Ethical Codes

As long as there have been professions there have been codes of ethics. These codes articulate the principles upon which a profession's duties and responsibilities are based. They help monitor professional behavior and at the same time protect the individuals in the profession.

Most people believe that professionals should render their services according to a set of guidelines that dictate appropriate and inappropriate behaviors. However, others believe that such codes are pointless and unnecessary. They believe that if professionals simply adhere to the moral behaviors and ethics of their culture, then their professional activities will be ethical and honorable. They further argue that professionals rarely turn to codes when they face a moral dilemma. Still other critics are skeptical about the effectiveness of a profession to police itself. In many cases, internal reviewers are reluctant to discipline a colleague and are therefore generous when claiming "reasonable doubt."

Proponents of professional codes of ethics maintain that codes play a major role in the professionalization of an occupational group and highlight the fact that the professional obligation is more than just an economic incentive. Codes of ethics are about recognizing a profession's obligation to society. Codes help create an environment in which ethical behavior is the norm.

Medical Codes of Ethics

One of the earliest codes of ethics is the *Code of Hammurabi*. It was written around 2000 BC and was an elaborate code of laws governing medical and surgical behavior. It set fees according to the social level of the patient and established punishments for malpractice. Clearly, early civilizations saw the need to be concerned for the general health welfare of the public.

The most famous code in the western world is the *Hippocratic Oath*, which was written around 500 BC. This code was the gold standard of behavior for many centuries. Ethical codes usually start with the *Hippocratic Oath* ("first, do no harm") and expand, including such things as (1) act in the best interest of the patient, (2) the patient has the right to refuse or choose treatment, (3) use fairness and equality when distributing scarce health resources, and (4) treat the patient with dignity. The predominance of the *Hippocratic Oath* has waned in modern times. Many doctors now believe that because social perceptions and values have changed, the oath should be adjusted. Today, there are a number of modernized oaths available for physicians (see Tyson [2001] for both the classical version and a modern version of the Hippocratic Oath).

Some codes of ethics were written for specific aspects of healthcare, for example, hospitals. In 1803, Thomas Percival wrote *Code for Medical Ethics*, which covers conduct in hospitals. In 1973, the American Hospital Association (AHA) adopted *A Patient's Bill of Rights* (see Annas, 1989). In 1992, it was revised to address the right of patients to review their medical records, disclosure of patient medical information, and responsibilities of both the patient and the hospital. In 2003, AHA replaced *A Patient's Bill of Rights* with the brochure *Patient Care Partnership*, which informs patients what to expect during their stay in a hospital.

The American Medical Association (AMA) has always maintained codes and principles of conduct. At its first meeting in 1847, the AMA adopted a code of ethics related primarily to medical education. In 1957, the Judicial Council of the AMA created *Principles of Medical Ethics*. This document was revised in 1980, mainly to eliminate references to gender. The latest revision was made in 2001. It emphasizes the preeminence of patients and advocates global access to healthcare. It includes a comprehensive nine-point list of principles of medical ethics. The principles are general tenets, for example, that physicians will be dedicated to providing competent care, that they will keep up to date with the latest developments in the field by personal study, and that they will make current and relevant information available to patients (American Medical Association, 2001). The AMA also adheres to its *Fundamental Elements of the Patient– Physician Relationship*, which includes opinions of the AMA's Council of Ethical and Judicial Affairs (American Medical Association, 1993). Most medical professional associations have a code of ethics.

A number of codes concern the use of humans in medical research. Two well-known examples are *The Nuremberg Code* and *The Declaration of Helsinki.*

The Nuremberg Code was published in 1948 as a response to the Nazi atrocities during World War II, especially regarding the use of human beings as experimental objects. The code is strong, reflecting society's reaction to what happened at Nuremberg. It presented ten points. The first point stated that the requirement for voluntary consent is absolute. There are no exceptions. The subsequent nine points spelled out the specific conditions for human research (National Institutes of Health, 1949).

The Declaration of Helsinki was adopted in 1964 in Helsinki, Finland by the Eighteenth World Medical Assembly. Since then it has been revised six times, the latest in 2008. *The Declaration of Helsinki* distinguishes between therapeutic and nontherapeutic experiments, giving researchers more moral leeway in therapeutic research (World Medical Organization, 1996).

Creating, applying, and following codes of ethics can be challenging. They provide professional directions and norms of behavior.

Ethical Concepts Regarding the Patient–Healthcare Provider Relationship

Across all aspects of healthcare, the patient–healthcare provider relationship is central. Successful healthcare outcomes depend to a large extent on a cooperative and effective relationship between the patient and the healthcare provider. The basic relationship includes five general concepts:

- Autonomy: the right of a person to make his or her health choices
- Beneficence: the obligation of the healthcare provider to act in the best interest of the patient
- Confidentially: the obligation of a healthcare provider to not carelessly and deliberately discuss information about a patient (implies that the healthcare provider must not distribute information regarding a patient unless the patient has signed a written consent or if the distribution is required by law)
- Informed choice: the patient decides whether to have a treatment or not only after being fully informed about and understanding the nature of the treatment

- Decision-making capacity: the patient has the ability to make decisions about his or her healthcare

The heightened media attention to medical matters in the last quarter of the twentieth century created new types of ethical situations for healthcare professionals. The media began covering new medical breakthroughs, devices, and procedures that in the past were mostly discussed among healthcare professionals. The information published was usually shallow, without details about warnings or side effects—specific information available only from healthcare providers.

This fortunately began to change with the advent of the Internet, which now provides consumers with extensive, *detailed* medical information. Patients now arrive at the doctor's office empowered with information; no longer is the healthcare enterprise or the government a gatekeeper of all medical information.

These changes have impacted the patient–healthcare provider relationship, and most patients have a new attitude toward healthcare in general. The paradigm now requires a more collaborative relationship between the patient and the healthcare provider. Joseph and Cook (2005: 198) express it this way:

> The physician has historically possessed more information than the traditional patient. This disparity has created a peculiar set of ethical issues for medical providers, based on their fiduciary responsibility to their patients. As with many relationships, the relationship between caregiver and patient changes, however, as information asymmetry diminishes. Relaxing the assumption that there is a significant difference in the information available to the physician and patient causes a new set of ethical issues to arise. In the extreme case, information inversion exists: the patient knows more about his or her condition than the attending medical personnel.

Joseph and Cook (2005: 2004) then elaborate on two types of ethical dilemmas that have been recast:

> **Traditional Dilemma 1:** How much time to spend on learning new medical techniques (since this was time that could otherwise be spent with patients); and

> **Traditional Dilemma 2:** Whether or not to discuss a medical innovation with a patient if the medical professional was not proficient with that innovation, or if that technology or innovation was not available locally.

Ethical concerns reach beyond individual healthcare providers. They affect the entire organization, including managers, administrators, and all staff. Hospitals and other health organizations deal with ethical concerns in formal and structured ways. Hospitals generally establish an ethics committee to handle ethical situations. Ethics committees are composed of members from a diverse range of professionals, including physicians and other healthcare providers, lawyers, clergy, and managers. These committees are also often willing to give advice to patients' families.

DISCLOSURE OF MEDICAL ERRORS

The increased emphasis on patient safety has been a driving force toward better disclosure of medical errors. Disclosing medical errors is difficult and has ethical and legal ramifications. The healthcare field is taking steps to see that institutions are developing and implementing policies and procedures for full disclosure of medical error.

Health information technologies, and especially the health electronic record, make it easier to track medical errors. It is the disclosure component that is being addressed more openly by healthcare providers, hospital administrators, medical ethicists, patients, medical safety experts, and accrediting organizations. The current theory is that error disclosure will lead to better understanding of medical errors and thus reduce them. Ultimately, this will enhance patient safety and the quality of health services.

STANDARDS OF CARE

Standards of care are closely related to the ethical relationship between the healthcare provider and the patient. A standard of care is a medical guideline that specifies treatment based on scientific medical evidence. Standards cover processes for diagnosis and treatment of specific illnesses and specific clinical care circumstances. In the legal arena, a standard of care is the minimal level of competency and judgment for which a healthcare provider can be held liable and legally accountable.

Evidence-based medicine is concerned with standards of care and therefore has a strong ethical aspect. If there is a "best evidence" to treat a health situation, then the clinician has an ethical responsibility to find that evidence. This is not a clear-cut issue, though, because having the "best" evidence does not necessarily mean that the "best" decisions will be made. Healthcare providers base their decisions on many factors, both scientific and personal, including "personal experience, personal biases and values, economic and political considerations, and philosophical principles" (Kerridge, Lowe, and Henry, 1998: 1151).

Ethics in Medical Research

Ethics impacts medical research in significant ways. According to Goodman and Cava (2008: 361–362), there are four main issues:

- Privacy, confidentiality, and best practices for data management
- Decision support, including the use of diagnostic and prognostic engines

- Loci of accountability and responsibility for duties ranging from database design and system evaluation to educational standards and patient awareness
- Use of intelligent machines in human subject's research to monitor, track, sort, randomize and otherwise perform operations on data about people

If human subjects are involved in a research study, the institution's Internal Review Board (IRB), also known as the Institutional Review Board, reviews the study first to ascertain the possible benefits and potential harm. The IRB concept is highly influential in the research environment. The objective is to protect the rights and welfare of the research subjects in terms of scientific, ethical, and regulatory aspects. The actual research project cannot begin without IRB approval. The IRB reviews research protocols, assesses the scientific merit of the proposed project, and ensures that prospective human subjects are capable of making decisions and fully understand the nature and risks of the research.

In recent years, IRBs have become even more scrupulous in their tasks and are viewed very seriously by researchers who are preparing research projects. Today's research is being monitored in an increasingly careful manner (Jordon, 2002). This reflects a growing awareness of ethical behavior in research and its importance to health informatics.

In the United States, the review boards are mandated by federal law. The first such law was the Research Act of 1974, passed in reaction to human research abuses earlier in the twentieth century. The law defines the nature of the review boards and stipulates that no research involving human subjects can be funded without passing through the IRB, including clinical trials of new drugs.

In the early 1900s, it was assumed that new knowledge gained by direct work with patients took priority over any personal impact on the patient's privacy or well being. The horrors revealed from World War II about inappropriate research brought an awareness of the deep ethical problems inherent in this attitude toward medical research.

New ethical concerns have arisen in modern times. A case in point is stem cell research, which has evoked passionate debate between those who see its powerful therapeutic possibilities and those who see its serious moral conflicts. Healthcare professionals cannot avoid being directly involved in ethical dilemmas. Information professionals also may have a conflict between their personal position on a subject and their profession's stance on that subject.

ETHICS AND INFORMATICS

Society generally understands the ethical aspects related to information. This is reflected in rules and regulations guiding advertisements, including political and prescription drug ads, and the one-sided "facts" that are published about emotional social issues. The creation, distribution, and use of information are often intertwined with the moral fiber of civilized behavior. The global explosion of information technologies and the saturation of the Internet into daily life have brought a new awareness of information ethics. Ethical issues related to information have existed since humans started communicating with each other, but the development and application of information technology have intensified the dimension of the ethical dilemmas.

In general, information ethics involves ownership of information, fairness and equitability, access, privacy, security, intellectual freedom, and accountability. Professions, such as healthcare, have their own specific information ethics issues. Ethics in health informatics has been discussed for decades. In fact, "informatics now constitutes a source of some of the important and interesting ethical debates in all the health professions" (Goodman and Miller, 2006: 380). A number of ethical issues are directly related to informatics—patient information, confidentiality, security, availability and access of data. Ethical questions are being asked about the use of diagnosis-making software, as this software is far from perfect. How far should a clinician go in relying on this software? Also, ethical questions are being raised about online consultation, remote prescribing, patient information systems, liability for patient care, the meaning of trust, patient consent, the compilation of global databases using private patient information, aggregated health data, and many others. Without doubt, ethics in health informatics involves technical, social, and political issues, all intertwined and complex and raising many questions.

MEDICAL LEGAL ISSUES

Healthcare organizations often have to deal with legal issues, varying in degrees of concern and complexity. Medical litigation has become so ubiquitous and at times unwarranted that legislation and referendums to reform the overall system are now common. At the same time, consumers need protection from harm and a recourse to justice.

Informed Consent

An informed consent is an agreement between a healthcare provider and a patient made for a medical procedure and/or participation in a clinical study. The agreement is made only after the patient clearly understands all the relevant medical facts and the risks that might be involved. Informed consent is derived from the premise of patient autonomy, that the patient has a right to make his or her own decisions.

At times, exceptions are made to the informed consent rule, such as during an emergency or when a patient is incompetent. To be considered competent, a patient must understand the options involved and understand the consequences of choosing among the options presented. Informed consent is a formal, legal process and is addressed by law in all 50 U.S. states.

Information Ownership

Information ownership is a complex issue, involving a number of interrelated factors, including legal and ethical issues related to the control of the information. The concept of "intellectual property," as regulated by copyright laws, guides our decisions about who owns what information. Copyright laws are aimed at preventing illicit use of someone else's work, be it a piece of art, music, writing, or software. Protection of intellectual property is essential if society wants people to keep creating products. It would be discouraging to spend years developing medical decision-making software that is then copied, reproduced, and sold without permission. Copyright and patent laws protect against this type of crime.

One of the numerous areas in healthcare where information ownership is an issue is the medical health record. The American Medical Association emphatically believes that the health record belongs exclusively to the health organization that created the record, while consumer groups and activists say that the record belongs to the patient or at least that there should be join ownership.

With continuously emerging electronic information technology and new forms of information on the horizon, copyright is getting even more complex. Sometimes it is not clear what is "free" on the Internet, especially when the copyright statements or instructions are muddled and difficult to understand. Significant changes in electronic copyright laws are being proposed all over the world that may strongly affect the way information is distributed, including health information.

Fortunately, librarians are usually well versed in copyright issues. According to Wood (2008: 175):

> All librarians are necessarily trained in copyright law and intellectual property issues, and this is no different in the health sciences. Increasingly in recent years, part of "virtual" information services has been the ability to provide scanned copies, such as PDF files, of full-text material from books, journals, and online resources. The librarian has no control over whether and how clinicians and researches share these among themselves.

Information ownership goes beyond the concept of intellectual property rights and presently it is interpreted to mean both possessing information and having responsibility for it. This implies not only the rights to create, modify, and sell information but also the right to say who can access and use the information. This involves many ethical, institutional, legal, and professional factors.

INFORMATICS IN ACTION! 11.1

Online Copyright Permission System

Location: Large medical research center

Problem: The researchers at the center are prolific in publishing their research, but they feel that they spend too much time obtaining copyright permissions for their manuscripts.

People Involved: A committee representing the research faculty and the electronic resources medical librarian in the center's library.

Action Taken: John, the electronic resources librarian, was contacted. The problem was not the lack of possibilities for online support for obtaining copyright permission. The situation was that there are numerous of such software and commercial sites. John approached the problem from several directions: (1) He analyzed the researchers' publications over the past three years and created a profile of the types of research conducted, primary formats, and so forth. (2) He compiled a list of copyright software and did extensive background reading on them. He included both user and manufacturer reviews. (3) He posted a message on professional blogs asking for informal recommendations from his colleagues based on their experiences. (4) John wrote a detailed report in which he recommended three software options. His report was forwarded to the faculty committee.

Takeaway: John familiarized himself with the materials published by the researchers. He was knowledgeable about software acquisition procedures and reviewed sources of software. He also enlisted help from professional networks.

Negligence/Malpractice

Medical malpractice may be an overt act or an omission by healthcare providers. It usually involves deviation from standard practice that results in injury to the patient. Lauren Pachman (2007), a medical litigation lawyer, lists four basic conditions for malpractice suits:

1. Doctor must have a duty to the patient
2. Doctor must have breached his duty to the patient
3. Patient has suffered an injury
4. Patient's injury must have been caused by the doctor's breach

Duty to the patient is usually implied when the patient puts his or her healthcare in the hands of the doctor and the doctor accepts the patient. As a result of this relationship, the doctor has an obligation to provide an established minimal level of care. Clearly, the patient must have been injured, and the injury must be tied to the doctor's breach of duty. Although the process seems straightforward, many medical factors involving documentation, witnesses, and subjective perceptions come into play.

Malpractice insurance is a major expense for healthcare providers. It covers legal judgments for negligent and/or improper treatment, unethical conduct, actual injury, and other situations. The cost of malpractice insurance keeps increasing because of the growing number and size of claims and changing economic and social factors.

Physicians claim that the cost of malpractice insurance affects their decision about where to practice medicine. Often physicians relocate to states where malpractice laws are more compatible with their economic well being. On the other hand, studies show that this may not be prevalent, but physicians may be limiting their practices because of high insurance cost. Cassels' (2008) study of neurosurgeons (a group with high malpractice insurance rates) shows that this group does limit its practice. Other research suggests that physicians do not tend to move out of areas where there is an excessive malpractice environment. Often the physicians chose to limit their services, sometimes drastically, rather relocating to other geographical areas. The idea is to limit their practice in order to limit their liability (Cassels, 2008). Without doubt, some physicians are moving to states with more palatable insurance laws, but others are taking different approaches to the way they practice.

Product Liability

The idea of product liability, "which holds manufacturers liable for injuries associated with their products in some circumstances, is among the most contentious domains of civil justice policy" (Garber, 2004). Product liability is based on the premise that manufacturers have a responsibility to make and market safe products. Tort laws mandate that manufacturers are held liable when they place something on the market that they know will not be inspected for defects and as a result humans are injured.

Product liability is not always based on manufacturer negligence. Liability can include such things as defects in the design or manufacturing and failures to warn of damage or danger.

Like malpractice, product litigation in healthcare has increased, particularly regarding pharmaceuticals and medical devices. Every day millions of people put their trust in a wide variety of medical devices and medications. Medical products are a large industry, with billions of dollars being spent each year on research, development, and marketing. In such an environment, risks can be high, so it is imperative that strict oversight be given to product safety. Unfortunately, the system is far from perfect. Defective medical devices affect thousands of people every year. Recent examples include defective infusion pumps, dialysis filters, hip replacements, pacemakers, stints, spinal discs, breast cancer testing kits, and heart values. There have also been high-profile cases of misrepresented medications.

Products can fail for many reasons, including poor design, production line error, human error, and manufacturer avarice. In the case of error, no matter how many safeguards, guidelines, and procedure policies are in place, human error will never be totally eliminated in the manufacturing process. In the case of avarice, there will always be manufacturers who will cut corners in order to raise profits or avoid loses. The research and development of new medical devices and/or drugs are extremely expensive. Delays mean less profit, and there may be pressure from customers to push for new devices or new drugs. This causes some companies to rush into sales before the product is ready to reach consumers. The process of obtaining patents and getting Food and Drug Administration approval of drugs and devices can be a very lengthy documentation process.

Fraud and Abuse

Fraud in healthcare is defined as "knowingly and willfully offering, paying, soliciting, or receiving remuneration to induce business that healthcare programs will reimburse. Healthcare fraud can result from internal corruption, bogus claims, unnecessary healthcare treatments, and unwarranted solicitations" (Armoni, 2000: 149). Fraud and abuse in the healthcare field are more than minor problems. In 2008, the *Washington Post* carried an article describing a situation in which Medicare paid as much as $92 million for wheelchairs and other home equipment in a scam where false prescriptions were ascribed to physicians who were dead. The Medicare ID for one doctor, dead for 9 years, appeared on 83 claims submitted by a Miami company (Lee, 2008). This is not an isolated case. In fact, the government established a joint Medicare Fraud Strike Force (MFSF) to address a problem that is estimated to cost taxpayers tens of billions of dollars annually.

Fraud and abuse in healthcare are not limited to schemes to take money from Medicare and insurance companies. Honest consumers spend billions of dollars each year on fraudulent products and services. Consumers hope to find cures for diseases, or want to improve their looks or longevity, and these desires lead them to spend large amounts of money on useless or bogus products and services.

The cost of fraud adds to the cost of care and to insurance premiums of both the healthcare provider and the consumer. Curbing health fraud is not just the responsibility of the healthcare industry and the government. It is the responsibility of every citizen and consumer.

PRIVACY AND CONFIDENTIALITY ISSUES

Healthcare is one of the fields most concerned about privacy and confidentiality, specifically as they relate to the collection, storage, and dissemination of patient information. As Felkey, Fox, and Thrower (2005: 345) state, "For both health care professionals and patients, privacy means being free from unauthorized intrusion and protecting personally identifiable information, including name, birth date, social security number, and financial data." Patient information may be shared with a host of people, including doctors and other healthcare providers, family, pharmacies, insurance companies, public health agencies, the government, researchers, schools, and employers. If patients fear too much for the security and privacy of their information, they may become too cautious about what they share with their healthcare providers. This would hinder proper treatment and thus negatively impact the patient.

To most people, privacy and the related issues of confidentiality and security are top priorities. Privacy usually refers to individuals, and confidentially refers to information. Privacy implies control over what can be known about us, confidentiality indicates control over the release of private information, and security refers to mechanisms for protecting privacy and confidentiality.

Privacy is based on the idea that individuals have the right to control information about themselves. If someone deliberately follows you and observes that every Monday you enter a psychiatrist's office at 2:00 p.m., and then he hacks into your psychiatrist's computer and gets a copy of your medical record, he has violated the *confidentiality* of your record (Goodman and Miller, 2006). Privacy is the right to be anonymous and protected from intrusions, and confidentiality is the control of who has access to the information. In healthcare this means that patients have control over how their health data are accessed and used. Although such control is not specifically designated in the U.S. Constitution, society looks at it as a basic right. Privacy violations existed long before the advent of computers, but the application of current information technologies has vastly increased the problem.

In general, healthcare professionals have always believed in the privacy of patient information. Policies and procedures for managing privacy have evolved over time, and the current high-speed, high-capacity information technology has intensified the concerns of privacy, confidentiality, and data security. Computerized systems make information more accessible to everybody—including those who should not have access. The healthcare community is keenly aware of the seriousness and importance of ethical and legal issues. Rodrigues (2000: e8) described it this way:

> Given the sensitive nature of health care information, and the high degree of dependence of health professionals on reliable records, the issues of integrity, security, privacy, and confidentiality are of particular significance and must be clearly and effectively addressed by health and health-related organizations and professionals.

Patient sensitivity to the privacy and confidentiality of their personal health information has become increasing apparent with the proliferation of the Internet, including the storage of health records on the Web. According to the American Medical Association (2008):

> The American Medical Association and many other healthcare associations have been very active in promoting the need to maintain privacy and con-

fidentiality of patient information. People using the Internet to search for medical information tend to value personal privacy highly, usually ranking it as the most important concern they have when searching online for medical information. Studies also conclude that, although many Internet health information sites provide privacy policies, very few of them actually follow the policies. This is a serious concern.

Secondary Uses of Patient Data

For decades, patient data have been used for purposes beyond the care of the individual patient. Cumulative patient data often form the basis of analysis, quality assessment, scientific research, and legal studies.

Much research is based solely on patient data. Descriptive research and time series studies rely on patient data–based research, sometimes called *retrospective, chart-based research*. Patient data–based medical research has a long and successful history of providing vital knowledge on the causes of disease and the effectiveness of treatments.

Patient data are of special interest for public health services, which need to study demographics trends. Usually, the data are combined to provide summary information and identify trends. Healthcare and social workers spend a lot of time and effort collecting and analyzing data. Also, in some legal situations health records are critical and serve as major pieces of evidence.

There are ethical concerns when data are shared in aggregated databases. It is essential that privacy and security mechanisms are established and that the patient's informed consent is clearly secured. Best practices need to be developed for sharing of data from different databases.

Without doubt, opportunities abound for the productive use of patient data on a meta level, beyond the immediate care of the patient, but protecting patient privacy and confidentiality is paramount. It is necessary to operate at intersections where medical privacy and confidentiality balance with the need for concrete data for research and decision making.

Health Grid Computing

In the past few years, grid computing has been increasingly applied to healthcare. Solomonides defines (2008: 140) grid computing as "a new technology enhancing services already offered by the Internet offering rapid computation, large-scale data storage, and flexible collaboration by harnessing together the power of a large number of commodity computers or clusters of basic machines." It is a form of distributed connections that enhances the aggregation and sharing of data and resources.

In health informatics, *health grid* describes grid infrastructures that use distributed computing power, databases, and medical expertise to manage and disseminate biomedical data. This technology enhances the aggregating and sharing of data on a large scale, serving clinics, public health officials, healthcare managers, movement agencies, and patients. At the same time it presents challenges for safeguarding privacy and confidentiality.

Health Insurance Portability and Accountability Act of 1996

The Health Insurance Portability and Accountability Act (HIPAA) passed in 1996 is set of rules mandated by the government on the appropriate use of individually identifiable health care information. Basically, the rules protect health information from misuse and inappropriate disclosure and set standards related to privacy, security, transactions, and identifiers.

The original impetus for creating HIPAA was to protect people's insurability when they changed jobs, but HIPAA was soon expanded to other areas, such as protection of personally identifiable health information. HIPAA limits the release and use of health records and gives patients more control over their personal health information. The safeguards covered in HIPAA are enforceable with civil and criminal penalties.

The section dealing with privacy is called the *Privacy Rule*, which regulates the use and disclosure of protected health information. This rule applies to any information that can be linked to a particular individual. This, of course, includes the medical record. It also provides the patient a means to correct inaccurate information in the medical record. The Privacy Rule requires that any use of information about the patient be reported to the patient, and HIPAA requires healthcare organizations to have specific administrative, physical, and technological safeguards for the security of the patient's information (Joseph and Cook, 2005: 220).

Becoming compliant with HIPAA is often difficult and sometimes required a major overhaul of system operations and significant changes in procedures and practices. As newer information technologies are implemented in healthcare organizations, the challenge becomes to increase network connectivity and enable access to key information without compromising confidentiality, security, integrity, or availability.

With the ubiquity of information technology and global connectivity, patients want to know where their information goes and who has access to it. They know that their information might be accessed anywhere in the world by anyone holding a mouse, and this concerns many patients. Fear can undermine their trust in the system. According to Joseph and Cook (2005: 222):

> Anyone seeking health-related information, products, or services has a right to expect that organizations and individuals who provide such information follow a set of guiding principles. If confidences are not kept, individuals will be less forthcoming with information, which in turn may impact the care they receive.

HIPAA is by no means the first or only government initiative to keep health information private and secure. Other federal and state laws have been passed. In addition, professional societies and associations as well as standards groups address the same issues. Because of the extensive litigation in modern times, organizations are developing stricter internal controls and procedures to secure privacy and confidentiality. Without doubt, HIPAA has changed the way health information is managed: "HIPAA is a turning point for the health care industry because it requires that the industry develop a set of national standards that will help bring the much needed data-standard unity to health care transactions and provide assurance that confidential patient information will be safe. . . " (Deshmukh and Croasdell, 2005: 228).

USA PATRIOT Act and Medical Privacy

The Uniting and Strengthening America by Providing Appropriate Tools Required to Intercept and Obstruct Terrorism (USA PATRIOT) Act was passed on October 26, 2001, and a second version was signed into law on March 9, 2006. One of the most contentious parts of the PATRIOT Act, Section 215, has a directive that affects the privacy and confidentiality of medical records. This part of the Act allows the government to require any person or organization to turn over "any tangible things," including medical information, that the government wants. The government does not have to show probable cause or even reasonable grounds for demanding the information. Furthermore, individuals whose information is being given to the government are not told about it.

Many doctors across the United States have protested Section 215 of the PATRIOT Act. They find it especially disturbing that they cannot even tell patients when the government has taken their medical information. Doctors not following the provisions in Section 215 can be prosecuted for obstruction of justice (Lenzer, 2006). The right balance between having the means to fight terrorism and protecting citizens against unreasonable search of their medical records is not likely to be found anytime soon.

ISSUES FOR HEALTH SCIENCES LIBRARIANS

Health sciences librarians are often involved when ethical and legal issues arise in healthcare. A number of codes of ethics for librarians address a variety of professional values. The most common values involve intellectual freedom, free and uncensored flow of information, free and equal access to information, and personal integrity and competence (Shachaf, 2005).

The health information professional, as a part of the healthcare team, is more than ever faced with the issues of what information to provide, how much information to provide, and when to give information access to consumers. Consumers of health services are demanding their rights to information for legal and ethical reasons. Information professionals are exposed to information management dilemmas more than ever.

The Medical Library Association's (1994) code of ethics for health sciences librarians lists five points where ethics intersect with the profession: (1) society, (2) clients, (3), institution, (4) profession, and (5) self. The Medical Library Association believes that health sciences librarians have their own ethical issues that go beyond those addressed in a general codes of ethics for librarians (such as the American Library Association's).

It is generally agreed that no code of ethics can address every specific case that might come up, but a good code makes clear the standards to be considered when addressing any of the specifics. Those who defend intellectual freedom and the right to privacy of citizens maintain these rights are *implied* in several places in the United States Constitution (1787), in particular the free speech rights in the First Amendment, the protection against military intrusion in the Third Amendment, unreasonable search and seizure in the Fourth Amendment, the protection against self-incrimination in the Fifth Amendment, and the due process clause in the Sixth Amendment (McCoy, 2003).

Health sciences librarians face critical privacy issues when dealing with patrons who may be patients or with healthcare providers who are caring for patients. A simple rule is that librarians provide requested information but do not *interpret* that information. In practice, this may not be as straightforward as it sounds. When librarians help create search queries and suggest specific information resources, they cannot avoid using a certain amount of subjective interpretation. It is impossible to formulate a good search query without having a concept of what the meaning is behind the question. Ethics are about human behavior in society, and health sciences librarians are keenly aware of what this means in their professional actions.

SUMMARY

A significant portion of ethical and legal issues in healthcare are related to information, particularly the privacy and confidentiality of data. The use of information technology in the practice of medicine and in biomedical research and the inappropriate implementation of information technology can lead to ethical and legal issues. Ethics and legal concerns related to health informatics and bioinformatics imply a major responsibility for health sciences librarians. There is a strong awareness of the immediate need to face these issues. "[T]here is a growing realisation that ethics must be a part of the planning process within biotechnology" (O'Mathúna, 2007: 115). The next chapter deals with bioinformatics and genomic medicine.

REFERENCES

American Hospital Association. "Patient Care Partnership." Chicago: American Hospital Association (2003). Available: www.patienttalk.info/AHA-Patient_Bill_of_Rights.htm (accessed December 23, 2008).

American Medical Association. "Fundamental Elements of the Patient–Physician Relationship." Chicago: American Medical Association (June 1993). Available: www.ama-assn.org/ama1/pub/upload/mm/Code_of_Med_Eth/opinion/opinion1001.html (accessed December 23, 2008).

American Medical Association. "Guidelines for Medical and Health Information Sites on the Internet." Chicago: American Medical Association (July 18, 2008). Available: www.ama-assn.org/am/Apu/Bcategory/1905.html (accessed December 27, 2008).

American Medical Association. "Principles of Medical Ethics." Adopted by the AMA's House of Delegates June 17, 2001. Chicago: American Medical Association (2001). Available: www.ama-assn.org/ama/pub/physician-resources/medical-ethics/ama-code-medical-ethics/principles-medical-ethics.shtml (accessed December 27, 2008).

Annas, George J. 1989. *The Rights of Patients: The Basic ACLU Guide to Patient Rights,* 2nd ed. Carbondale, IL: Carbondale Southern Illinois University Press.

Armoni, Adi. 2000. *Healthcare Information Systems: Challenges of the New Millennium.* Hershey, PA: Idea Group Publishing.

Cassels, Caroline. "Aggressive Malpractice Environments Dictate How, Not Where, Neurosurgeons Practice." New York: Medscape (May 1, 2008). Available: www.medscape.com/viewarticle/573903 (accessed December 26, 2008).

Deshmukh, Pooja and David Croasdell. 2005. "HIPAA: Privacy and Security in Health Care Networks." In *Information Ethics: Privacy and Intellectual Property* (pp. 219–237), edited by Lee A. Forman and A. Graham Peace. Hershey, PA: Information Science Publishing.

Felkey, Bill G., Brent I. Fox, and Margaret R. Thrower. 2005. *Health Care Informatics: A Skills-based Resource.* Washington, DC: American Pharmacists Association.

Garber, Steven. 2004. "Should We Give Up on Medical Product Liability?" *RAND Review* (Summer). Santa Monica, CA: RAND. Available: www.rand.org/publications/randreview/issues/summer2004/38.html (accessed December 27, 2008).

Goodman, Kenneth. 1998. *Ethics, Computing, and Medicine: Informatics and the Transformation of Health Care.* Cambridge: Cambridge University.

Goodman, Kenneth W. and Anita Cava. 2008. "Bioethics, Business Ethics, and Science: Bioinformatics and the Future of Healthcare." *Cambridge Quarterly of Healthcare Ethics* 17: 361–372.

Goodman, Kenneth and Randolph A. Miller. 2006. "Ethics and Health Informatics: Users, Standards, and Outcomes." In *Biomedical Informatics: Computer Applications in Health Care and Biomedicine* (pp. 379–402), 3rd ed., edited by Edward H. Shortliffe and James J. Cimino. New York: Springer.

Institute of Medicine. Committee on Quality of Health Care in America. 2000. *To Err Is Human: Building a Safer Health System.* Washington, DC: National Academies Press.

Jordon, Theresa J. 2002. *Medical Information: A User's Guide to Informatics and Decision Making.* New York: McGraw-Hill.

Joseph, Jimmie L. and David P. Cook. 2005. "Information Imbalance in Medical Decision Making: Upsetting the Balance." In *Information Ethics: Privacy and Intellectual Property* (pp. 197–218), edited by Lee A. Forman and A. Graham Peace. Hershey, PA: Information Science Publishing.

Kerridge, Ian, Michael Lowe, and David Henry. 1998. "Ethics and Evidence Based Medicine." *British Medical Journal* 316, no. 7138 (April 11): 1151–1153.

Lee, Christopher. "Billings Used Dead Doctors' Names." Washington, DC: *Washington Post*, July 9, 2008. Available: www.washingtonpost.com/wp-dyn/content/article/2008/07/08/AR2008070802340.html (accessed December 27, 2008).

Lenzer, Jeanne. "Doctors Outraged at Patriot Act's Potential to Seize Medical Records." British Medical Journal 332, no. 69 (January 14, 2006). Available: www.bmj.com/cgi/content/full/332/7533/69 (accessed December 27, 2008).

McCoy, Michael R. 2003. "Freedom, Security, Patriotism: An Ethical Dilemma." *Kentucky Librarian* 67, no 3: 20–24.

Medical Library Association. "Code of Ethics for Health Sciences Librarianship." Chicago: Medical Library Association (1994). Available: www.mlanet.org/about/ethics.html (accessed December 27, 2008).

National Institutes of Health. Office of Human Subject Research. Regulations and Ethical Guidelines. "Nuremberg Code." Reprinted from *Trials of War Criminals before the Nuremberg Military Tribunals under Control Council Law 10, no. 2: 181-182.* Washington, DC: U.S. Government Printing Office (1949). Available: http://ohsr.od.nih.gov/guidelines/nuremberg.html (accessed March 20, 2009).

O'Mathúna, Dónal P. 2007. "Bioethics and Biotechnology." Cytotechnology 53, no. 1–3: 113–119.

Pachman, Lauren. "Medical Malpractice Litigation." *Contingencies* (January–February, 2007). Available: cache.search.yahoo-ht2.akadns.net/search/cache?ei=UTF-8&p=medical+litigation&fr=moz2&u=www.contingencies.org/janfeb07/policy.pdf&w=medical+litigation&d=YhFzmi72Q9fm&icp=1&.intl=us (accessed December 8, 2008).

Percival, Thomas. 1803. *Medical Ethics; or, a Code of Institutes and Precepts, Adapted to the Professional Conduct of Physicians and Surgeons.* Manchester, UK: S. Russell.

Rodrigues, Roberto J. 2000. "Ethical and Legal Issues in Interactive Health Communications: A Call for International Cooperation." *Journal of Medical Internet Research* 2, no. 1 (January–March): e8.

Shachaf, Pnina. 2005. "A Global Perspective on Library Association Codes of Ethics." *Library & Information Science Research* 27, no. 4: 513–533.

Solomonides, Anthony E. 2008. "Compliance and Creativity in Grid Computing." In *Ethical, Legal, and Social Issues in Medical Informatics* (pp. 140–155), edited by Penny Duquenoy, Carlisle George, and Kai Kimppa. Hershey, PA: IGI Global.

Stedman's Online Medical Dictionary, 27th ed. Philadelphia: Lippincott Williams & Wilkins (2009). Available: www.stedmans.com/section.cfm/45 (accessed January 29, 2009).

Tyson, Peter. "The Hippocratic Oath Today" Public Broadcasting Service—NOVA Online. Survivor, MD. (March, 2001). Available: www.pbs.org/wgbh/nova/ doctors/oath.html (accessed December 3, 2008).

The United States Constitution. "The U.S. Constitution Online." (September 17, 1787). Available: www.usconstitution.net/const.htm l (accessed December 8, 2008).

Wells, Ken R. 2006. "Medical Ethics." In *The Gale Encyclopedia of Nursing and Allied Health* (pp. 1693–1696), 2nd ed., vol. 3, edited by Jacqueline L. Longe. Detroit: The Gale Group.

Wood, Elizabeth H. 2008. "Information Services in Health Sciences Libraries." In *Introduction to Health Sciences Librarianship* (pp.161–178), edited by M. Sandra Wood. Binghamton, NY: The Haworth Press.

World Medical Organization. 1996. "Declaration of Helsinki." *British Medical Journal* 313, no. 7070 (December 7): 1448–1449.

Chapter 12

Bioinformatics and Genomic Medicine

Bioinformatics and genomic medicine will dominate the world of biomedical sciences in the coming years. Informatics professionals and enlightened health sciences librarians, working hand in hand, can be closely involved in the new frontier of molecular information. It is imperative that anyone working in the health information professions become knowledgeable about bioinformatics. This chapter covers the basics of bioinformatics and suggests ways that information professionals can play a role.

DEFINING BIOINFORMATICS

Bioinformatics, sometimes called *biological information science*, is interdisciplinary in nature, involving a number of fields of study including biology, biochemistry, mathematics, computer science, information science, and health informatics. According to the National Center for Biotechnology Information (2004), bioinformatics is "the field of science in which biology, computer science and information technology merge to form a single discipline." It is a specialized area of informatics that focuses on the management of information related to the underlying basic biological sciences.

Bioinformatics differs from clinical health informatics in that it starts at the molecular level; clinical informatics is more generic and deals with information directly related to healthcare delivery. Bioinformatics is the art and science that deals with the acquisition and application of biomedical knowledge at the basic level in order to improve healthcare services.

Altman and Mooney (2006: 763) define bioinformatics as "the study of how information is represented and analyzed in biological systems. . . ." The underlying concept in all the definitions is *information*. Bioinformatics looks at the understanding of biological processes as an information problem, and its procedures utilize information technology to uncover biological processes.

Bioinformatics evolved from the work of scientists who studied biological processes at the subcellular level, particularly at the information processing level—hence the term *bioinformatics*. Knowledge management became the focus because of the massive amounts of data this type of research generates. In the beginning, bioinformatics concentrated on collecting and organizing sequencing information and in constructing databases for the distribution of this information. Today bioinformatics has moved beyond this to include analyzing, interpreting, and applying the information.

Bioinformatics professionals devoted much time and effort to develop procedures and information structures to efficiently handle the data. Now, researchers have turned their attention to translating the growing data store into applications. This is called *translational bioinformatics* and is composed of two primary stages. The first one is to process basic biological discoveries and apply them to human biology. The second is to translate this information into actual benefits for the health of the population (Butte, 2008).

According to the American Medical Informatics Association (2007) part of translational bioinformatics concerns "the development of storage, analytic, and interpretive methods to optimize the transformation of increasingly voluminous biomedical data into proactive, predictive, preventative, and participatory health." Translational bioinformatics is basically an information challenge, and a cross-section of professionals are becoming involved, including bioinformatics professionals, computer experts, clinicians, and health sciences librarians.

AREAS OF BIOINFORMATICS STUDY

Bioinformatics includes a broad range of fields, including DNA sequence alignment, genome structuring, computational biology, genomic analysis (including the human genome sequencing and nonhuman genomes), proteomics, and pharmacogenomics. *Sequence alignment* is a technique for lining up DNA-related data, usually in a table or matrix form, to show relationships among the data. The relationships may be based on functional, structural, or evolutionary factors.

Genome structuring deals with the physical arrangement of macromolecular materials, generally proteins, using computational tools. *Computational biology* involves the analysis of genetic information stored in databases, often very large databases, to find genes, understand the structures of proteins, and acquire other DNA sequence information. *Genomics analysis* deals with genetic information from specific species. Gene analysis allows the researcher to compare newly found genes with previously analyzed ones in order to determine how the new gene's protein sequence functions. For example, genes in cancer cells are compared with genes in healthy tissue to see how they differ.

Proteomics deals with proteins. A *proteomic* is the protein complement expressed by the genome. The functions and interactions of proteins are complex. There are more than a million proteins in the human body.

Pharmacogenomics uses genetic information to develop new drugs. Pharmaceutical companies believe genome projects will open up new avenues of research and development and at a much faster pace than in the past. Others are cautious about how long this will take to really develop. "The extent to which genomics will actually be able to help identify validated drug targets is uncertain. Genomics and bioinformatics are still young areas, and the drug development cycle can take up to ten years" (Howard, 2000: 59).

Howard (2000) identified five major activities associated with bioinformatics: data acquisition, database development, data analysis, data integration, and analysis of integrated data. *Data acquisition* is concerned with the direct collecting of data, usually from the laboratory. Many specialized instruments have been developed or adapted for this type of data capture. Most labs use information management systems to handle the data. *Databases* are developed to organize and store the captured data. This is not an easy task because the information exists in many formats and users have a broad range of needs. Once again, the basic tenet of information service arises: What do the users need and in what form do they need it? Good database design will allow the user to easily retrieve the data and perform *data analysis*. The next step is to *integrate* the data with other databases to look for similarities and differences. Finally, the *integrated data* are analyzed for new insights into the functions of living organisms.

Bioinformatics is opening avenues for understanding the role of genetics in health, specifically by studying the fundamentals of information in biological systems from the molecular level up. Today, bioinformatics is undergoing a rapid evolution, primarily because of the development and applications of genomics and related tools. Environmental cleanup and agricultural produce enhancement are two examples.

Bioinformatics applications moved early into the healthcare field. The first product to be approved by the Food and Drug Administration was insulin, in 1982. This led to a number of genetically engineered products, such as growth hormones, clot-dissolving agents, proteins for stimulating the production of blood, and the anticancer drug interferon (Encyclopedia Britannica, 1994).

DEOXYRIBONUCLEIC ACID: THE INFORMATION KEY TO LIFE

The key to all life (plants and animals) on earth is information and this information is processed and passed on by a chemical information system known as *deoxyribonucleic acid* (DNA). DNA, a chained information molecule, is a sequence of chemicals defining the genetic material that guides the structuring and processing of life. We call it the key to life because each DNA molecule contains chemically coded instructions for building, operating, and maintaining the organism that contains it. DNA is one of the most powerful and complex information systems in the natural world. It is the book of an organism's life. The study of bioinformatics closely involves DNA.

Genes and Genetics

Genes carry biochemical information in the cells of living organisms. They are discreet information units encoded in the DNA sequence. Genetic information comes from both parents and is the basis for all organisms' characteristics, such as a rabbit's eye color, a pea plant's height, or a human's specific talent. In the nucleus of each cell is a complete copy of who or what the organism is.

The field of genetics is based on the research of Gregor Mendel (1822–1884), whose work unfolded quietly in a monastery in what was then Brünn, Austria. He experimented with peas for seven years in a small strip of garden in the monastery. During those years he asked (and answered) many questions about cross-breeding plants. He would take pollen from one kind of plant and put it into the flowers on another. Mendel cross-bred tall plants and short plants to see what would result. He probably expected to get middle-sized plants, but they all turned out to be tall. When he planted the seeds from the second-generation plants, he got another surprise: about one plant in four of the third generation was short. Clearly, information about how tall to grow had been passed to the second-generation seeds even if it did not affect the height of the plants themselves.

Growing thousands of seeds and carefully recording the characteristics of the plants and seeds in each generation, Mendel formulated some basic principles of genetics. He published an article in 1865, in the journal of the local natural science society, but practically no one read it. Mendel never discovered what part of the seeds carried the information behind his discoveries, and he didn't give it a name. It was not until 1909 that Danish botanist Wilhelm Johannsen coined the word "gene" for the basic unit of inheritance. You might say that in Nature's recipe for making a dog, a person, a cockroach, a cauliflower plant, or any other living creature, the step-by-step instructions are carried in genes.

Genetics has become an important aspect of daily life, including healthcare. Work is being done to genetically alter bacteria in order to mass-produce useful medical products, such growth hormones for young people afflicted with growth disorders. Many disorders are being approached with gene therapy, which is basically replacing malfunctioning genes with healthy ones. One of the most exciting projects is The Human Genome Project, discussed later.

The Genome

The total collection of genes in an organism is called the *genome*. Sometimes the difference between *genetics* and *genomics* is misunderstood. Genetics is the study of single genes and their characteristics; genomics is the universal study of the functions and interactions of the complete set of genes in a genome. According to Guttmacher and Collins (2002: 1513):

> Genomics has a broader and more ambitious reach than genetics. The science of genomics rests on direct experimental access to the entire genome and applies to common conditions, such as breast cancer and colorectal cancer, human immunodeficiency virus (HIV) infection, tuberculosis, Parkinson's disease, and Alzheimer's disease.

The human body has about 1,000 trillion cells, and in the nucleus of each of those cells is a complete copy—the genome—of what the person is. All genomes are similar. We all have a large number of genes that make us human, plus a few genes that give us different traits from each other.

In the nineteenth century, Mendel laid the groundwork for genetic science. Since Mendel's time genetics flourished, and in 1953 the secret world of DNA was revealed by James Crick and Francis Watson when they modeled the double helix. Another major milestone was reached a few years ago when the human genome was mapped.

Genome Mapping

Genome maps, also called *linkage maps*, are constructed to help researchers navigate through the genome complex. Like any kind of map, the genome map has landmarks that tell researchers where they are and help them find what they are looking for. "One could say that genetic maps serve to guide a scientist toward a gene, just like an interstate map guides a driver from city to city" (National Library of Medicine, 2004). These "landmarks" can be a number of things, such as DNA sequences, switching sites that turn genes on and off, or actual genes. Genome maps often chart a new frontier, helping researchers both locate known genes and find new ones.

In medical research, genome maps help researchers identify which genes are involved in specific human diseases, trace patterns of inheritance, and zero in on the regions where specific genes are located. Genetic mapping can provide firm evidence that a disease transmitted from parent to child is linked to one or more genes; provide clues about which chromosome contains the gene and precisely where it lies on that chromosome; help locate the single genes responsible for relatively rare inherited disorders like cystic fibrosis and muscular dystrophy; and guide scientists to genes that are believed to be involved in common disorders like asthma and heart disease (National Human Genome Research Institute, 2008).

Genomic maps orient sequence information and make gene hunting faster and more efficient. In the early days of genomic research, scientists had to tediously manually map the genomic region under study, but today information technology, access to the Internet, and genomic database maps are all that are required.

The Human Genome Project

The Human Genome Project, an international effort co-sponsored by the U.S. Department of Energy and the National Institutes of Health, began in 1990 and was completed in 2003. Its purpose was to identify all of the human genes and make this information available for biological studies. The stated project goals were to

- *identify* all the approximately 20,000–25,000 genes in human DNA,
- *determine* the sequences of the 3 billion chemical base pairs that make up human DNA,
- *store* this information in databases,
- *improve* tools for data analysis,
- *transfer* related technologies to the private sector, and
- *address* the ethical, legal, and social issues (ELSI) that may arise from the project. (U.S. Department of Energy, 2008)

Before the project, it was thought that the human genome contained 60,000 to 80,000 genes. As the project neared completion, it became apparent that there are closer to 30,000 to 35,000 genes. On the other hand, some scientists say that we may have missed thousands of genes "hidden" deep down in the information codes.

One might ask, "Why do we want to decode the human genome?" The answer is because it will provide us with detailed information with which to understand how chromosomes are able to structure, organize, and use DNA. This knowledge will lead to a better understanding of how life is structured.

Mutations in DNA coding sequences cause diseases. Faults in the human genome are related to at least 1,500 diseases, ranging from cancer to kidney failure to birth defects. The connections between gene mutations and diseases will become much clearer now that the entire human genome has been mapped and sequenced. Much exciting work lies ahead with the study of genomes. Dr. David K. Gifford, a computer scientist at the Massachusetts Institute of Technology, said in the *New York Times* (October 25, 2002) that "[t]he human genome project produces a parts list and we can now move on to the question of how those parts talk to one another" (Wade, 2002).

By no means is the Human Genome Project the only genome mapping project to be conducted. Efforts to map the genome exist in many research settings around the world, varying in size, complexity and goals. One example is the Personal Genome Project at Harvard. This project focuses on the individual and coordinates the data obtained with other personalized data, such as imaging and laboratory tests and medical history. This is in contrast to the Human Genome Project, which focused on the genome as an entity (Mason, Seringhaus, and Sattler de Sousa e Brito, 2008).

The Human Genome Project has provided immense amounts of nucleotide sequencing data to researchers around the world. The sharing of such data was one of the mandated purposes of the project, and this certainly has been accomplished. Links to the databanks holding the genomic data exist in MEDLINE and may be accessed via PubMed (Lindberg and Humphreys, 2008).

The completion of the Human Genome Project was a major milestone in bioinformatics. Attention is now turning toward how genomes vary in specific individuals. This frontier of research may culminate in the day when healthcare is individually tailored based on the patient's specific genetic makeup.

Stem Cell Research

Stem cells are unspecialized cells that reproduce for a long time by cell division. These cells can be prompted to turn into specialized cells, such as muscle.

In the past few years scientists have perfected how to isolate stem cells from a human embryo and grow them in the laboratory. Embryonic stem cells are preferable over adult stem cells for research because embryonic cells can stay alive and reproduce for a year or more. The first challenge is to find out how they work. Once there is an understanding of the basic mechanisms of stem cells, then advances can be made toward applications.

Stem cell research is another facet of the quest to conquer diseases. By understanding how stem cells work, genomic scientists are learning the root causes of disease and body malfunctions. Related to this is the possibility of individualized treatment and disease prevention.

There is enthusiasm for the possible applications of DNA knowledge, but there are scientific, legal, and ethical concerns as well. Some scientists believe that we must tread softly until we have a better understanding of the implications of DNA research and applications. Questions have been raised about the safety of recombinant food, and many people object to cloning because of personal, religious, or cultural beliefs.

All indications are that science is on the edge of a vast new frontier with the development of stem cell research. There is great hope for new possibilities in understanding and conquering diseases across a wide range. The goal of stem cell research is to find and understand the intrinsic, natural information hidden in the cells of all living things. The information gained will be organized, stored, and retrieved with systems developed and managed by information professionals who are trained to handle this highly specialized type of information.

Genetic Testing

Gene-based testing is steadily moving into the public and commercial sectors. One well-known application is in the field of criminal investigation and identification. Like fingerprints, each of us has a unique DNA makeup. More and more law enforcement agencies are using DNA identification, and it is important to many court cases. DNA mapping was used extensively to identify people who lost their lives in the attacks on September 11, 2001.

DNA can be used to prove a person guilty or innocent of a crime. An outstanding example of this purpose is the Innocence Project at the Benjamin N. Cardoze School of Law at Yeshiva University in New York City. The Innocence Project is a nonprofit legal clinic that handles cases where postconviction DNA testing of evidence can yield conclusive proof of innocence. This project clearly shows that DNA testing is a major factor in providing scientific proof that can clear innocent people convicted of a crime. This is a dramatic example of the use of genetic testing, and there are hundreds of lesser-known examples.

One of the most common medical uses of genetic testing is carrier screening, which involves identifying unaffected individuals who carry one copy of a gene for a disease that requires two copies for the disease to be expressed. Others uses are preimplantation genetic diagnosis (procedures performed on embryos prior to implantation), prenatal diagnostic testing, newborn screening, presymptomatic testing for estimating the risk of developing adult-onset cancers and Alzheimer's disease, confirmational diagnosis of a symptomatic individual, and forensic identity testing (National Human Genome Research Institute, 2007).

Gene testing has brought up questions and instigated debates in a number of areas. The most common question is: How much information should be given to an individual about his or her genetic predisposition for a disease or condition? It should be pointed out that genetic tests can determine the risk of certain diseases but usually do not have much predictive power. In others words, individuals can be told that their genes show a presence of risk, but the test cannot predict with certainty that the individual will have the disease. Over the past few years, genetic tests services (23andMe.com and DecodeMe.com) have sprung up on the Internet. In the future, it is expected that more tests will be commercially available as new technologies for genomic analysis enter the market and more "genetic epidemiology data are generated that facilitate interpretation" (Wilfond and Ross 2008: 1).

The general public has concerns that go beyond the science involved in genetic testing. Certainly, the public is interested in the array of medical potentials, but at the same time they are concerned about the ethical, privacy, and confidentiality issues as well as the potential misuse of personal genetic data. This remains a mystifying area of research and speculation. Consumers read about the breakthroughs, along with the hype, and wonder about the social and political impacts. Perhaps one of the challenges facing health sciences librarians is to help consumers access and evaluate this kind of information.

Genetic Engineering and Cloning

Understanding the DNA information systems not only is leading to a comprehension of the very basics of life but also is opening doors for a multitude of practical and powerful applications. One that comes to mind right way is *genetic engineering*.

Genetic engineering and cloning are two concepts that are very much in people's minds today. Although both of these techniques are related to the manipulation of the information codes in DNA, they are two quite different and distinct ideas and should not be confused.

Genetic engineering is the altering of genetic information in cells or organisms to enable them to make new substances or perform new functions. The cells are not exactly duplicated, as in cloning. The information in the genes is altered, not replicated.

Some successful applications of genetic engineering have been to use altered DNA to fight crop destruction by plant viruses, eat up garbage, dissolve blood clots in patients with heart attacks, stimulate red blood cells in people with chronic anemia, and synthesize interferon, an anticancer drug. The list of improved food products and critically important medicines continues to expand.

Cloning is the use of specialized techniques and technology to make exact copies of a single gene, a segment of DNA, an entire cell, or a complete, genetically identical organism. The information in the genes is replicated. In 1996, cloning caught the world's attention when scientists at the Roslyn Institute in Scotland cloned a sheep named Dolly from a cell that had been taken from the mammary gland of an old ewe and then grown in culture. This was the first mammal ever to be cloned from an adult body cell. It should be emphasized that, in general, cloning researchers are not particularly interested in cloning complete organisms; rather, they are interest in cloning genes and cells to be used in research, especially in medical research.

There are still great mysteries concerning DNA. Despite all that we have learned about what it is and how it works, there is still much to understand. Will scientists come to a complete understanding of DNA and show how mutations and natural selection explain every part of the development of life on this planet? As research advances, we continue to be intrigued and amazed at what DNA shows about the marvels of life, but it is much more than just curiosity that has lead us into this frontier of science. There is a great potential for improving the quality of life.

GENOMIC DATABASES

Development of databases has gone hand-in-hand with the development of bioinformatics. Genomic data are stored in databases, and therefore bioinformaticians must know how to manage and work with large databases. "The sheer scale of data involved in genomic research is mind-boggling and the field of bioinformatics has grown up to help provide the computational tools required" (Taylor, 2006: 34).

Genomic databases are large and complex. Molecular scientists use them to analyze biochemical properties and structures and to trace the evolutionary histories of organisms. Researchers can search for information in the databases by forming queries that match DNA sequences in the databases. These databases are growing rapidly, doubling every 15 months or so. At the same time, more and more people are using the systems, and the number of queries is increasing dramatically (Williams and Zobel, no date).

Bioinformatics data and information are so diverse and complex that no single, totally comprehensive databases has yet been created. Most databases are free and open to the public, although some require fees. The following are examples of bioinformatics databases:

- GenBank®. Available: www.ncbi.nlm.nih.gov/Genbank (accessed January 18, 2008). The National Institutes of Health maintains GenBank®. This is an annotated collection of all publicly available DNA sequences. There are approximately 85,759,586,764 bases in 82,853,685 sequence records in the traditional GenBank® divisions and 108,635,736,141 bases in 27,439,206 sequence records in the Whole Genome Shotgun division as of February 2008.
- European Bioinformatics Institute—Genomes Pages. Available: www.ebi. ac.uk/genomes (accessed January 18, 2008). This contains the European Molecular Biology Laboratory (EMBL) database, which was the first completed genome for viruses, phages, and organelles in the early 1980s. Since then, hundreds of complete genome sequences have been added, including those from archaea, bacteria, eukaryote, organelles, plasmids, and viroids.
- Ensembl. Available: www.ensembl.org/index.html (accessed January 18, 2008). Ensembl is a cooperative project that aims at developing a system for automatic annotation of vertebrates and large eukaryotic genomes. Ensembl presents up-to-date sequence data and the best possible automatic annotation for metazoan genomes. Available now are human, mouse, rat, fugu, zebrafish, and mosquito genomes.
- DNA Databank of Japan (DDBJ). Available: www.ddbj.nig.ac.jp/intro-e. html. (accessed January 18, 2008). DDBJ is the sole DNA databank in Japan officially certified to collect DNA sequences from researchers and to issue the internationally recognized accession number to data submitted. The database was established in 1986 and from the beginning functioned as one of the leading international DNA databases. It includes the databases of the European Bioinformatics Institute (EBI) in Europe and National Center for Biotechnology Information (NCBI).
- Genomes Online Database (GOLD). Available: www.genomesonline.org (accessed January 18, 2008). GOLD is a comprehensive Web-based database for information regarding genome projects around the world. It pro-

vides the largest available and most detailed monitoring of genome sequencing projects.

- Karyn's Genomes. Available: www.ebi.ac.uk/2can/genomes/genomes.html (accessed January 18, 2008). This database contains general information about organisms whose genomes are completely sequenced. The main aim of the database is to provide a short and concise explanation as to why it is important to obtain these organisms' genomic sequences, including publication data for where the sequences can be found.
- Mouse Phenome Database (MPD). Available: phenome.jax.org/pub-cgi/phenome/mpdcgi?rtn=docs/aboutmpd (accessed January 18, 2008). MPD is a comprehensive international database resource for the laboratory mouse, providing integrated genetic, genomic, and biological data to facilitate the study of human health and disease.
- National Center for Biotechnology Information (NCBI). Available: www.ncbi.nlm.nih.gov (accessed January 18, 2008). The NCBI, at the National Library of Medicine, is considered to be the world's largest biomedical research center, with ten different genetic databases available for research, including GenBank®, described earlier.
- National Human Genome Research Institute (NHGRI) Policy and Legislation Database. Available: www.genome.gov/PolicyEthics/LegDatabase/pubsearch.cfm?CFID=818183&CFTOKEN=83786403. This database includes federal and state laws and statutes. The materials focus on the privacy and confidentiality of genetic information, genetic testing, and commercialization and patenting.

Because of the growing interest in bioinformatics and the development of high-throughput devices for capturing data, the amount of data being created is causing an even bigger growth in databases and in the resources needed to manage them. This enormous amount of incoming data is presenting challenges to biotechnology companies, pharmaceutical companies, informaticians in the bioinformatics field, and also general areas of health informatics.

BIOINFORMATICS APPLICATIONS

Bioinformatics is no longer viewed as an esoteric academic pastime, as it was through most of the twentieth century. It is perceived as a very viable specialty with untold potential for applications (Guttmacher and Collins, 2002). Hoyt, Sutton, and Yoshihashi (2007: 215) list several immediate applications of bioinformatics:

- Diagnosing the 3,000–4,000 hereditary diseases that exist today
- Protein research to discover more targets for future drugs

- Pharmacogenomics to personalize drugs based on genetic profiles
- Complete genetic profiles will lead to better preventive medicine tests
- Gene therapy to treat diseases such as cancer. The most common way to achieve this is to use genetically altered viruses that carry human DNA. This approach, however, has not been proven to be helpful and not approved by the FDA
- Microbial genome alterations for energy production (bio-fuels), environmental cleanup, industrial processing and waste reduction
- Genetically engineered drought and disease resistant plants
- In spite of these interesting areas, it is estimated that less than 0.01% of microbes have been cultured and characterized. As an exception, the complete genome for the common human parasite Trichomonas vaginalis was report in the January 2007 issue of the journal *Science*

GENOMIC MEDICINE

Genomic medicine uses techniques and discoveries from genomic research. It is based on understanding how individual genes and the entire genome are related to disease and health. Taking advantage of basic biological processes is not a modern phenomenon. It goes back thousands of years to when we learned to make rising bread, beer, and cheese (Encyclopedia Britannica, 1994), but never with the depth, scale, and understanding like what is happening today.

Recognizing that genes define health risks for people is also not a recent idea. Before the DNA era, it was known that family traits and family medical histories played a role in predicting ones health conditions, but DNA-related discoveries are making these observations more scientific. The molecular causes of disease are becoming understood because of the insights provided by genetic models of the pathophysiologies involved. There are complex interactions among and between genes and the environment that contribute to disease (Burke, 2003).

Personalized Medicine

A major goal of genomic medicine is to use DNA to better diagnose disease and to detect genetic predispositions to disease. This will lead to *gene therapy* and the creation of drugs based on molecular information. Researchers are studying ways to correlate DNA variants with the treatment responses of patients with the objective of developing tailor-made medications. This is called *personalized medicine.*

The concept of personalized medicine is to analyze a patient's genotype data, determine how the disease affects specifically this patient, and then select a therapy and/or medication based on the data. The diagnosis and treatment plan does not depend solely on the DNA analysis, but the analysis is integrated into the traditional clinical work up, including medical history, laboratory tests, and imaging results. The objective of personalized medicine is to give the most appropriate care possible on a highly individualized basis, increasing the accuracy of the diagnosis and treatment proposed, and deliver treatment in a fast and efficient way.

The idea of personalized medicine is beginning to show real possibilities of becoming a meaningful part of healthcare. Pharmacogenomics is one of the personalized medicine applications. It deals with the integration of genomics technologies, advances in clinical medicine, and patient and family histories in order to tailor therapeutics to individual patients. Pharmacogenomics can help tailor prescriptions to subpopulation as well as to specific, individual patients. In the end, this will help improve the effectiveness and safety of drugs (Issa, 2007).

Personalized medicine appears to have a great potential, but it must first overcome some challenges. Matching genotype data to desirable drug responses is a complex task and requires advanced and effective information technologies, high-quality databases, and appropriate treatment algorithms (Issa, 2007). This underscores one of the important roles that the information professional plays in bioinformatics.

Societal Concerns

There is no doubt that new frontiers are being encountered in genetic research, including real potentials in understanding and curing diseases. However, the new data and possibilities are also raising some new concerns, particularly legal and ethical ones. For example, if a DNA profile shows that someone has a potentially incurable disease, should that person be told? Can this information cause discrimination, such as in job applications or insurance coverage? What should the boundaries and rules be for stem cell research? To what extent should genetic information become a part of a patient's health record?

The U.S. government addressed concerns about indiscriminant gene testing when Congress passed the *Genetic Information Nondiscrimination Act of 2008,* which was signed into law on May 21, 2008. Basically, the law is designed to guard against the improper use of genetic information in health insurance and employment situations. The law states that health insurance premiums cannot be based on genetic predisposition to a disease. Regarding employment, genetic data cannot be used in decisions about hiring, job placement, promotion, or firing.

Impact and Hopes

The sequencing of the human genome truly opened the door to genomic medicine. Liebman (2002: 201) observes that medicine is at a significant crossroads:

> Although many innovations in technology have made the "practice" more efficient and effective, nothing has yet had the potential for revolutionizing the "science" more than the results of the human genome project and its continuing generation of information and knowledge about disease processes and individual differences.

It is anticipated that the continuing development of genomics will impact the current standards of care for treatment of disease. Genomics promises powerful tools for diagnosis, prognosis, and prevention and is therefore relevant to healthcare informatics. The challenges and opportunities have just begun. Genetics and genomic medicine depend on information technology, and health informatics is supporting this rapidly growing field of medicine.

Of particular importance to health sciences librarians is that genomic research and progress is producing a volume of biological information that "at once contains secrets to age-old questions about health and disease and threatens to overwhelm our current capabilities of data analysis. Thus, bioinformatics is becoming critical for medicine in the twenty-first century" (Altman and Mooney, 2006: 765). Clearly, the effects of genomics on biology and medicine cannot be underestimated.

ROLE OF THE HEALTH INFORMATION PROFESSIONAL

Genetic research is yielding a profusion of microdata and thereby creating a need for new information management techniques and technologies. For the health information professional, the challenge is to represent, integrate, and store enormous amounts of data and develop user-friendly systems for then retrieving and displaying the data.

The field of genomics and bioinformatics is in its embryonic stage, but it is rapidly developing; it certainly behooves health sciences librarians to take stock of what they can do to become a part of this major medical frontier. It is clear that health sciences librarians have the potential to provide a wide range of biological and genomic informational services, but they must enhance their knowledge and expertise of this new field if they wish to provide high-quality services (Lyon et al., 2004).

Health sciences librarians have many options. Bioinformatics includes the subareas of the biosciences, health informatics, and allied information professions. Computer technology, database design, and database searching are important aspects of all the subareas, and health sciences librarians are well versed in information technology and database management. Health sciences librarians can help design databases with high levels of interoperability, standardize biomedical vocabularies, create knowledge representations, and explore the best ways to construct internal associations of data and then devise effective data querying techniques (Miller, 2000). For an example of how health sciences librarians can be involved in DNA database management, see Information Action! 12.1.

Bioinformatics faces some of the same challenges that any information service situation faces. These include, according to Hemminger (2005: 437), identifying "What are the best methods to represent and organize data that

INFORMATICS IN ACTION! 12.1

DNA Property Rights

Location: Biotechnology research center

Problem: The head of a task force working on a network for global sharing of DNA sequencing data becomes concerned that the members of the team have a poor understanding of intellectual property rights related to data sharing on a global scale, particularly proprietary and commercial DNA data. Violation of privacy is also an issue.

People Involved: The head of the task force, the knowledge manager of the center's library, and other members of the task force.

Action Taken: Fred, the knowledge manager, suggested a simple but sensible solution: a short course, required for the task force team, on the issues and nuances of intellectual property rights and the privacy of personal DNA data. He focused on current laws and policies regarding DNA data management and individual privacy. He was given approval to design and deliver the course. The course covered the basics of intellectual property rights, including issues that have arisen in the networking and distant communication environment with the rapidly growing interchange of DNA data.

Takeaway: By training and experience, Fred was well versed in intellectual property issues. Also, he was prepared by being up to date on new laws, issues, and international agreements that have come to the forefront in the global networking environment and in the management of DNA data.

---

facilitates knowledge extraction; how to relate information acquired from many different disciplines; [and] how to search disparate types of information captured from a plethora of heterogeneous resources."

The idea of librarians being involved in bioinformatics is not new. As mentioned earlier, some of the largest and most prestigious bioinformatics databases were created with the aid of librarians at the National Library of Medicine. Health sciences librarians continue to be involved in searching and teaching others to search these databases. Generally, librarians with a science background or a liaison relation with a science or information technology department find it easier to develop these roles (Alpi, 2003).

Alpi (2003) also identified three basic areas where health sciences librarians can be of immediate service to bioinformaticians: (1) teach molecular biology and clinical genetics information workshops to students, researchers, clinicians, and librarians; (2) create Web-based guides to molecular biology and clinical genetics resources for a variety of audiences, including consumers; and (3) provide searching and reference support and partner with clinicians and researchers.

In an earlier chapter of this book, we discussed the information specialty called *the informationist*. The idea of an informationist is that a person has expertise in both information management and in a subject domain. Bioinformatics is an area where the health sciences librarian can pursue this concept. An information professional with a strong biomedical background would be in a unique position to join the bioinformatics team.

Of special interest to health sciences librarians working in bioinformatics is the Molecular Biology and Genomics SIG of the Medical Library Association (http://medicine.wustl.edu/~molbio/). This special interest group exchanges information about molecular biology, genome projects, and clinical genetics information resources and promotes communication and collaboration in the development and delivery of information services related to bioinformatics.

SUMMARY

Bioinformatics is one of the leading areas of science in the twenty-first century. New information technology and procedures continue to evolve to support this field. Without doubt, bioinformatics is closely tied to healthcare, and health sciences librarians have emerging opportunities to play a vital role in this booming field.

REFERENCES

Alpi, Kristine. 2003. "Bioinformatics Training by Librarians and for Librarians: Developing the Skills Needed to Support Molecular Biology and Clinical Genetics Information Instruction." *Issues in Science & Technology Librarianship* 37 (Spring). Available: www.istl.org/03-spring/article1.html (accessed December 27, 2008).

Altman, Russ B. and Sean D. Mooney. 2006. "Bioinformatics." In *Biomedical Informatics: Computer Applications in Health Care and Biomedicine* (pp. 762–789), 3rd ed., edited by Edward H. Shortliffe and James J. Cimino. New York: Springer.

American Medical Informatics Association. *AMIA Strategic Plan*. Bethesda, MD: The American Medical Informatics Association (March 2007). Available: www.amia.org/inside/stratplan (accessed January 19, 2009).

Burke, Wylie. 2003. "Genomics as a Probe for Disease Biology." *New England Journal of Medicine* 349, no.10 (September 3): 969–974.

Butte, Atul J. 2008. "Translational Bioinformatics: Coming of Age." *Journal of the Medical Informatics Association* 15, no. 6 (November–December): 709–714.

Encyclopaedia Britannica Online. "Biotechnology." Chicago, IL: Encyclopaedia Britannica Online (1994). Available: http://www.britannica.com/ (accessed March 20, 2009).

Guttmacher, Alan E. and Francis S. Collins. 2002. "Genomic Medicine—A Primer." *New England Journal of Medicine* 347, no. 19 (November 7): 1512–1520.

Hemminger, Bradley M. 2005. "Introduction to the Special Issue on Bioinformatics." *Journal of the American Society for Information Science and Technology* 55, no. 5 (March): 437–439.

Howard, Ken. 2000. "The Bioinformatics Gold Rush." *Scientific American* 283, no. 1: 58–64.

Hoyt, Robert, Melainie Sutton, and Ann Yoshihashi. 2007. *Medical Informatics: Practical Guide for the Healthcare Professional.* Pensacola: University of West Florida.

Issa, Amalia. 2007. "Personalized Medicine and the Practice of Medicine in the 21st Century." *McGill Journal of Medicine* 10, no.1 (January): 53–57.

Liebman, Michael. 2002. "Biomedical Informatics: The Future for Drug Development." *Drug Discovery Today* 7, no. 20: s197–s203.

Lindberg, Donald A.B. and Betsy L. Humphreys. 2008. "Rising Expectations: Access to Biomedical Information." *Yearbook of Medical Informatics.* Heidelberg, Germany: International Medical Informatics Association, 3, no. 1: 165–172.

Lyon, Jennifer, Nunzia B. Guise, Annette Williams, Teneya Koonce, and Rachel Walden. 2004. "A Model for Training the New Bioinformationist." *Journal of the Medical Library Association* 92, no. 2 (April): 188–195.

Mason, Christopher E., Michael R. Seringhaus, and Clara Sattler de Sousa e Brito. 2007. "Personalized Genomic Medicine with a Patchwork, Partially Owned Genome." *Yale Journal of Biology and Medicine* 80, no. 4 (December): 145–151.

Mendel, Gregor. 1865. "Versuche uber Pflanzen-Hybriden" ["Experiments on Plant Hybrids"]. *Verhandlungen des naturforschenden den Vereines* [Brünn, Austria] 4: 3–47.

Miller, Perry L. 2000. "Opportunities at the Intersection of Bioinformatics and Health Informatics: A Case Study." *Journal of the American Medical Informatics Association* 7, no. 5 (September–October): 431–438.

National Center for Biotechnology Information. *A Science Primer.* Bethesda, MD: National Library of Medicine, National Institutes of Health (March 29, 2004). Available: www.ncbi.nlm.nih.gov/About/primer/Bioinformatics.html (accessed December 29, 2008).

National Human Genome Research Institute. *Gene Testing.* Bethesda, MD: National Institutes of Health (July 24, 2007). Available: www.ornl.gov/sci/techresources/Human_Genome/medicine/genetest.shtml (accessed December 29, 2008).

National Human Genome Research Institute. *Genetic Mapping.* Bethesda, MD: National Institutes of Health (July 23, 2008). Available: www.genome.gov/10000715 (accessed December 29, 2008).

National Library of Medicine. *Genome Mapping: A Guide to the Genetic Highway We Call the Human Genome.* Bethesda, MD: National Library of Medicine, National Institutes of Health (March 29, 2004). Available: www.ncbi.nlm.nih.gov/About/primer/mapping.html (accessed December 29, 2008).

Taylor, Paul. 2006. *From Patient Data to Medical Knowledge: The Principles and Practice of Health Informatics.* Malden, MA: Blackwell Publishing, Ltd.

U.S. Department of Energy, Office of Science and Office of Biological and Environmental Research. 2008. "What Is the Human Genome Project?" Washington, DC: U.S. Department of Energy Office of Science and Office of Biological and Environmental Research. Human Genome Program (August 19, 2008): Available: www.ornl.gov/sci/techresources/Human_Genome/project/about.shtml (accessed December 27, 2008).

Wade, Nicholas. "Gains in Understanding Human Cells." *New York Times,* October 25, 2002. Available: http://query.nytimes.com/gst/fullpage.html?res=9B01E3DC

103CF936A15753C1A9649C8B63&scp=1&sq=David+K.+Gifford&st=nyt (accessed December 28, 2008).

Wilfond, Benjamin and Lainie Friedman Ross. 2008. "From Genetics to Genomics: Ethics, Policy, and Parental Decision-making." *Journal of Pediatric Psychology* (July 22, Epub ahead of print): 1–9.

Williams, Hugh E. and Justin Zobel. "Indexing and Retrieval for Genomic Databases." Melbourne, Australia: Department of Computer Science, Royal Melbourne Institute of Technology (no date). Available: http://goanna.cs.rmit.edu.au/~jz/fulltext/ieeekade02.pdf (accessed December 27, 2008).

Chapter 13

The Age of Health Informatics

Health informatics evolved slowly over the last 40 years of the twentieth century, and, in the new millennium, it has blossomed into a robust and vital part of healthcare endeavors. For a profession, such as health informatics, to remain viable, it must maintain strong educational and research components. This final chapter discusses the educational and research aspects of health informatics as well as the current trends and future promise of the profession within the infrastructure of health informatics.

EDUCATION, RESEARCH, AND CAREER PATHS

The foundation of a profession is shaped and guided by a formal educational structure and an extensive, continuing research endeavor. The educational component ensures there will be a continuity of professionals in the field, and research verifies and expands the knowledge domain of the discipline.

Education is the pillar of a profession, and it is how the basic systematic knowledge and fundamental proficiencies are instilled in the professional. The educational requirements are usually established by the practitioners of the profession and are often regulated by professional bodies with accreditation control and/or examinations of competence. Legal mandates may also require some professionals to obtain a license. With health informatics, the application areas are widely diversified, so practitioners must be competent in many areas. The interdisciplinary nature of health informatics, while highly necessary, raises the level of complexity of the educational structures.

Educational Pathways

Health informatics professional societies, educators, and individuals have always been concerned about the education of health informaticians, particularly with the perception that too many practitioners have limited education and training specifically related to what they do. This, of course, is the result of people transitioning into informatics to fill the suddenly significant need for skilled professionals in the field. For example, the International Medical Informatics Association (IMIA) noted that many health care professionals lacked sufficient knowledge of data processing technology and how to use it in medical decision making. The IMIA (2000: 3) suggested that "through improved education of health care professionals and through an increase in the number of well-trained workers in health and medical informatics that this lack of knowledge and associated skills can begin to be reversed."

In all developing fields, it takes time to work out the necessary educational foundation. In health informatics, professionals question and discuss the nature of the programs of study and where they should be developed and delivered. The interdisciplinary nature of health informatics makes it even more difficult to answer these questions. Because of the overlapping disciplines within health informatics and the lack of common jobs in the field, there is no set health informatics curriculum. As Hersh (2002: 77) states, "The lack of a common skill set and curriculum is different from librarianship or medicine, where there are basic skills that all library science or medical degrees, respectively, can be expected to have." Hersh and others have pointed out that there is a need for a core curriculum for health informatics, and this issue is still being discussed in the profession. Most recently, Hersh (2008) detailed the challenges faced in describing the education and workforce needs in health informatics.

Education programs and curricula are based on the theoretical foundations of the field, its applications, and the profession's perception of the competencies needed. As a field emerges, practitioners need to identify the competencies that they require, which usually spurs debate in the profession. As mentioned, health informatics is a broad, interdisciplinary field, with a wide range of applications and theoretical constructs. Any detailed list of health informatics competencies will be long and broad, but the competencies can be distilled into some general concepts. The IMIA (2000) lists three major classes of desired competencies:

1. Methodology and Technology for the Processing of Data, Information and Knowledge in Medicine and Health Care
2. Medicine, Health and Biosciences, Health Systems Organization
3. Informatics/Computer Science, Mathematics, Biometry

In 2005, the American Health Information Management Association and the AMIA released a joint report stressing the importance of standardizing a set of competencies to develop curricula for informatics to build a strong workforce In 2007, Huang investigated the competencies needed for health informatics by analyzing the curricula of health informatics programs; he found that the common competencies taught were research methods, health information systems, and informatics/computer science methods.

Health informatics curricula are still young and remain a mixture of interdisciplinary areas. Educational courses and programs in health informatics exist in many forms and are offered by academic institutions, professional associations, government agencies, healthcare facilities, and others. These offerings have varied from single courses to comprehensive informatics programs that offer different types of degrees. The AMIA (2007) lists the following types of health informatics programs that are generally available:

- Associate degree in informatics
- Undergraduate degree in informatics
- Masters degree in informatics
- PhD degree in informatics
- Informatics specialization within other degree programs
- [National Library of Medicine]–sponsored postdoctoral fellowships
- Other postdoctoral research fellowships
- Certificate programs

There are avenues outside of traditional academia for the education and training of health informaticians. For example, the National Library of Medicine has strongly supported health informatics since the inception of the field. This support has taken many forms, including database information resources, research grants, training grants, and a variety of training programs. The U.S. Department of Health and Human Services (2008) lists the following examples of training programs:

- Postdoctoral research
- Training for graduate and medical students
- Research program for visiting scientists
- Clinical elective for medical and dental students
- [National Library of Medicine] rotation for medical informatics trainees
- Postdoctoral research in biomedical image processing and document image analysis.

Other government agencies also provide health informatics education. In 1995, the U.S. Department of Veterans Affairs (VA) started its VA Advanced Fellowship Program in Medical Informatics because of its concern about the small number of medical informatics experts within its own organization. The purpose of the program was to give advanced training to those already working in informatics in the VA and to recruit and retain other professionals to work in the VA. Basically, it is a two-year postresidency/postdoctoral research and educational learning program, with the fellows spending their time in activities relevant to the VA (U.S. Department of Veterans Affairs, 2008).

An example of the involvement of professional associations in education is the AMIA's 10 × 10 program. The basic idea is to bring together course content from various informatics training programs, with an emphasis on distance learning. The training is application focused and offered at academic institutions, professional meetings, in the workplace, and elsewhere. The goal is to train 10,000 healthcare professionals in informatics by the year 2010.

Continuing Education

Most professions need a strong mechanism for continuing education in order to keep up with current research and development. Health informatics is evolving rapidly, with new knowledge and technologies supplanting the old. Like other professionals, health informaticians need to be lifelong learners in order to continually adapt to the changing times.

There are many avenues for continuing education in health informatics. Almost all university-based informatics programs include continuing education courses, ranging from short courses to full certifications. Another avenue is professional associations, which often offer continuing education courses at meetings and online.

The requirement for recertification has spawned many continuing education offerings in health informatics. For example, some states require 30 contact hours of continuing education in some informatics fields to retain licensure. This requirement can be met by any combination of courses taken in accredited university programs and approved courses of professional associations. Also, health informaticians who have licenses in certain health or other fields are required to take continuing education courses in those fields. The good news is that information technology is providing healthcare information professionals with new tools and methods for self-directed continuing learning, allowing immediate access to vast resources for updating and keeping informed.

Health Informatics Research

Because of the interdisciplinary nature of health informatics, its research cuts across many fields. Health informatics research methods are both quantitative and qualitative, and research is both application driven and theoretically based.

Initially, health informatics research centered on developing models and subsequent computer-based systems that delivered professional knowledge and current information to healthcare providers. Research included studies on how computer-based systems impacted the reasoning and behavior of healthcare providers and how the systems affected patient care and organizational management.

Health informatics research focuses evolved over time. In 2006, the *Handbook of Research on Informatics in Healthcare and Biomedicine* was published, which included chapters on current research topics in the field. Its table of contents reflects the most popular research areas at that time. Some of the areas are electronic health records, security in information systems, chronic disease registers, standards, health classification systems, virtual reality, modeling biological systems, brain mapping, information processing in clinical decision making, knowledge management in medicine, telemedicine systems, semantic Web services in healthcare, artificial intelligence in medicine, and genomic databanks (Lazakidou, 2006). Clearly, research in health informatics is diverse, and there are many frontiers for future investigators as well as many areas of opportunities for health sciences librarians.

Career Opportunities

The major application areas in health informatics discussed in Chapter 4 parallel the available career opportunities. Health informatics careers are open to individuals with a broad range of backgrounds, including librarianship, computer science, medical specialties, management, and education. There are many career options and job opportunities, and the needs will inevitably increase as the field develops. According to Hersh (2008), although there is no "succinct" definition of informatics and little data on the nature of the existing workforce, there are substantial career opportunities. Specifically, opportunities in the specialty areas of informatics, such as clinical informatics as they relate to patient safety, are growing (Kilbridge and Classen, 2008).

Because of the dynamic nature of the terminology in the health informatics field, it would be a challenge to compile a complete list of position job titles. Many titles do not include *health informatics* or *medical informatics*, although the positions clearly are in areas of informatics. Instead, the titles and descriptions of the positions reflect activities in a particular work environment. Remember that any profession or occupation is defined by its *activities*, not necessarily by its name, and this certainly is the case at the present time with health informatics. The AMIA (2005) gives examples of career options:

> People coming out of degree programs may be managers, project designers, researchers, programmers, systems analysts, or educators; the settings in which they work can range from hospitals and health systems to health information technology system vendors to health companies to insurers to academic departments.

It is useful to sort job positions into two general categories: (1) specialties and (2) areas of employment. Examples of specialties include, among others:

- Academic teaching and educational support
- Data quality management
- Privacy and security of medical information
- Health information systems management
- Health information technology
- Clinical data management
- Clinical information systems management
- Medical research and development
- Health sciences librarianship

Examples of areas of employment include, among others:

- Academia: Opportunities would usually require candidates to have an advanced degree and some experience in teaching.
- Consulting companies: These companies usually advise and assist healthcare organizations with development and implementation of information systems and provide knowledge management solutions.
- Corporate research and development: The heart of the modern healthcare industry is research and development of new products. Activities in this area involve extensive and complex information management, from the research lab to marketing.
- Government and nongovernment agencies: These agencies are involved in health planning and analysis of information on a wide scale, ranging from local to global initiatives.
- Hospitals and other healthcare facilities: As more healthcare organizations utilize electronic medical records systems, they need professionals to implement and manage these systems.
- Insurance industry: Opportunities in this area would usually involve the analysis of health insurance claims and health records.
- Medical software companies: These companies require individuals with strong programming skills and knowledge of the healthcare sector.
- Pharmaceutical companies: Health informatics professionals are needed to aid in the research and development processes as well as in the analysis of drug use information.
- Public health organizations: Individuals working in these organizations are needed to collect and analyze data on populations and communities. The design and implementation of surveillance systems, disease reporting systems, and databases are also areas of opportunities.

Professional Associations

Professional societies and associations play an important role in all professions. These organizations offer members opportunities to network with other individuals in the field, learn about new developments, promote education, and codify ethical standards.

HEALTH INFORMATICS ASSOCIATIONS

Following are examples of health informatics professional associations:

- American Medical Informatics Association (AMIA). Available: www. amia.org (accessed December 31, 2008). AMIA was founded in 1990. Its membership is composed of physicians, nurses, dentists, pharmacists, other clinicians, health information technologists, computer scientists, medical librarians, educators, and industry representatives. According to the Web site, AMIA members "advance the use of informatics in clinical care, personal health management, public health/population, and research with the ultimate objective of improving health." The organization is the official United States representative to the International Medical Informatics Association.

- American Nursing Informatics Association (ANIA). Available: www.ania.org (accessed December 31, 2008). ANIA was formed in 1992, and members include healthcare professionals working with clinical information systems, educational applications, data collection/research application, and other applications. According to the Web site, ANIA's objective is to provide "professional networking opportunities for nurses working in healthcare informatics and a forum for the advancement of nursing and nursing professionals in informatics."
- Canada's Health Informatics Association (COACH). Available: www.coachorg.com (accessed December 31, 2008). COACH was formed in 1975. Its membership is composed of physicians, nurses and allied health professionals, healthcare executives, educators, information technology vendors, and others interested in technology systems for the effective use of health information in healthcare decision-making. According to the Web site, COACH "believes in the importance and the value of strategic alliances with other organizations involved in the field of health informatics in Canada and internationally. It is committed to building a strong international network in health informatics through international organizations, such as the International Medical Informatics Association (IMIA), and other national associations around the world."
- European Federation for Medical Informatics (EFMI). Available: www.efmi.org (accessed December 29, 2008). EFMI, founded in 1976, is federation of a number of European countries. According to the Web site, "All European countries are entitled to be represented in EFMI by a suitable Medical Informatics Society." The objectives of the federation are to advance international cooperation and dissemination of information on medical informatics on a European level. Also, EFMI promotes research, development, application, and education in medical informatics.
- International Medical Informatics Association (IMIA). Available: www.imia.org (accessed December 30, 2008). IMIA began in 1967 as Technical Committee 4 of the International Federation for Information Processing (IFIP) and in 1989 was officially established by law in Switzerland. Its membership consists of national, institutional, and affiliate members and honorary fellows. IMIA's goal is to serve as a bridge connecting health informatics groups around the world. In this respect, it has close ties with the World Health Organization (WHO) as a Non Government Organization (NGO). One of its well-known activities is the triannual meeting World Congress on Medical and Health Informatics.

Examples of related associations with membership crossing over to health informatics include the following:

- American Health Information Management Association (AHIMA). Available: www.ahima.org (accessed December 30, 2008). The beginnings of the AHIMA go back to 1928 when the Association of Record Librarians was established by the American College of Surgeons. Over the years the organization has undergone several name changes, reflecting the evolution of information management, arriving at its present name in 1991. The organization has always based its activities on the premise that medical record quality is essential to patient care and research.
- American Society for Information Science and Technology (ASIS&T). Available: www.asis.org (accessed December 30, 2008). ASIS&T was founded in 1937. Its members come from diverse backgrounds, such as computer science, linguistics, management, librarianship, engineering, law, medicine, chemistry, and education. According to the Web site, it "has been the society for information professionals leading the search for new and better theories, techniques, and technologies to improve access to information. ASIS&T brings together diverse streams of knowledge, focusing what might be disparate approaches into novel solutions to common problems."
- Healthcare Information and Management Systems Society (HIMSS). Available: www.himss.org (accessed December 30, 2008). HIMSS focuses on information technology and management systems. It was founded in 1961, with both individual and corporate members. According to the Web site, HIMSS' mission is to "lead change in the healthcare information and management systems field through knowledge sharing, advocacy, collaboration, innovation, and community affiliations."
- Medical Library Association (MLA). Available: www.mlanet.org (accessed December 29, 2008). The MLA, founded in 1898, includes both individual and institutional members. According to the Web site, the MLA is "committed to educating health information professionals, supporting health information research, promoting access to the world's health sciences information, and working to ensure that the best health information is available to all." The MLA includes an informatics special interest group.

TRENDS AND HORIZONS IN HEALTH INFORMATICS

Health informatics is one of the most exciting areas of healthcare. Current trends are leading toward new horizons in theoretical understanding and innovative applications.

Advances in Health Informatics Technologies

The future of health informatics will be defined by changes in the healthcare environment and advances in technology. Healthcare and health informatics will continue to rely on technology.

Fickenscher (2007) identified eight categories of change impacting healthcare, including (1) standardization, (2) digitization, (3) nanotization, (4) de-tethered networks, (5) peripheral intelligence, (6) integrated biogenomics, (7) noninvasive medicine, and (8) robotics. Each of these categories is discussed elsewhere in this book, and they provide a good framework for reviewing the technologies on the horizon of health informatics.

Standardization refers to processes and agreements for developing formats and guidelines to ensure the consistency, accuracy, and transportability of health information. Further standardization will improve quality of care and safety of patients, reduce costs, and streamline the flow and exchange of healthcare information. At the heart of this is the need for terminologies and coding systems that are technologically compatible and globally interoperable so that the systems will work seamlessly throughout all networks. New interchange platforms are being developed for this, such as Web 3.0. In a digitized environment, standardization is absolutely essential.

Digitization refers to the acquiring, storing, and transporting of information in digital formats. The move toward universal digitization of healthcare information is accelerating in all areas of health informatics applications. Digitized imaging techniques are giving physicians new, in-depth views of the human body in both real-time and simulated situations. Picture archiving and communication systems are being refined and integrated into electronic health records, networks, and other communication devices.

Digitization allows faster, more inclusive navigation through images. These new techniques allow better diagnostics and less invasive procedures, making it easier on the patient and providing more accurate information to the physician. Methods for integrating diagnostic imaging and therapies are being enhanced, and some are being applied to nuclear medicine.

Digital image management and the evolving related enhanced technologies are making the dream of a national electronic health information system become a reality. A number of agencies and organizations are pursing this, including, among others, the Department of Health and Human Services, the Institute of Medicine, and the Healthcare Information and Management Systems Society.

Nanotization in medicine has accelerated in the past few years and without doubt is leading to new medical technologies. Ray Kurzweil, the entrepreneur and futurist, believes that robust integration of nanotechnology into medical practice is a given certainty. He stated that "remote sensors will measure and report data daily to a physician's digital database and when a problem is detected the doctor is alerted" (Milken Institute, 2005). Nanotechnology is also being integrated into molecular therapeutics. For example, nanoparticle technology has the promise of zeroing in on the exact spot of a tumor and delivering the exact amount of chemotherapy needed. It may be possible to place machines the size of red blood cells into diabetic patients that will release insulin when they need it. This kind of therapy control has the potential to increase drug effectiveness and decrease drug dosage to alleviate harmful side effects.

De-tethered mobile networks are increasingly popular and far reaching. Improved, sophisticated satellite phones continue to appear on the market, and healthcare professionals are embracing them. Internet-based communications via the short message service (SMS) of mobile phones are being used to remind patients of appointments and to manage chronic diseases. Global positioning systems (GPS) are potentially useful, such as locating wandering Alzheimer's patients. Text messaging is the method of choice for a large part of the population, including healthcare providers and their patients. New technologies are making text messaging much easier and more convenient.

Peripheral intelligence sensors are being placed on hospital beds, and computer chips may soon be implanted in patients. Sensors will be connected to a wide range of medical devices throughout the healthcare organization and in the patient's home to monitor vital signs. This type of new and promising technology is exciting, with the potential to be integrated into some types of treatments, for example, for diabetes and tumor control.

Integrated biogenomics is emerging with the development of bioinformatics. As genomic medicine advances, genomic research and clinical research will intersect and merge. The National Library of Medicine predicts that, by 2025:

> [E]very patient will be a potential Visible Man or Woman, with imaging data that can be viewed interactively. As the Visible Human Project begins to incorporate physiology, biochemistry, and other necessary components of life, scientists and healthcare practitioners will be able to see proteins unfolding, DNA in operation, the nanoscale activities that are at the very heart of life itself. (U.S. Department of Health and Human Services, 2006: 13)

Prevention and treatments will be specific and routinely personalized to individuals.

Noninvasive modalities, such as virtual reality, will use three-dimensional and four-dimensional viewing to allow healthcare providers to plan their work, tailored to the individual characteristics of the patient. This type of virtual simulation is also enhancing and changing teaching methods in medical education.

Robotics technology is becoming more sophisticated with new sensors and voice recognition applications. Robots are now used to perform both major surgeries and minimally invasive surgeries. At a different level, robots retrieve supplies, deliver reports and mail, and fill pharmaceutical orders. Robotic devices will soon dispense medications at all points of care, such as clinics, patient care units, and operating rooms, providing medications immediately when needed with superior accuracy and therefore with fewer medical errors.

Health Informatics and an Innovative Internet

The Internet has impacted healthcare by empowering consumers, supporting telehealth, connecting global health information and resources, creating cyberspace healthcare business ventures, and opening new communication pathways. The Internet is now part of the healthcare infrastructure. Clinicians use the Internet to provide patient care. Health records are stored in cyberspace, and both healthcare professionals and health consumers take advantage of the Internet's vast amount of information.

The advent of Web 2.0, soon to be followed by Web 3.0, has created a method of open communication, with decentralized authority and freedom to share. Web 2.0 concepts are about creating communities of participation, sharing, and open source software, along with sophisticated multimedia tools. Web 2.0 has spawned offshoots, such as Health 2.0. "Through Health 2.0 Web sites a patient can do amazing things: search for and obtain tailored, high quality medical information, medical diagnoses, personal medical record keeping, exhaustive SNP [single nucleotide polymorphisms] analysis of their own genome, and even some do-it-your epidemiology" (Bleicher, 2008: 38). All of these developments have brought in a new term, *cybermedicine*, which refers to the application of global networking and the Internet to the health sciences. Future medicine is arriving everyday, and, in terms of informatics, it is primarily cyberspace based.

Finally, it should be noted that the ubiquity of the Internet and the promises of the Web 2.0 platform have helped usher in the concept of wellness. The traditional paradigm of healthcare was treating the sick, giving emergency service, and being reimbursed for services. "Medicine is a classic supply and demand system. The simple principal drive of the system today is illness" (Ball, 2003: 76). The Internet is changing the paradigm by empowering people around the global to take charge of their health and be aggressive participants in their own wellness.

Emerging Health Informatics Specialties

In the years ahead, new specialties in health informatics will emerge in response to changes in healthcare and to societal pressures. An excellent example of this is disaster informatics.

Not only is information important in the delivery of healthcare, but it is critical in emergency and disaster situations. Because medical care in these situations is a paramount concern, it follows that health informatics has an essential role to play, especially in the integration of medicine, public health, information, technology, and humans in an emergency. The terrorist attacks and natural disasters in the past decade have highlighted areas that lack efficient and coordinated communication systems, which caused confusion, misinformation, and, in some cases, chaos. Health informaticians must assume a role in helping to mitigate such inefficiencies. The National Library of Medicine has taken a lead role in creating the Disaster Information Management Research Center (DIMRC) to help with national emergency preparedness and response efforts. A corollary specialty is developing, called *disaster informatics*, which studies the need and uses of information and related technology in disaster and emergency preparation, response, and recovery efforts.

A FINAL WORD

Health informatics began with the interest and need to develop computer applications for medicine and healthcare. Over four decades, it has developed into a complete discipline with a theoretical foundation, research component, and refined set of application theorems. It continues to be one of the most exciting areas of healthcare and to offer health sciences librarians in health informatics intriguing opportunities.

INFORMATICS IN ACTION! 13.1

Emergency Preparedness Information

Location: Large metropolitan hospital

Problem: The hospital's chief information officer (CIO) requested an emergency preparedness plan to be expanded to address bioterrorism, including information protocols for the hospital staff.

People Involved: The committee on bioterrorist emergency preparedness and the informationist from the hospital library.

Action Taken: Blanche, the informationist, knows that the Internet has many links to terrorism preparedness resources, such as the ones at the National Library of Medicine and the Center for Disease Control and Prevention. She and her assistant reviewed numerous sites, selecting ones that might be useful. Next, she conducted a random survey of the hospital staff to identify their information needs. After consulting with the committee chair, Blanche designed a bioterrorism preparedness kit, including, among other things, a list of procedures to be followed in case of an attack, leaflets with suggestions, and a bibliography of resources.

Takeaway: Clearly, the informationist was aware of the existing resources. Her professional knowledge provided her with a starting point, and her familiarity with the needs of healthcare personnel helped her to create the bioterrorism preparedness kit.

With the exponential use of the Internet and the rising health awareness of the general public, health information is becoming one of the largest sought-after information segments in our society. Health-related Web sites continue to grow, and, according to the National Library of Medicine, one-third of all MEDLINE searches are conducted by the general public. Along with this are the rapidly evolving and changing information technologies and their applications to healthcare. These factors foretell a golden age of health informatics on the horizon.

Health informatics is not an end in itself. Its purpose is to provide information for the care of patients in all circumstances. Bad information will generate poor quality of care; good information will support quality care. This simple concept highlights the critical role of the healthcare information professions in all their forms. The future of health informatics is an open frontier with unlimited potentials.

Without a doubt, this is the age of health informatics. Health information technology is big business, permeating the entire field. In developed countries, around 10 percent of the gross domestic product is devoted to healthcare, and approximately 5 percent is devoted to information and communication technology. The information technology in health care is a considerable economic factor (Haux, 2006).

The amount of information processed in the healthcare endeavor is staggering. Haux (2006) analyzed a typical large hospital and compiled some enormous statistics for one year of operation. The hospital had 50,000 inpatients and 250,000 outpatients. There were 20,000 operations reports, 250,000 discharge letters, 20,000 pathology reports, 100,000 microbiology reports, 200,000 radiology reports, 800,000 clinical chemistry reports, and around 400,000 new patient records (Haux, 2006). Modern healthcare is information driven, and health informatics is critical to its entire infrastructure.

Finally, health sciences librarians should ask themselves the question: What role do I want to play in health informatics? Throughout this book the point was repeatedly made that there is a role for health sciences librarians in health informatics, but librarians have to be proactive in seeking these opportunities.

In Chapter 2, the concept of an informationist was defined as an information specialist who has received graduate training and practical experience providing them with an interdisciplinary background in a medical or biological science and in information sciences/informatics. The concept of an informationist continues to evolve and has come to be called the *Informationist Specialist in Context* (ISIC). The idea is still in its infancy, but it reflects a change in the environment of health sciences information and the involvement of health sciences librarians. The evolving horizons of health informatics, as discussed in this chapter, offer this type of information specialists an avenue to become a standard part of the health informatics team.

The shifting information infrastructure paradigms in healthcare reflect changes in healthcare and the advent of robust information technologies. Health sciences librarians need to follow these changes closely to understand the potential impacts on their work environment and to be able to forecast the changes necessary to support their community of users. Healthcare structures, intelligent information technology, computing devices, communication networks and devices, medical advances mainly in genomic medicine, and government legislation to support health information technology are emerging as major elements in the paradigm shifts. Healthcare organizations, including educational institutions, will be more flexible and virtual, with new channels of communications among units in the organization. Knowledge management will be focused, with new ways to integrate and personalize data into knowledge-based paradigms. The advanced versions of the Internet are going to increase the presence of communities of professionals sharing data, knowledge, and experience. New economic models for managing and marketing information will be implemented, and new care models will focus on personalized medicine and prevention of disease (Goldstein et al., 2007).

The U.S. government is supporting these paradigm changes. Congress just passed The American Recovery and Reinvestment Act of 2009, allocating billion of dollars for developing and implementing health information technologies such as universal electronic health records. This bill will impact the healthcare industry, particularly health informatics.

Health sciences librarians are poised to be a major force in the changes in healthcare if they understand the basic tenets of health informatics. It is not necessary for health sciences librarians to become technical experts in health informatics, but they do need to grasp the intersections of health informatics and health sciences librarianship. In order to become respected members of the health informatics team, health sciences librarians need to know and apply the basics of health informatics, aggressively seek ways to integrate health informatics initiatives in their organizations, and demonstrate their value to the health informatics community. The premise of this book is that this can be done.

REFERENCES

American Health Information Management Association and American Medical Informatics Association. "Building the Work Force for Health Information Transformation." Chicago: American Health Information Management Association (2005). Available: www.ahima.org/emerging_issues/Workforce_web.pdf (accessed December 30, 2008).

American Medical Informatics Association. "Degree Programs, Certificate Programs, Fellowships, and Short Courses." Bethesda, MD: American Medical Informatics Association (November 29, 2007). Available: www.amia.org/informatics/acad& training/index.asp (accessed December 29, 2008).

American Medical Informatics Association. "FAQ." Bethesda, MD: American Medical Informatics Association (2005). Available: www.amia.org/inside/faq/#3 (accessed December 31, 2008).

Ball, Marion J. 2003. *Consumer Informatics: Applications and Strategies in Cyber Health-care.* New York: Springer-Verlag.

Bleicher, Paul. "Health 2.0: Do It Yourself Doctoring." *Applied Clinical Trials* (October, 2008). Available: http://appliedclinicaltrialsonline.findpharma.com/appliedclinical trials/Technology+Viewpoint/Health-20-Do-It-Yourself-Doctoring/ArticleStandard/ Article/detail/556205?ref=25 (accessed December 31, 2008).

Fickenscher, Kevin. 2007. "Expert Forewords." In *Medical Informatics 20/20 Quality and Electronic Health Records Through Collaboration, Open Solutions, and Innovation* (pp. xv– xvii), edited by Douglas Goldstein, Peter J. Groen, Suniti Ponkshe, and Marck Wine. Sudbury, MA: Jones and Bartlett.

Goldstein, Douglas, Peter J. Groen, Suniti Ponkshe, and Marc Wine. 2007. *Medical Informatics 20/20 Quality and Electronic Health Records Through Collaboration, Open Solutions, and Innovation.* Sudbury, MA: Jones and Bartlett.

Haux, Reinhold. 2006. "Health Information Systems—Past, Present, Future." *International Journal of Medical Informatics* 75, no. 3–4 (March –April): 268–281.

Hersh, William. 2002. "Medical Informatics Education: An Alternative Pathway for Training Informationist." *Journal of the Medical Library Association* 90, no. 1 (January): 76–79.

Hersh, William. 2008. "Health and Biomedical Informatics: Opportunities and Challenges for a Twentieth-first Century Profession and its Education." In *IMIA Yearbook of Medical Informatics.* Heidelberg, Germany: International Medical Informatics Association.

Huang, Qi Rong. 2007. "Competencies for Graduate Curricula in Health, Medical and Biomedical Informatics: A Framework." *Health Informatics Journal* 13, no. 2: 89–103.

International Medical Informatics Association. Working Group 1: Health and Medical Informatics Education. 2000. "Recommendations of the International Medical Informatics Association (IMIA) on Education in Health and Medical Informatics." *Methods of Information in Medicine* 39, no. 3 (August): 267–277. Available: www.imia.org/pubdocs/rec_english.pdf (accessed March 20, 2009).

Kilbridge, Peter M. and David C. Classen. 2008. "The Informatics Opportunities at the Intersection of Patient Safety and Clinical Informatics." *Journal of the American Medical Informatics Association* 15, no. 4: 397–407.

Lazakidou, Athina A. 2006. "Table of Contents." In *Handbook of Research on Informatics in Healthcare and Biomedicine.* Hershey, PA: Idea Group Reference.

Milken Institute. 2005. *Bits, Biology & Bionics: Medicine in 2005.* Santa Monica: Milken Institute Global Conference. Available: www.milkeninstitute.org/presentations/ slides/gc05_bits_bio_bionics.pdf (accessed December 30, 2008).

U.S. Department of Health and Human Services, National Institutes of Health, National Library of Medicine. 2006. *Charting a Course for the 21st Century: NLM's Long Range Plan 2006–2016.* Bethesda, MD: National Library of Medicine.

U.S. Department of Health and Human Services, National Institutes of Health, National Library of Medicine. "Training Opportunities." Bethesda, MD: The Lister

Hill National Center for Biomedical Communications (May 14, 2008). Available: http://lhncbc.nlm.nih.gov/lhc/servlet/Turbine/template/training%2CTraining oppor.vm (accessed December 31, 2008).

U.S. Department of Veterans Affairs. "VA Advanced Fellowship Program in Medical Informatics." Washington, DC: U.S. Department of Veterans Affairs (November 8, 2008). Available: www.va.gov/oaa/specialfellows/programs/SF_MedicalInformatics. asp?p=8 (accessed December 30, 2008).

Glossary

admission-discharge-transfer (ADT): The systematic management of the complete cycle of processes that patients go through during a hospital stay from admission to discharge.

Advanced Research Projects Agency Network (ARPANET): A wide-area computer network that promoted the free exchange of information and eventually became the basis for today's Internet. It was created in the 1960s by the U.S. Department of Defense.

adverse event: Any unexpected or dangerous medical occurrence that may transpire during the provision of healthcare. The event may or may not be related to the specific treatment being given.

alert message: A warning of a medical situation that needs attention. The alert is computer generated and is based on a set of specified criteria related to physical reactions and/or on the presence of any abnormal condition recorded from lab tests or other empirical observations.

ambulatory medical record system (AMRS): A patient medical record generated for clinical outpatients. It includes the same basic information as any medical record, such as patient history, billing information, test results, and treatment protocol.

ambulatory monitoring: The physiological monitoring of a patient who is moving about and is engaged in normal physical activities.

angiography: An X-ray technique that produces increased contrast resolution images of the internal structures of arteries and veins. It is used to diagnose blood vessel problems. The images can be presented in several formats, such as still images, screen displays, film, or motion images.

applications research: Research that is concerned with solving immediate application problems, usually of a physical nature. This is in contrast to basic research, which has a goal of advancing the theoretical foundation of a subject by enhancing its general knowledge base.

archival storage: Any system for storing data and information for future use. The archive may be used for future operations and/or provide documentation for legal purposes. Traditionally, the actual physical format was paper based and was stored in library-type storage bins, but now archival storage usually implies a computer-based system, similar to electronic back-up systems.

artificial intelligence (AI): An area of study that attempts to program computers to emulate human reasoning and actions.

automated indexing: Using a computer to construct indexes. Most methods are based on frequency of use and surrounding context of nontrivial words in a text. While far from perfect, research consistently shows that automated indexing is a viable method, most evidenced by the successful use of automatic indexing by Internet search engines.

bedside terminals: Computer terminals, usually stationary, used by healthcare providers to manage patient information at the point of care. Common tasks include accessing information, placing orders, and updating records.

behaviorism: The theory that psychologists can know all about a patient by observing his or her behavior rather than by searching for deep, underlying mechanisms. Understanding gained by observation provides the framework for modifying the patient's behavior.

bibliographic control: The processes by which records of materials in libraries and other information systems are generated and organized for effective retrieval. Ultimately, it facilitates intellectual access to knowledge.

bibliographic database: An electronic collection of records containing information about books, journals, and other information resources. The collection is organized and structured with uniform descriptions and formats and is accessed with query software, resulting in pointers to the literature in a field.

bioinformatics: A specialized area of informatics that focuses on the management of information related to the underlying basic biological sciences. It is interdisciplinary in nature, involving a number of fields of study including biology, biochemistry, mathematics, computer science, information science, and health informatics.

biomedical engineering: The application of engineering tools to the medical field, mostly concerned with the development of instruments and devices for healthcare. It is a combination of engineering, health sciences, biological sciences, and a host of other application fields.

biomedical informatics: A field of study related to the management and applications of biomedical information, with a strong emphasis on information technology. Previously called *medical computing* and *medical informatics*.

bit map: A technique for storing images in a computer. The images are represented by an array of dots. Each dot is stored as one or more bits in memory. Black and white images can be represented by one bit per dot, but color requires more bits. When the array of dots is output on a computer screen or printed, the collected dots appear to the human eye as an image.

Bluetooth: A wireless protocol for short-range, low-power radio transmission and reception. It is used in a wide range of applications, including cordless telephones and other short-distance, fixed, or mobile devices.

case management: The coordinating and monitoring of a patient's progress during a healthcare situation, across a wide range of settings, including acute and long-term care, managed care, worker's compensation, private practice, and occupational health.

Centers for Disease Control and Prevention (CDC): The U.S. Department of Health and Human Services agency that is responsible for protecting the health and safety of citizens by investigating health problems, reporting incidence and trends in infectious disease, promoting disease prevention and control, and providing general public health information.

chromosome: A very long DNA molecule, found in cells, that provides portions of the hereditary information of an organism. The chromosomes come in pairs, and the human body contains 23 pairs, or 46 total chromosomes, one half from the mother and one half from the father.

classification: The process of bringing like things together on the basis of similarities and differences. A systematic arrangement in sets or categories according to established criteria.

clinical decision-support system: An interactive computer system that helps healthcare professionals with patient-related decision making.

clinical guidelines: Systematically developed recommendations for the treatment and care of patients, particularly in the clinical areas. The guidelines are based on the latest available evidence for care, applied with consideration of individual health circumstances.

clinical information system (CIS): A structured system for managing the full range of activities and processes related to the delivery of patient care, including the health record, scheduling of appointments, billing, tests and medication orders, and treatment planning.

clinical research: Research and experimentation related to the medical sciences and application procedures used by clinicians in caring for patients.

clinical trials: The amalgamation of collective data on individual patient interactions to new treatments, tests, or drugs in order to ascertain the safety and efficacy of these new approaches.

coding: The use of numbers, letters, or other symbols to represent information concepts. The concepts may be index terms, sets of diseases, procedures, or symptoms. Codes are shorthand mechanisms that save space and time and reduce the risk of misunderstanding.   ·

community health information network (CHIN): Computerized system for exchanging health information among a variety of health organizations and individuals, such as clinics, hospitals, physicians, and public health agencies.

computed radiography: A cassette-based imaging technique in which the tape is fed through a computer scanner to read and digitize the image. Software is used to enhance and manipulate the resulting image.

computed tomography (CT): The use of an X-ray beam to take a cross-sectional picture of the body, including the soft tissues and blood vessels. The X-ray beam is mounted on a wheel that rotates around the subject. Because it is taking pictures from all angles, bones and soft tissues do not block the view.

confidentiality: The assurance that patient information will be accessible only to those authorized to view and use the information; pertains to access to, use of, and release of private information.

consumer health informatics (CHI): The application of information technology to provide the general public with information about health and the healthcare services available to them.

context: The placement of a word, data, or information in a document in order to determine the intended meaning and related circumstances.

continuity of care: The management of a patient's care over time and across several healthcare points and care providers.

contrast radiography: An imaging technique that uses contrast compounds to highlight the differences in photographic density in a radiograph.

controlled vocabulary: A vocabulary in which only an approved list of words can be used as terms; used to manage synonyms and near-synonyms to bring together semantically related terms.

credentialing: The recognition by a professional authority of the quality or qualifications of an individual organization or a resource.

critical care: Close attention and care of patients with complications or unstable conditions, usually in an intensive care unit, by specially trained healthcare providers.

database: A structured collection of information records that is managed with computer software, allowing easy access and updating. There are different types of databases, including bibliographic, full text, numerical data, and image.

database management system (DBMS): Computer software that organizes, stores, updates, and retrieves information from a database or a collection of databases.

data standard: Documented agreements on how data are represented, structured, and formatted to ensure internal consistency when exchanging or transferring data.

data warehouse: A large repository of databases, holding archived information, structured for easy retrieval; the information is used for research analysis, reporting, planning, and historical documentation.

decision-support system: Computerized information system for helping users make decisions. These systems are usually interactive, offering suggestions and alternatives and incorporating feedback in order to identify the best decision from a set of possibilities.

deoxyribonucleic acid (DNA): A complex molecule that contains chemically coded instructions for building, operating, and maintaining a living organism. It is structured like a spiral-shaped ladder, with two twisted rails joined by a series of rungs, known as the *double helix*. The rungs are the simple molecules adenine, thymine, cytosine, and guanine, abbreviated A, T, C, and G, respectively.

DICOM (Digital Imaging and Communications in Medicine): A widely used standard for processing, storing, transferring, and displaying medical imaging information. The basic elements of the standard are format definition and networking communication protocol.

digital acquisition of images: The capturing or converting images to digital format for archiving and retrieval electronically. Images are acquired from a variety of devices, either directly in digital format, or on film, which can be converted to digital form.

digital image: An image that is stored in computer memory as a bit array, with each tiny picture pixel represented by one or more bits of computer memory.

digital library: A collection of information artifacts in electronic format stored and organized for optimal retrieval with a computer.

digital radiography: The processes and procedures of producing and storing medical images in digital format for retrieval, transfer, and use.

direct entry: The process of entering data directly into a computer information system, usually by the person who collected the data.

distributed computer system: A structurally and logically independent set of computers that share information and some physical resources.

DNA sequence database: Large, accessible databases of DNA sequences, sometimes with context information, that promote the exchange of sequence information among researchers in genomics and bioinformatics.

electrocardiogram (ECG): A device that records the electrical activity of the heart over a period of time. A heart beat is trigger by an electrical impulse that travels through the heart. An ECG measures the parameters of the impulse in both the top and lower chambers of the heart.

electroencephalography (EEG): A device that measures the electrical activity in a brain.

electronic health record (EHR): A computer-based health record. The patient's medical information is stored in digital form and can be viewed on computers, easily accessible from many points by authorized personnel involved in the care of the patient.

electronic textbook: A textbook stored online. It may be either a replica of a print textbook or it may be electronically created and available only in electronic form.

endoscope: A medical device, inserted into the patient, that allows observation of the inside of the body with a minimum invasiveness.

Entrez: A multifunctional search engine for searching databases from the National Center for Biotechnology Information (NCBI). It includes PubMed.

epidemiology: The study of the factors related to the incidence, distribution, and causes of illness in a population.

ethics: Societal norms of conduct. The concept goes beyond what is strictly right, wrong, or legal. It includes a sense of what is good for oneself and for others.

evidence-based guidelines: A list of consensus approaches based on the principles of evidence-based medicine, with emphasis on the latest and best evidence from the published medical research literature.

evidence-based practice (EBP): The idea that clinical decision making should be based on the best available evidence related to the medical situation at hand. It is a method for linking individual clinical expertise with the current research related to a specific health event.

expert system: A computer system that is designed and programmed to accomplish tasks that experts accomplish using their intelligence and experience.

fee for service: A healthcare payment model in which the health provider is free to recommend most services thought necessary, without regard to insurance plan control. The insurance plan pays for what is covered, and the patient pays the remainder.

fluoroscopy: An X-ray–based technique that allows real-time images to be seen by the healthcare provider. The patient is placed between an X-ray source and a fluorescent screen. An X-ray beam moves through the patient and strikes a fluorescent plate, which is amplified for on-the-spot viewing.

Food and Drug Administration (FDA): The U.S. Department of Health and Human Services agency that is responsible for regulating food, drugs, medical devices, and cosmetics. The agency also approves the use of new medical devices and drugs.

full-text database: A database that contains the full text of a document, along with the citation. The database is organized and searchable by computer systems.

functional magnetic resonance imaging (fMRI): An advanced version of MRI that functions in real time, showing living tissues in action, not just as static pictures.

gene: The basic unit of heredity. Each cell has a complete set of all the genes that determine the characteristics of an organism.

gene therapy: A variety of techniques for correcting the defective genes responsible for disease.

genome: The total collection of DNA in an organism.

genomics: The study of the entire genome.

genomics database: A large database containing gene sequencing information, protein characteristics, and other data collected from genomic research.

genotype: The genetic makeup of a cell, an organism, a group of organisms, or an individual. Genotype does not refer to the physical appearance of the organism but to its genetic information.

Health Insurance Portability and Accountability Act (HIPAA): In 1996, the U.S. Congress passed a law establishing the rules governing appropriate use of individually identifiable healthcare information. The rules protect health information from misuse and inappropriate disclosure; encompass the issues of privacy, security, transactions, and identifiers; and protect health insurance coverage for workers when they change or lose their jobs.

Health Level Seven (HL7): A data interoperability standard for sharing and exchanging healthcare information, particularly in clinical and administrative areas.

health maintenance organization (HMO): A type of health plan in which a group of independent practitioners form a medical practice and contract with patients who pay in advance according to a continuing fixed period basis.

hospital information system (HIS): An integrated information system that handles the administrative, financial, and clinical operations of a hospital. The system guides the daily activities of a hospital, including patient tracking and coordination of clinical functions.

Human Genome Project: Started in 1990 as an international effort co-sponsored by the U.S. Department of Energy and the National Institutes of Health and completed in 2003, its purpose was to document all of the human genes and make them accessible for further biological study.

hypermedia: An extension of the concept of hypertext, allowing a nonlinear connection among information resources for graphics, audio, video, and text.

image compression: The procedures for reducing redundancy in an image with the purpose of optimizing the storage and/or transmission of the image. Data compression algorithms are used to help accomplish this, but image compression has its own special problems.

image database: A database made up of medical imaging files of various formats, available for immediate clinical use, as an archive, and for educational purposes.

image enhancement: The use of computer-based software to improve the appearance of images, such as color quality, sharpness, contrast, and size.

image integration: The coordination of related information in order to enhance the interpretation and management of images.

image management: Techniques, policies, and procedures for organizing, storing, retrieving, transferring, displaying, and using images.

imaging informatics: An area of informatics that deals with the full range of techniques for acquiring and managing images.

imaging modality: Different devices and methods for acquiring images of the body.

implementation phase: The penultimate step in the system analysis process when the system hardware, software, and documentation are put into place. The final stage is to evaluate the operation of the system.

information need: A set of information entities that a person requires to solve a problem or make a decision. It may turn out that the perceived need of the user may not be the actual need for the solution of the targeted problem, and this is often the root of an information retrieval failure.

information retrieval: The technique of storing and retrieving recorded knowledge. Specifically, it is the process of selecting bibliographic citations, abstracts, full text, numeric data, and images from databases using a variety of access points, such as subjects or authors.

intellectual property: The ownership of a creative product, such as books, journal articles, software programs, music, art, Internet pages, and many other things. Such endeavors are protected by copyright laws and patents.

Internet: Interconnected networks appearing to be a single, worldwide network, with gateways to communicate with one other, providing access to many millions of text and multimedia documents.

Internet2: A nonprofit consortium of universities, industry, and government formed to promote, develop, and implement an advanced application of leading-edge network technologies and capabilities.

knowledge-based system: A database that, in addition to containing facts in the form of numeric, text, or images, incorporates rules for manipulating and integrating new input with stored information to create new knowledge. The rules may come from experts in the field who provide insight and advice to the topic under discussion.

knowledge record: A physical object that conveys information over time by symbols, sounds, or sights. It may be printed on paper, digitized on computer storage devices, imprinted on microforms, or chiseled on stone.

laparoscope: A medical device used to perform surgery through a small incision. A tiny camera and externally controlled small surgical devices are inserted to perform surgery.

local area network (LAN): A geographically limited data network, typically implemented by a single organization.

magnetic resonance imaging (MRI): An imaging modality that involves a mixture of magnets, atoms, radio frequency, and computers. MRI captures detailed images of the structure and functions of the subject from any plane or viewpoint. Instead of using radiation detection, MRI scanners create a strong magnetic field around the subject, and those forces spin hydrogen atoms in the body's tissues to align themselves with the magnetic field and send radio frequency pulses to imprint the image.

malpractice: An overt act or an omission by healthcare providers that results in injury to the patient. Such incidents usually involve deviation from standard practice.

managed care: A approach to medical care aimed at healthcare organizations and providers, with the objective of reducing the cost of healthcare.

medical computer science: An early name for *health informatics.*

medical datum: A single piece of standalone information, usually of value only when combined with a significant amount of related data.

medical imaging: The use of specialized instruments and techniques to take pictures of the interior of the body.

medical information science: A subarea of information science that focuses on medical information and related subjects.

Medical Literature Analysis and Retrieval System (MEDLARS): An electronic bibliographic database developed in the 1960s by the National Library of Medicine, initially as an electronic version of its long-running and well-known Index Medicus.

medical record: A file, either paper or electronic, that contains pertinent information about a patient, collected during healthcare encounters, usually over a period of time.

Medical Subject Headings (MeSH): Developed by the National Library of Medicine, this specialized vocabulary has over 18,000 terms related to the biomedical literature and has become the primary tool for subject cataloging and indexing.

MEDLINE: An online bibliographic database produced by the National Library of Medicine, with over 16 million references to the journal literature in the life sciences, particularly in biomedicine. It is considered the premier bibliographic database produced by the National Library of Medicine.

MedlinePlus: A version of MEDLINE that primarily provides the consumer with health information.

metathesaurus: A vocabulary database within the Unified Medical Language System that ties many vocabularies together, including the concepts, their various names, and the relationships among them.

MYCIN: An early AI-based, computer-assisted decision-support system for recommending therapies for patients with infections.

nanotechnology: The creation of products at very small atomic and molecular levels, using nano-sized materials. This technology holds promise for the healthcare field.

National Center for Biotechnology Information (NCBI): A national resource for molecular biology information developed as a unit of the National Library of Medicine in 1988.

National Health Information Infrastructure (NHII): An initiative to improve the healthcare system in the United States, with a focus on information technology, including technology, systems, standards, applications, and related laws and policies. The facilitator of the initiative is the U.S. Department of Health and Human services, whose task is to bring together private and publics sectors in order to achieve the initiative.

neuroinformatics: A subarea of health informatics that focuses on the creation, analysis, and management of data collected about the nervous system. Its techniques draw on such areas as neuroscience, computer science, the physical sciences, and statistics.

nursing informatics: A subarea of health informatics that deals with information problems related to the field of nursing.

occupational health: Focuses on health and safety related to the work environment.

ontology: A semantic model of what is known in a field of knowledge, for example, medicine.

pathology: The study of the causes and nature of disease.

patient monitor: Electronic medical device that captures and displays a patient's physiological signs. Such devices measure a wide range of parameters and come in many sizes, from compact and mobile to large and complex.

personal digital assistant (PDA): A small, lightweight, handheld computer, with audio capabilities, used as personal organizers and capable of connecting as a mobile phone. Newer models are coming with enhanced features.

personal health record (PHR): A record that belongs exclusively to a patient, who is responsible for building and maintaining the record and has complete control over who can access the record.

pharmacogenomics: The application of individual genetic information to optimize drug therapy for particular patients. The word represents the combination of the concepts of genetics and pharmaceuticals.

pharmacy information system: A system that supports all of the activities in a pharmacy, such as maintaining customer files, filling orders, controlling inventory, and managing personnel and daily operations.

physiology: A branch of science that deals with the normal functions of plants and animals while they are living.

picture-archiving and communication systems (PACS): Electronic information systems that store, retrieve, distribute, and present images for healthcare services and research. PACS are now part of the fundamental technological infrastructure supporting radiology practice in the digital age.

point-of-care system: Devices, often wireless, that permit patient data to be input and retrieved at the patient's bedside.

positron emission tomography (PET): An imaging modality in which isotopes are injected into the patient, enabling three-dimensional color pictures. The radioactive isotopes give off a positron, a tiny piece of antimatter. When this positron collides with an electron in the tissues, the two particles annihilate each other and give off a gamma ray, a very powerful electromagnetic pulse that can be detected by a nearby scanner.

preferred-provider insurance (PPI): A type of managed care whereby an insuring company contracts a large group of providers that are not usually related to each, except in terms of the PPI grouping.

preferred-provider organization (PPO): A type of health provision plan that involves advanced selective contracting of services, with negotiated fees for a wide range of services.

primary care: The initial level of care usually encountered by a patient.

privacy: The concept that individuals have the right to control information about themselves. It is the right to be anonymous and protected from intrusions.

public health: Deals with the general health of a population and includes methods for promoting good health in society at large.

public health informatics: A subarea of health informatics that focuses on the information needed to provide a profile of the general health and welfare of a society and on the systems for collecting data and converting them into information. Data are gathered from disparate sources and then compiled, organized, and synthesized.

PubMed Central: A free online service archive of biomedical and life sciences journal literature from the National Library of Medicine.

search strategy: A plan or method for systematically identifying useful data or documents in an information storage file.

Semantic Web: An enhanced Web site that associates ideas among information resources rather than just collecting documents on a topic. The association leads the user through various databases, driven by the commonality of the ideas.

sequencing: Determining the order of the four basic nucleotide bases in a DNA string.

systematic review: A formal, structured method for reviewing a research report that critiques the way the research was conducted and assesses the validity of the data and results.

Systematized Nomenclature of Medicine–Clinical Terms (SNOMED–CT): A comprehensive, unified medical terminology system created by the American College of Pathologists. Presently, it is owned by the International Health Terminology Standards Development Organization (IHTSDO). It is a licensed standardized vocabulary system made available free of charge in the United States by the National Library of Medicine.

telehealth: A general term for the delivery of healthcare from a distance using communication technology and networking.

telerobotics: Robotic manipulation from a distance.

tertiary care: The third level of care, usually provided in a medical center or at a research-focused site, usually referred to by primary and secondary care providers.

time-oriented medical record: A medical record with the data arranged chronologically as acquired.

ultrasound imaging: The use of sound waves and their echoes to create images. The scanners create images of muscles and internal organs in real time by bouncing high-frequency sound waves off the body structures being targeted for examination.

Unified Medical Language System (UMLS): A unifying terminology tool from the National Library of Medicine.

wide area network (WAN): A network with a broad geographical range, usually involving a number of different organizations.

World Wide Web (WWW): A hypermedia-based interface to the Internet, commonly referred to as the Web.

Index

A

Accountability, 218
Administrative support systems, 174–175
Admission-discharge-transfer, 173–174
AI. *See* Artificial intelligence
Algorithms, 48, 144, 202
Alternative medicine. *See* Complementary and alternative medicine
Ambulatory care, 35, 64, 144
American College of Physicians, 66, 67
American Dental Association, 28, 118
American Health Information Management Association (AHIMA), 155, 250, 256
American Medical Informatics Association (AMIA), 11, 232, 254–255
Angiography, 196–197
Artificial intelligence, 144–145
Atlases, 207–209

B

Basic research, 32
Behavioral informatics, 69–70
Best practice, 56–57
Bibliographic control
  cataloging, 127
  classification, 127
  indexing, 128–130
  Library of Congress Subject Headings (LCSH), 127
  Medical Subject Headings (MeSH), 125, 127, 130
  semantic network, 130
  SPECIALIST, 130
  subject vocabularies, 127–128
  Unified Medical Language System (UMLS), 130
Billing, 153

Bioinformatics, 73
  applications, 241–242
  areas of, 232–233
  biological information science, 232
  cloning, 238–239
  definition, 231–232
  deoxyribonucleic acid (DNA), 233–234
  genetic engineering, 238–239
  genetic testing, 237–238
  genome, 234–235
  genome mapping, 235
  human genome project, 236–237
  and medicine (*see* Genomic medicine)
  role of health information professional, 244–246
  stem cell research, 237
  translational bioinformatics, 232
Biological information science. *See* Bioinformatics
Biomed Central, 126
Biomedical databases, 138–139
Biomedical engineering, 27
Biomedical informatics. *See* Health informatics
Biomedical journals. *See* Medical literature

C

CAM. *See* Complementary and alternative medicine
Care delivery, 15, 17, 57, 112, 134
Career opportunities, 29, 253
CAT scans, 195
Cataloging. *See* Bibliographic control
CDC. *See* Centers for Disease Control and Prevention
Centers for Disease Control and Prevention (CDC), 35, 71–72

Change, management of, 88–89, 161, 178, 183, 185–187
CHI. *See* Consumer health informatics
Chief Medical Information Officer (CMIO). *See* Health information systems
Chiropractors, 27
Classification. *See* Bibliographic control; Medical terminology
Clinical decision-support systems, 17, 66, 69, 172
Clinical expert systems, 145–146
Clinical guidelines, 66–67
Clinical informatics, 65, 231, 253
Clinical information systems, 65–66
Clinical laboratory technologists, 27
Cloning. *See* Bioinformatics
CMIO (Chief Medical Information Officer). *See* Health information systems
Cochrane Database of Systematic Reviews, 55
Code of Hammurabi, 213
Coding systems, 115–118
Complementary and alternative medicine, 36
Computational biology, 732
Computed tomography, 77, 195–196
Computer science, 97, 250–251
Computer-based patient records. *See* Electronic health records
Computerized physician order entry (CPOE), 163
Connectivity and interoperability, 148–149
Consumer health informatics, 77
Consumer health terminology, 78
Continuing education, 252
Controlled vocabulary, 128, 129, 201
Copyright, 219–220
CPOE. *See* Computerized physician order entry (CPOE)

D
Data. *See* Medical data
Data analysis, 233
Data mining, 104
Database management systems, 138
Databases, 112, 136–139, 233, 244. *See also* Genomic databases
DBMS. *See* Database management systems
Decision-making process, 47–48
Dental assistants, 28
Dental hygienists, 28
Dental informatics, 68–69

Dentists, 28
Deoxyribonucleic acid (DNA), 233–234
Diagnosis, 23, 197, 238
DICOM. *See* Digital Imaging and Communications in Medicine
Digital images, 200, 257
Digital Imaging and Communications in Medicine (DICOM), 199
Digital radiography, 205
Distance learning, 69, 252
DNA (deoxyribonucleic acid). *See* Deoxyribonucleic acid (DNA)
Doctor of Osteopathic Medicine. *See* Physicians
Documenting healthcare operations. *See* Medical data

E
EBM. *See* Evidence-based medicine
Educational pathways, 249–252
Edwin Smith Papyrus, 5
e-health. *See* Telehealth
EHRs. *See* Electronic health records
e-journals. *See* Medical literature
Electronic health records (EHRs)
    basic functions, 159
    challenges, 157–158
    data entry by physicians, 163
    definition, 156
    ideal EHR, 159–160
    implementation of, 161
    information ownership, 163–164
    issues and caveats, 162
    need for, 156–157
    privacy and confidentiality, 162
    security, 162
    selection of, 160
    terminology standards, 162
    trends of, 164–165
    universality of, 157
    user interfaces, 160–161
    versus paper records, 158–159
    Web-based systems, 161–162
Endoscopy, 197
Entrez system, 125, 270
Ethics
    disclosure of errors, 216
    and informatics, 217–218
    levels of, 211
    medical codes, 213–214

in patient relationships, 214–216
in practice of medicine, 211–212
professional codes, 212–213
in research, 216
standards of care, 216
Evidence-based guidelines. *See* Evidence-based
  medicine
Evidence-based medicine
  critics of, 56, 98
  goals of, 98
  guidelines for, 55–56
  and librarians, 97–98
  linking to best practice, 56–57
  in medical school curricula, 57
  procedures, 54–55
  rise of, 53–54
Expert systems, 145–146

F
FDA. *See* Food and Drug Administration
Fluoroscopy, 196
fMRI. *See* Functional magnetic resonance
  imaging
Food and Drug Administration (FDA), 24,
  118, 222
Fraud and abuse. *See* Medical legal issues
Functional magnetic resonance imaging, 76,
  193, 195

G
GENBANK database, 240
Genetic engineering and cloning. *See*
  Bioinformatics
Genetic testing. *See* Bioinformatics
Genome. *See* Bioinformatics
Genomic analysis, 232
Genomic databases, 239–241
Genomic medicine, 242, 243–244,
Genomic structuring, 232
Grid computing, 224–225
Group medical practice, 34
Guidelines, 47–48, 55–56, 59, 66–67, 212

H
Health grid computing, 224–225
Health informatics
  careers, 254
  competencies, 250–251
  continuing education in, 252
  definition, xiii, 8–10

as a discipline, 10–11
education pathways, 249–252
emerging specialties, 259–260
extent of, 17
impacting healthcare, 43
major applications areas, 63
as a profession, 11
professional associations, 254–256
research in, 252
skills and competencies, 38–39
technology advances, 257–259
trends, 256
Health information infrastructure, 148–150
Health information systems
  chief medical information officer (CMIO),
    171
  clinical information systems, 172
  complexity of, 170
  hospital information systems, 173–176
  information resources management (IRM),
    171
  and the Internet, 37
  laboratory systems, 176
  as part of healthcare, 169
  pharmaceutical systems, 177
  radiology systems, 176
  resources management, 171
  supportive health information systems,
    176–178
Health information technology
  barriers, 14–15, 133–134
  benefits, 135t
  challenges, 13–16
  changing healthcare environment, 14
  communication improvement, 17
  error reduction, 17
  expectations, 134–136
  industry, 14, 15
  mobile, 142
  PDAs, 143
  and people, 16
  radio frequency identification, 143
  role of, 11, 17
  and societal changes, 16, 18
  ubiquity of, 12
  wearable, 142
  wireless, 142
Health informationists, 28–29, 99–100
Health Insurance Portability and
    Accountability Act (HIPAA), 225–226

Health Level 7 (HL7), 199–200
Health literacy, 79–80
Health maintenance organizations, 34
Health records
    access to, 57
    and computers, 13
    electronic (*see* Electronic health records)
    evaluation of, 52–53
    nature of, 153
    need for, 3
    people factor, 53
    personal, 155
    problem-oriented, 154
    relation to healthcare, 4
    ubiquity of, 4
Health sciences librarians
    definition, 86
    and evidence-based medicine, 97
    intellectual base, 94
    and knowledge management, 104–105
    new roles, 95, 166
    operational theorems, 94–95
    partnerships, 103–195
    relationship to health informatics, 85, 93–94
    and research, 101–103
    and technology, 96–97
Health sciences libraries
    and bioinformatics, 100
    changing environments, 88–89
    description of, 86
    education roles, 100–101
    impact of technology, 89–90
    Medical Library Assistance Act (MLAA),
        90–91
Healthcare
    industry, 14–15, 24, 74, 134, 262
    new paradigm, 22–23
    people in, 24
    teams, 23
    universality of, 21
Healthcare industry. *See* Healthcare
Healthcare informatics. *See* Health informatics
Healthcare providers, 91–93
Healthcare systems, 23, 24
HIPAA. *See* Health Insurance Portability and
    Accountability Act
Hippocratic Oath, 213
HL7. See Health Level 7
Home-care nurse. *See* Registered nurses
Hospital nurse. *See* Registered nurses

Hospitalists, 26–27
Human Genome Project. See Bioinformatics
Human–computer interfaces, 184
Hypothetic-deductive method, 47–48

I
ICD. *See* International Statistical
    Classification of Diseases and Related
    Health Problems
Identifying services, 140
    innovation, 259
    and integrated medical information
        systems, 37
    negative concerns, 141
    as social platform, 140
    Web 2.0, 259
    Web-based healthcare information systems,
        141
Imaging informatics, 76–77
Imaging management, 198
Immunization registries, 72
Implementation phase, 161, 183–185
Index Medicus, 87
Indexing, 201–203
Informatics, 8
Information
    age of, 7
    challenges, 6
    definition, 6
    extraction, 203, 147
    intellectual problem, 5–6
    management of, 169–171, 173, 176–178
    nature of, 7
    ownership, 163–164, 219
    properties, 6
    and quality care, 48
    role in systems, 7
    storage and retrieval, 200 203–205
Information explosion, 7
Information Resources Management (IRM).
    See Health information systems
Information retrieval, 127–128
Information seeking behavior, 91–93
Information specialist in context, 100, 261
Information technology, 4, 11–23, 52, 261
Informationist, 28–29, 99–100, 245–246,
    261–262
Insurance, 23–24, 36–37, 220–221, 225
Integrated medical information systems.
    See Health information systems

Intellectual property, 219
International Statistical Classification of
  Diseases and Related Health Problems,
  117
Internet, 139, 259
Interoperability. See Connectivity and
  interoperability
Intranet, 175
IRM. See Health information systems

J
Johns Hopkins Pathology Data Warehouse, 75
Journals. See Medical literature

K
Knowledge management, 104

L
Laboratory informatics, 75–76
Laboratory management systems, 176
Legal issues. See Medical legal issues
Library of Congress Subject Headings
  (LCSH), 127
Libraries. See Health sciences libraries
Licensed practical/vocational nurses, 29
Long-term care, 35

M
Magnetic resonance imaging (MRI), 195
Malpractice. See Medical legal issues
Mammography, 197
Managed care, 22, 25, 33, 34
Medical classification, 127, 115
Medical coding systems, 117–121
Medical computing, 8–9
Medical computing science, 8–9
Medical data
  desirable characteristics, 44–45
  documenting operations, 45
  gathering, 44–45
  nature and importance, 44
  sources for, 46
Medical databases, 137, 138–139, 137
Medical decision making, 43–44, 47
Medical education, 26, 143
Medical errors
  accessing blame, 51–52
  in medication, 50
  and poor communication, 50
  and safety, 50

  solutions, 52
  types, 50
Medical imaging
  access, 203
  acquisition, 194
  angiography, 196–197
  background, 191–192
  basics, 192–193
  computed tomography, 195
  digital, 193–194
  education and research, 198
  emerging technologies, 206
  endoscopy, 197
  fluoroscopy, 196
  and health sciences librarians, 207
  indexing of, 200–203
  mammography, 197
  manipulation, 198–199
  and medical practice, 194
  nuclear modalities, 195–196
  picture archiving and communication
    system (PACS), 205–206
  quality of, 205
  transport, 199–200
  ultrasound, 196
  uses of, 197
  X-rays, 194–195
Medical imaging informatics, 76–77
Medical informatics, 9
Medical knowledge, 101, 112
Medical legal issues
  fraud and abuse, 222
  information ownership, 219–220
  informed consent, 218–219
  issues for librarians, 226–227
  malpractice, 220
  negligence, 220
  privacy and confidentiality, 222–224
  product liability, 221–222
Medical Library Assistance Act (MLAA),
  90–91
Medical Library Association (MLA), 103,
  227, 256
Medical libraries. See Health sciences libraries
Medical literature
  e-journals, 123–124
  indexing of (see Bibliographic control)
  journals, 121–123
  open access, 124–125
  origins of, 4–5, 120

Medical literature *(continued)*
reference books, 121
textbooks, 121
types, 120
Medical Literature Analysis and Retrieval
Systems (MEDLARS), 13
Medical practice, 22–24, 33–34, 194
Medical records. *See* Health records
Medical research, 32–33
Medical Subject Headings (MeSH), 125, 127,
130
Medical terminology
classification, 115–118
coding, classes of, 117
definitions, 114
examples of, 117–118
importance of, 101
ontologies, 115
registries, 118–119
Medicare, 24, 164–165, 222
Medication errors, 51, 74
MEDLINE, 125
MEDLINEplus, 34, 124–125
MeSH. *See* Medical Subject Headings
Metathesaurus, 130
Mobile technology. *See* Health information
technology
Molecular biology, 233
Monitoring, 57, 58, 143
MRI. *See* Magnetic resonance imaging
MYCIN, 13

N
Nanotechnology, 257–258
National Coordinator for Health Information,
157
National Health Information Infrastructure,
149
National health record, 165–166
National Institutes of Health, 24, 125, 214,
236, 240
National Library of Medicine (NLM), 86–88
National Network of Libraries of Medicine
(NN/LM), 91
Natural language processing, 147
Negligence. *See* Medical legal issues
Networking, 136, 175
Nomenclature, 114–115, 130
Nuclear medicine modalities, 195–196
Nurse practitioners, 29

Nursing, 31, 117, 211, 255
Nursing informatics, 67–68

O
Occupational health nurse. *See* Registered
nurses
Office nurse. *See* Registered nurses
Open access. *See* Medical literature
Outpatient care, 35

P
PAs. *See* Physician assistants
PACS. *See* Medical imaging
Paper records, 158–159
Paramedics, 29–30
Pathology informatics, 75
Patient, role of, 34–35
Patient care
changes in, 48
consumer services, 98–99
hospital admission, 173–174
hospital discharge, 173–174
issues, 49
levels of, 64
quality of, 48–49
safety in, 49–50
standards for, 50
Patient Care Partnership, 213
Patient monitoring, 58–59
Patient safety, 49–51
Patient's Bill of Rights, 213
PCP. *See* Physicians
PDAs. *See* Health information technology
Personal health record. *See* Health records
Personalized medicine, 242–243
PET. *See* Positron emission tomography
Pharmaceutical informatics, 74–75
Pharmaceutical management systems, 177
Pharmacists, 30
Pharmacogenomics, 232, 233, 243
Physician assistants, 30–31
Physicians, 24, 25–26
Picture archiving and communication system
(PACS). *See* Medical imaging
Podcasting, 12
Positron emission tomography (PET),
195–196
Primary care informatics, 63–64
Primary care physicians (PCP). *See* Physicians
Principles of Medical Ethics, 213

Privacy, 222–223
Problem-oriented health record. *See* Health records
Product liability. *See* Medical legal issues
Professional associations, 254–256
Proteomics, 233
Public health informatics, 70–72
Public health nurse. *See* Registered nurses
PubMed, 125–126

Q
Quality care, 48–49

R
Radio frequency identification (RFID), 143
Radiological informatics. *See* Medical imaging informatics
Radiology information system (RIS), 176–177
Records. *See* Health records
Registered nurses (RNs), 31
Registries, 115, 118–120
RFID. *See* Radio frequency identification (RFID)
RIS. *See* Radiology information system (RIS)
RNs. *See* Registered nurses
Robotics, 146–147

S
Security, 162
Semantic Web. *See* Web 2.0
Sequence, 232, 234–235, 240–241
Shared Pathology Informatics Network (SPIN), 75
Smith, Edwin, 5
SNOMED-CT (Systematized Nomenclature of Medicine–Clinical Terms), 118
SPECIALIST. *See* Bibliographic control
Speech recognition, 147
SPIN. *See* Shared Pathology Informatics Network
Standard of care, 50, 216
Stem cell research. *See* Bioinformatics
Subject vocabularies. *See* Bibliographic control
Systems analysis
    basic rules, 179
    and design, 178–179
    determine needs, 180
    evaluation of, 186–187

human–computer interfaces, 184
implementation, 183–184
managing change, 185–186
quality checklist, 184–185
role of library, 187
selecting technology, 180–183

T
Telecare. *See* Telehealth
Telecommunications, 58, 136
Telehealth, 58–59
Telehomecare. *See* Telehealth
Telemedicine. *See* Telehealth
Terminologies, 114–115, 130, 257
Training, 148, 161 207, 251
Translational bioinformatics. *See* Bioinformatics
Triage nurse. *See* Registered nurses
Two-dimensional image processing, 194

U
Ultrasound, 196
UMLS. *See* Bibliographic control
Unified Medical Language System (UMLS). *See* Bibliographic control
Uninsured people, 36–37
USA PATRIOT Act, 226
User interface, 160–161, 184

V
Veterinarians, 31–32
Veterinary informatics, 72–73
Virtual reality, 147–148
Visible Human Project, 87
Vocabulary, 116, 120, 127–128, 129, 202

W
Wearable technology. *See* Health information technology
Web 2.0, 90, 123, 137, 140, 259
Web-based healthcare information systems. *See* Internet
Wellness, 33
Wireless technology. *See* Health information technology
World Wide Web, 17

X
X-rays, 191, 194–195

About the Authors

Ana D. Cleveland, PhD, is Regents Professor and Director of the Health Informatics Program, University of North Texas, Denton, Texas. Dr. Ana D. Cleveland holds degrees in mathematics, health sciences, and information sciences. She has taught medical librarianship and health informatics for over 30 years. Her areas of research include indexing and retrieval, information-seeking behavior, digital libraries, and Web 2.0, all in relation to health informatics. Under her leadership, the University of North Texas, Health Informatics Program was ranked third in the nation by *U.S. News and World Report*. She has held faculty appointments in the Department of Family Medicine and the School of Public Health, University of North Texas–Health Sciences Center, Ft. Worth, Texas. Dr. Ana D. Cleveland has received numerous grants in areas related to health informatics, and she has presented papers in the United States, Europe, South America, the Caribbean, and Mexico. She has served as a consultant to the National Institutes of Health, National Library of Medicine, National Network of Libraries of Medicine/South Central Region, Medical Library Association, National Endowment of the Humanities, Organization of American States, U.S. Department of Education, as well as many local and statewide libraries. She has also served on a number of advisory boards, both nationally and regionally. Dr. Ana D. Cleveland has received many awards, including the Lucretia W. McClure Excellence in Education Award from the Medical Library Association.

Donald B. Cleveland, PhD, is Professor Emeritus, University of North Texas, Denton, Texas. Dr. Donald B. Cleveland holds degrees in computer science, library science, and information science. His consulting assignments have focused on scientific information networks, application of information technologies, and medical indexing and retrieval. He has served as a consultant to a number of governmental agencies and private organizations, including the National Institutes of Health, National Library of Medicine, World Health Organization, Cleveland Foundation, and American Heart Association. He has had numerous international assignments in Africa, Europe, South America, the Caribbean, and Mexico. In addition to scholarly papers and books, Dr. Donald B. Cleveland has published a book on the brain for young people and just completed another children's book on communication to be published in the fall of 2009.

Drs. Don and Ana Cleveland have several joint publications, including three editions of the textbook *Introduction to Indexing and Abstracting.*